NUTRITION
and the
STRENGTH
ATHLETE

NUTRITION in EXERCISE and SPORT

Edited by Ira Wolinsky and James F. Hickson, Jr.

Published Titles

Exercise and Disease,
Ronald R. Watson and Marianne Eisinger

Nutrients as Ergogenic Aids for Sports and Exercise,
Luke Bucci

Nutrition in Exercise and Sport, Second Edition,
Ira Wolinsky and James F. Hickson, Jr.

Nutrition Applied to Injury Rehabilitation and Sports Medicine,
Luke Bucci

Nutrition for the Recreational Athlete,
Catherine G. Ratzin Jackson

NUTRITION in EXERCISE and SPORT

Edited by Ira Wolinsky

Published Titles

Sports Nutrition: Minerals and Electrolytes,
Constance V. Kies and Judy A. Driskell

Nutrition, Physical Activity, and Health in Early Life:
Studies in Preschool Children,
Jana Pařizková

Exercise and Immune Function,
Laurie Hoffman-Goetz

Body Fluid Balance: Exercise and Sport,
E.R. Buskirk and S. Puhl

Nutrition and the Female Athlete,
Jaime S. Ruud

Sports Nutrition: Vitamins and Trace Elements,
Ira Wolinsky and Judy A. Driskell

Amino Acids and Proteins for the Athlete—The Anabolic Edge,
Mauro G. DiPasquale

Nutrition in Exercise and Sport, Third Edition,
Ira Wolinsky

Published Titles Continued

Gender Differences in Metabolism: Practical and Nutritional Implications, Mark Tarnopolsky

Macroelements, Water, and Electrolytes in Sports Nutrition, Judy A. Driskell and Ira Wolinsky

Sports Nutrition, Judy A. Driskell

Energy-Yielding Macronutrients and Energy Metabolism in Sports Nutrition, Judy A. Driskell and Ira Wolinsky

Nutrition and Exercise Immunology, David C. Nieman and Bente Klarlund Pedersen

Sports Drinks: Basic Science and Practical Aspects, Ronald Maughan and Robert Murry

Nutritional Applications in Exercise and Sport, Ira Wolinsky and Judy Driskell

Nutrition and the Strength Athlete, Catherine G. Ratzin Jackson

NUTRITION
and the
STRENGTH ATHLETE

edited by

CATHERINE G. RATZIN JACKSON

CRC Press
Boca Raton   London   New York   Washington, D.C.

Library of Congress Cataloging-in-Publication Data

Nutrition and the strength athlete / edited by Catherine G. Ratzin Jackson
     p. cm. — (Nutrition in exercise and sports series)
     Includes bibliographical references and index.
     ISBN 0-8493-8198-3 (alk. paper)
     1. Athletes—Nutrition. 2. Physical fitness—Nutritional aspects. 3. Weight training. I.
Jackson, Catherine G. Ratzin. II. Nutrition in exercise and sport.

TX361.A8 N83 2000
613.2'024'796—dc21   00-057962

Visit the CRC Press Web site at www.crcpress.com

Series Preface

The CRC series, Nutrition in Exercise and Sport, provides a setting for in-depth exploration of the many and varied aspects of nutrition and exercise, including sports. The topic of exercise and sports nutrition has been a focus of research among scientists since the 1960s, and the healthful benefits of good nutrition and exercise have been appreciated. As our knowledge expands, it will be necessary to remember that there must be a range of diets and exercise regimes that will support excellent physical condition and performance. There is not a single diet-exercise treatment that can be the common denominator, or the single formula for health, or panacea for performance.

This series is dedicated to providing a stage upon which to explore these issues. Each volume provides a detailed and scholarly examination of some aspect of the topic.

Contributors from any bona fide area of nutrition and physical activity, including sports and the controversial, are welcome.

We welcome the contribution *Nutrition and the Strength Athlete* by Catherine Ratzin Jackson. This is the second book contributed by her to the series, the first being *Nutrition for the Recreational Athlete*. Separately or together they constitute an extremely useful reference source in the area of sports nutrition.

Ira Wolinsky, Ph.D.
Series Editor
University of Houston

Dedication

To my children, Blair Thomas, Brent Mathew, Bryce Robert, and Marissa Cathryn, who adopted strength training as part of their lifestyle at very young ages. They are *my* role models for health, fitness, and wellness.

Preface

This volume is part of a miniseries of special topics in the CRC series on Nutrition in Exercise and Sport. The series has become a highly regarded source of accurate, up-to-date information in the field of sport and exercise nutrition. The subject matter of this particular volume covers a topic fraught with controversy and misconception. It is intended that only scientifically based information be presented on the topic and that myths surrounding resistance training be dispelled.

By way of introduction to the volume it is necessary to define several terms and set the stage for the importance of the topic area. Progressive resistance training is also referred to as strength training; the intent of this mode of exercise is to improve the strength of muscle with the use of submaximal and repetitive stimuli. Strength training is frequently used to reduce the risk of injury, maximize bone density and bone health, rehabilitate injury, and in general improve the quality of life. Weight training is also a mode of progressive resistance training. However, the desired result is an increase in muscle mass or bulk; the intent of this mode of exercise is to increase muscle size and power through the use of a minimal number of repetitions with high resistance. The distinctions between the two are not necessarily finite, as most athletes use a combination of both.

The importance of strength and weight training cannot be emphasized enough. It is recognized by the American College of Sports Medicine that this mode of exercise is necessary to maintain a high quality of life. It is also recognized that strength training is of benefit to the young (Appendix A), healthy adults (Appendix B), older adults (Appendix C), and adults with or at risk for osteoporosis (Appendix D).

This book begins with an extensive review of the parameters within which resistance training is defined. Subsequent chapters cover areas of known interest to those who participate in resistance training. The book concludes with a practical chapter of applications to a particular sport. Each chapter has been written by experienced and highly regarded researchers and practitioners in the area of this mode of exercise. All of the authors participate in some form of strength training as part of their lifestyle. It is the intent to have made this volume informative, interesting, and practical.

Catherine G. Ratzin Jackson, Ph.D.
July 2000

The Editor

Catherine G. Ratzin Jackson, Ph.D., F.A.C.S.M., is professor and chair of Kinesiology at California State University, Fresno. She received her B.A. degree in chemistry and physics and her M.A. in chemistry from Montclair State University, Montclair, New Jersey. Her Ph.D. in exercise physiology was from the University of Colorado, Boulder. As part of her Ph.D. training she attended the University of Colorado School of Medicine, Denver. Dr. Jackson has served in research and teaching positions in higher education for the last 18 years. She has also conducted basic research into long-term spaceflight by means of faculty fellowships at NASA Ames Research Center, Moffett Field, California, through the NASA/ASEE program at Stanford University, Stanford, California, and was a NASA/JOVE fellow.

Dr. Jackson is a fellow of the American College of Sports Medicine (ACSM), twice a former President of the Rocky Mountain Chapter of ACSM, and has served the College on national committees. Other avocations have included the presidency of the Western States Association of Faculty Governance and 18 years as a competitor in the sport of fencing. She was twice the State of Colorado Womens' Champion. She was also trained in management at the Harvard Graduate School of Education, Cambridge, Massachusetts.

Dr. Jackson is a frequent contributor to the CRC Series on Nutrition in Exercise and Sport. Her first book, published by CRC Press, was *Nutrition for the Recreational Athlete.*

Contributors

Michael G. Coles, Ph.D.   Department of Kinesiology, California State University, Fresno, California

Keith C. DeRuisseau, M.S.   Department of Nutrition, Food and Exercise Sciences, Florida State University, Tallahassee, Florida

Emily M. Haymes, Ph.D., F.A.C.S.M.   Department of Nutrition, Food and Exercise Sciences, Florida State University, Tallahassee, Florida

Catherine G. Ratzin Jackson, Ph.D., F.A.C.S.M.   Chair, Department of Kinesiology, California State University, Fresno, California

William J. Kraemer, Ph.D., F.A.C.S.M.   Director, The Human Performance Laboratory, Ball State University, Muncie, Indiana

Jacobo O. Morales, Ph.D.   Department of Kinesiology, California State University, Fresno, California

Nicholas A. Ratamess   The Human Performance Laboratory, Ball State University, Muncie, Indiana

Tracey A. Richers, M.A.   Denver Public Health, Denver Health and Hospital Authority, Denver, Colorado

Tausha Robertson, M.S.   Center for Healthy Student Behaviors, University of North Carolina, Chapel Hill, North Carolina

Martyn R. Rubin   The Human Performance Laboratory, Ball State University, Muncie, Indiana

Shawn R. Simonson, Ed.D., C.S.C.S.   Department of Wellness and Movement Sciences, Western New Mexico University, Silver City, New Mexico

Ann C. Snyder, Ph.D., F.A.C.S.M.   Director, Exercise Physiology Laboratory, Department of Human Kinetics, University of Wisconsin, Milwaukee, Wisconsin

Jeff S. Volek, Ph.D., R.D.   The Human Performance Laboratory, Ball State University, Muncie, Indiana

M. Brian Wallace, Ph.D.   Senior Vice President, Director, Human Performance Laboratory, Evolution Sport Science, Boston, Massachusetts

Contents

1

Basic Principles of Resistance Training

William J. Kraemer, Nicholas A. Ratamess, and Martyn R. Rubin

CONTENTS

1.1 Introduction

Improving health and performance during resistance training is a multidimensional concept. For example, optimizing the training stimulus is one factor conducive to improving performance. However, training cannot be optimal if either recovery between workouts or nutritional intake is not adequate. Recovery periods enable the body to adapt to the training sessions and prepare for subsequent workouts. Nutritional intake (i.e., macro and micronutrients, caloric intake) plays a complementary role to training for growth, repair, and energy supply and is discussed elsewhere in this book. Thus, acute muscular performance and subsequent training adaptations may be limited if both factors are not properly addressed. This concept becomes increasingly important during long-term resistance training because the rate of progress decreases considerably compared to initial improvements. Therefore, optimizing nutritional intake, recovery, and training are mandatory requirements of any strength and conditioning program if the desired level of physical development and performance is to be reached.

The primary focus of this chapter will be to give the reader a basic understanding of how to develop and optimize a resistance training program. An optimal resistance training exercise prescription will more effectively meet the training goals of the individual and result in more effective exercise stimuli and better training adaptations. The design of resistance training programs is based on the correct manipulation of program variables, some of which include exercise selection, order, load, and volume, in accordance with the needs and goals of the individual. The outcome is the improvement in one or more training goals, such as muscular strength, power, endurance, or hypertrophy.

In general, the human body adapts favorably to stresses placed upon it. However, the period of adaptation to a specific program is short, so continual variation and progressive overload are necessary for increases in muscular fitness. An understanding of the interaction of the acute program variables involved in resistance training program design is very important for optimal progression beyond the initial phase of adaptation. Therefore, the purpose of this chapter is to discuss each program variable and provide recommendations based on current resistance training literature. In addition, the importance of training variation, termed *periodization*, is discussed in relation to manipulating the variables for long-term improvements in physical conditioning.

1.2   Basic Principles of Resistance Training

Resistance training is a general term that encompasses several modalities of exercise. For example, any type of activity performed against an external resistance (i.e., plyometrics, environmental factors, sport-specific devices, manual labor, certain sporting events) may increase muscular strength, power, local muscular endurance, and/or hypertrophy. Of these different modalities, weight training (i.e., barbells, dumbbells, weight machines) is most effective for increasing muscle size and strength because it provides great variability as to the movements performed and is easily quantifiable such that progression is easily monitored and prescribed. Thus, the remainder of this chapter focuses upon weight training.

Perhaps the most important concept in weight training is "program design." Program design encompasses the systematic manipulation of training variables in order to maximize the benefits associated with weight training. The first step in program design is to determine training goals via a needs analysis. A needs analysis consists of answering questions based on what is expected from weight training. It also ensures that the program is individualized. For example, some common questions are:

- Are there health or injury concerns that might limit the exercises performed or the load lifted?
- To which type of equipment does one have access?
- What is the training frequency and are there any time constraints that may affect workout duration?
- What muscle groups need to be trained?
- What are the targeted energy systems (i.e., aerobic or anaerobic)?
- What type of muscle actions are needed?
- If training for a sport or activity, what are the most common sites of injury?
- What are the goals of this training program? Is it to increase muscle size, strength, power, speed, endurance, balance, coordination, and/or flexibility? Is it to reduce percent body fat, or to improve normal physiological function (i.e., lower blood pressure, strengthen connective tissue, reduce stress), or is it a combination of these factors?

Once the weight training program has been properly designed and initiated, progression becomes the primary consideration. Thus, further modifications of the program are needed in order to introduce different stimuli to the body, forcing it to adapt. Perhaps the three most important concepts in weight training are: progressive overload, specificity, and variation.

1.2.1 Progressive Overload

Progressive overload is a general term that refers to the gradual increase of the stress placed on the body during training. A Greek strongman, Milos of Crotona, has been credited with the first use of progressive resistance exercise. It is reported that Milos carried a young calf across his shoulders every day until the beast was fully grown. Eventually he carried a 4-year-old heifer the length of the stadium at Olympia, a distance of almost 200 meters. In reality, the human body has no need to develop large and strong muscles unless it is forced to do so. Thus, increasing the demands placed on the body is paramount for progression. There are several ways in which overload can be increased during a weight training program. For example, for strength, hypertrophy, endurance, and power improvements: (1) load may be increased; (2) repetitions may be added to the current workload; (3) repetition speed may be altered according to goals such as increased speed with current workload for power improvements; (4) rest periods may be shortened for hypertrophy and/or endurance improvements; and (5) volume may be increased within reasonable limits. Special care must be taken when volume is increased. It has been recommended that volume be increased only in small increments of 2.5 to 5% to avoid overtraining.[1] In addition, several advanced techniques such as heavy negatives (eccentric work) or partial repetitions have been used as supplemental methods to help provide workout variations and overload the musculoskeletal system.[1,2]

1.2.2   Specificity

Specificity is the paramount principle when designing resistance training programs. All training adaptations are specific to the stimulus applied. For example, the physiological adaptations to training are specific to the (1) muscle actions involved; (2) speed of movement; (3) range of motion; (4) muscle groups trained; (5) energy systems involved; and (6) intensity and volume of training.[1,3] Although there are some carryovers of training effects, the most effective weight training programs are those designed to target specific training goals.

1.2.3 Variation

Variation in training, called periodization, is a very important concept for weight training. In particular, "periodization" becomes increasingly important over long-term training periods when continual progression is the ultimate goal. Variation implies that alterations in one or more of the acute program variables such as volume or intensity are systematically included in the design of the weight training program. Planned rest and recovery from training is also a vital factor. Periodization was developed among the former Eastern European weightlifters and field athletes as a means of varying training to optimize both performance and recovery.[3] The former Eastern European coaches and sport scientists carefully observed the training patterns of their successful athletes, who typically trained with higher volume initially and gradually decreased volume with increases in intensity as the competition season approached. These observations formed the basis of the classic model of periodized training for athletes. However, training variation is not limited to athletes or advanced training in general. These applications have currently been extended beyond that of the athlete population and now form the basis of training among individuals with diverse training needs. In addition to sport-specific training of athletes,[4–6] periodized training has been shown to be effective for recreational[7–9] and rehabilitation[10] training goals.

The underlying concept of periodization is Selye's general adaptation syndrome (Figure 1.1). Selye's theory proposes that the body adapts via three phases when confronted with stress: (1) shock, (2) adaptation, and (3) staleness. *Shock* represents the response to the initial training stimulus in which soreness and performance decrements are produced. Performance then increases during the second stage, *adaptation*, in which the body adapts to the training stimulus. Once the body has adapted, no further adaptations will take place unless the stimulus is altered. This produces the third stage, *staleness*, in which a training plateau is encountered. This model demonstrates the importance of periodization because training plateaus are inevitable, and those who experience the greatest benefits in resistance training are those who are able to either limit or train through plateaus.

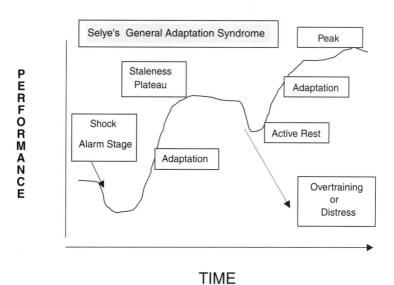

TIME

FIGURE 1.1

Selye's General Adaptation Syndrome Model is a theoretical model. Alarm or shock is the first stage in the introduction of a resistance training program. The next phase is the adaptation phase, in which the body adapts to the stress. Then a training plateau can occur, which represents a subsequent need for program modification. This could be the highest peak for that period of time unless an active rest period is utilized that results in a reduction in performance. Then, if a new program is started, a new adaptation phase results, and at some point peaking occurs in relationship to the individual's genetic upper limits. Overtraining can result if no active rest is allowed or if the training program is not varied.

Weight training programs can be varied in an infinite number of ways. However, one specific model of periodization has been the focus of several investigations (Table 1.1). This system has been called the "classical model of periodization." In 1981 in the United States, Stone, O'Bryant, and Garhammer[9] developed a hypothetical model for strength and power sports based on the model used by Eastern European weightlifters. This model divided a macrocycle (whole year of training) training phase into five meso-cycles: hypertrophy, strength, power, peak, and active rest. The hypertrophy phase is characterized by high-volume, low-to-moderate intensity training with the goals of increasing muscle mass and improving tolerance to training during subsequent mesocycles. The major goals of the strength and power phases are to bring about gradual increases in strength and power. Each phase entails an increase in intensity and a subsequent decrease in volume. The peaking phase entails maximizing strength and/or power for a competition. This peaking phase, or tapering, has been shown to be effective for perfor-mance enhancement.[11] The further reduction in volume helps compensate for the high intensity. The active rest phase consists of low-intensity activity and is intended to allow recovery from previous high-intensity training. It has been suggested[1] that this phase may be the most important for reducing the risk of overtraining. In addition, recent evidence has suggested that if you can go through these cycles three or four times in a given year (macrocycle), the benefits are even greater. This further supports the concept that variation in training is a vital component of optimization of the adaptational response.[12]

TABLE 1.1

Classic Model of Periodization

	Hypertrophy	Strength	Power	Peaking	Active Rest
Sets	3–5	3–5	3–5	1–3	Light
Reps	8–20	2–6	2–3	1–3	Activity
Intensity	Low	High	High	Very high	

Another popular model of periodization is a nonlinear (undulating) model. It is called nonlinear because of the dramatic change in the loads used. For example, an individual may train using 8 to 10 repetition-maximum (RM) loads on Monday, 3 to 5 RM loads on Wednesday, and 12 to 15 RM loads on Friday for 12 weeks followed by a period of active rest; the cycle is repeated. This model of periodization has been shown to be as effective as the classical model[13] over short-term training periods. In addition, one can have a power day (e.g., 30% of 1 RM) and the variation of the training intensities and vol-umes progresses on a weekly or biweekly basis, depending upon the number of distinct training zones. An active rest is usually taken every 12 weeks before another building phase is undertaken.[12]

A number of studies have investigated periodized weight training in both untrained men and women (Table 1.2). All of these studies have reported sig-nificant strength improvements during periodized training. In addition, peri-odized training has shown greater improvements than low-volume, single-set training.[14-17] Several of the cited studies directly compared periodized to nonperiodized training. The duration of training was relatively short for the majority of these studies (6 to 15 weeks), whereas one study[17] was 6 months in duration. Stone et al.[9] and O'Bryant et al.[18] reported that periodized training was superior to nonperiodized training, while Herrick and Stone,[19] McGee et al.,[15] and Baker et al.[13] did not report much difference between the two modes of training. It does appear that similar improvements may be obtained during short-term training periods. However, variation becomes increasingly important over long-term training periods. Marx et al.[17] studied single-set vs. periodized multiple-set training in previously untrained women during 6 months of training. They reported similar improvements in strength for both types of training during the first 3 months. However, only the periodized multiple-set group continued to improve during the last 3 months. Therefore, previously untrained individuals may respond favorably to both periodized and nonperiodized training, but alterations in program design are warranted in order to obtain further improvements in muscular fitness.

A number of studies have examined periodized training in resistance-trained individuals. Kraemer[5] reported periodized multiple-set training superior to nonperiodized single-set training in college football players. Kramer et al.[20] reported superior strength increases with periodized training compared to single-set training but did not report much difference between periodized and nonperiodized multiple-set training over 14 weeks. Baker et al.[13] reported similar strength improvements between classic and nonlinear periodization, both of which were only slightly better than nonperiodized training over 12 weeks. Schiotz et al.[21] reported greater increases in the bench press during periodized training but not the squat following 10 weeks of training. Studies in advanced or elite weight lifters during long-term training periods have shown periodized training to be superior.[22–24] Thus, similar improvements in strength may be obtained with either periodized or nonperiodized resistance training in trained individuals during short-term periods of 12 to 14 weeks. However, training over long periods requires program variation.

1.3   Acute Program Variables

The basis of weight training program design is an optimal prescription of the acute training variables. In doing so, the most effective programs are those that are designed specifically for individual training goals. Common goals associated with weight training are increased muscular strength, power, endurance, speed, coordination and balance, hypertrophy, and reduced percent body fat.[1] Several studies have reported the efficacy of weight training for improving these health and performance parameters. In addition, a positive carryover effect to motor performance, exercise performance, and normal activities of daily life has been observed which has direct impact on improving athletic performance and the quality of life in general. Thus, maximizing the benefits of weight training is best accomplished by manipulating the variables in a systematic manner in relationship to the training goals.

TABLE 1.2

Comparisons of Different Studies in the Literature Using Periodization (UT = untrained, TR = trained, M = men, F = women)

Reference	Gen.	Exp.	Program	Exercises	Freq.	Duration	Strength Increase
Dolezal & Potteiger[8]	M	UT	3 × 4–15RM - periodized	13 ex. TB	3×/week	10 weeks	BP = 24%; SQ = 23%
Herrick & Stone[19]	F	UT	a) 3 × 6RM b) 3 × 10–2RM - periodized	6 ex. TB	2×/week	15 weeks	BP: a = 25.2%; b = 32% SQ: a = 46.3%; b = 53.5%
O'Bryant et al.[18]	M	UT	a) 3–5 × 10–2RM - periodized b) 3 × 6RM	8 ex. TB	3×/week	11 weeks	SQ: a = 39.2%; b = 29.4%
Stone et al.[9]	M	UT	a) classic periodization b) 3 × 6RM	6 ex. TB	3×/week	6 weeks	SQ: a = 31kg; b = 23kg
Kraemer[5]	M	T	a) 1 × 8–10RM b) 2–5 × 10–1RM - periodized	8 ex. TB	3×/week	14 weeks	BP: a = 3.4%; b = 11.2%
Kraemer[5]	M	T	a) 1 × 8–12RM b) 2–4 × 15–3M - periodized	20 ex. TB	3–4×/week	24 weeks	LP: a = 6.1%; b = 20.3%
J. B. Kramer et al.[20]	M	RT	a) 1 × 8–12RM; b) 3 × 10RM c) 1–3 × 10–2RM - periodized	7 ex. TB	3×/week	14 weeks	SQ: a = 12%; b = 25.6%; c = 22%
Marx et al.[17]	F	UT	a) 1 × 8–12RM b) 3 × 15–3RM - periodized	10 ex. TB	3–4×/week	6 months	BP: a = 13.6%; b = 45.5% LP: a = 11.6%; b = 32.6%
McGee et al.[15]	M	UT	a) 1 × 8–12RM; b) 3 × 10RM c) 3 × 10–3RM - periodized	7 ex. TB	3×/week	7 weeks	SQ: a = 6%; b = 10.4%; c = 8.1% SQ reps: a = 46%; b = 74%; c = 71%
Sanborn et al.[16]	F	UT	a) 1 × 8–12RM b) 3 × 10–2RM - periodized	8 ex. TB	3×/week	8 weeks	Avg. 1RM: a = 24.2%; b = 34.7%
Stowers et al.[14]	M	UT	a) 1 × 10–12RM; b) 3 × 10–12RM c) 5–7 × 3–10RM - periodized	7 ex. TB	3×/week	7 weeks	BP: a = 7.8%; b = 9.5%; c = 8.4% SQ: a = 14.7%; b = 21%; c = 27.6%
Baker et al.[13]	M	MT	a) 3–5 × 6–8RM; b) 3–5 × 3–10 (classic) c) 3–5 × 3–10 nonlinear periodization	8 ex. TB	3×/week	12 weeks	SQ: a = 26.1%; b = 27.7%; c = 28.4% BP: a = 12.5%; b = 11.6%; c = 16.4%

Bell et al.[144]	MF	MT	3–6 × 2–10(65–85% 1RM) - periodized	7 ex. TB	3×/week	16 weeks	LP: M = 34.9%; F = 80.5% BP: M = 26.6%; F = 29%
Häkkinen et al.[23]	M	EWL	Periodized volume/intensity	OL, SQ, Str	5×/week	1 year	Isom KE = 3.5%; S = 1.2%; CJ = 1.7%
Häkkinen et al.[97]	M	EWL	Periodized volume/intensity	OL, SQ, Str	5×/week	1 year	Isom = 3.5%; S = 1.5%; CJ = 2.0%
Häkkinen et al.[24]	M	EWL	Periodized volume/intensity	OL, SQ, Str	5×/week	2 years	Isom = 4.9%; WL total = 2.6%
Schiotz et al.[21]	M	T	a) 3–4 × 6–15RM - constant b) 3–5 × 10–1RM - periodized	9 ex. TB	4×/week	10 weeks	BP: a = 5.0%, b = 8.3% SQ: a = 11.2%; b = 9.7%
Willoughby[22]	M	ADV	a) 5 × 10RM; b) 5 × 6–8RM c) classic periodization	BP, SQ	3×/week	16 weeks	S:BW ratio: BP: a = 0.07; b = 0.08; c = 0.22 SQ: = 0.15; b = 0.25; c = 0.43

KEY (in alphabetical order):

1. ADV = Advanced Lifters
2. BP = Bench Press
3. CJ = Clean and Jerk
4. EWL = Elite Weight Lifters
5. Isom = Isometric
6. LP = Leg Press
7. MT = Moderately Trained
8. OL = Olympic Lifts
9. RT = Recreationally Trained
10. S = Snatch
11. S:BW = Strength to Body Weight Ratio
12. SQ = Squat
13. STR = Structural Lifts
14. TB = Total Body
15. WL = Weightlifting Total

The acute program variables associated with weight training are muscle action, load, volume, frequency, muscle grouping, exercise selection and order, rest periods, and repetition speed. The alteration of one or several of these variables will change the training stimulus and will force the body to adapt accordingly.

1.3.1 Muscle Action

Concentric, eccentric, and isometric muscle actions influence the adaptations to weight training. Generally, most weight training programs consist predominantly of dynamic muscle actions (i.e., a concentric and eccentric component to each repetition). However, isometric exercise has been shown to increase muscular strength[25] and, in addition, has been a popular testing modality for strength gains associated with weight training.[3,26] In general, greater force is produced during eccentric actions.[27] They are more efficient neurologically,[27,28] less metabolically demanding,[29,30] most conducive to hypertrophy,[31] and most conducive to delayed-onset muscle soreness[32] compared to concentric actions. In addition, increasing dynamic strength is most effective when eccentric actions are included.[33,34] Thus, the inclusion of both concentric and eccentric actions in weight training is important for increasing dynamic muscular strength, increasing muscle size, and reducing the effects of detraining.[33,34]

Isometric exercise drew the attention of the American public in the early 1950s based on the research conducted by Hettinger and Muller.[35] They suggested that strength gains of 5% per week were attainable by one daily 6-second isometric contraction at 67% of maximal voluntary contraction (MVC). Although subsequent studies have shown that isometric training produces significant strength gains, albeit considerably less than that suggested by Hettinger and Muller, it is an often overlooked form of training and is far less common than traditional dynamic resistance exercise. In addition, isometric training may be performed relatively cost-free because any immovable object (i.e., wall, heavy-loaded barbell,) or partner-resisted movement can be used as the resistance.

Studies have shown that isometric training increases muscular strength most specifically at the joint angles trained, a concept known as *angular* specificity.[25,36] In addition, some studies have shown that strength increases transfer to nontrained angles by approximately $\pm$ 30° of the trained angle,[25] with the greatest magnitude of carryover taking place at joint angles corresponding to greater muscle lengths.[36] Factors such as the intensity,[37] number of contractions,[1] duration,[26,38] frequency,[38,39] volume,[1] and rest periods[38] affect the magnitude of strength improvement. It has been generally recommended that maximal or near-maximal contractions be performed for at least 3 to 5 seconds in duration, using at least 15 to 20 contractions daily at multiple joint angles.[1] In addition, the performance of isometrics with free weights, functional isometric training, has been shown to be effective for increasing muscular strength[40] and appears effective for enhancing dynamic 1 RM strength, especially if the contractions are performed at the sticking region of an exercise.

1.3.2 Load

Load represents the amount of weight lifted per repetition or set and is highly dependent upon other variables such as exercise order, volume, frequency, muscle action, repetition speed, and rest period length. Generally, loads corresponding to 90% of one-repetition maximum (1 RM) or greater are considered heavy, 70 to 90% of 1 RM are considered moderate, and below 70% are considered light. Altering the training load can significantly affect the acute metabolic,[22,41–43] hormonal,[44–46] neural,[47–50] and cardiovascular[51,52] responses to training.

Training status is an important determinant of load prescription. Loads of at least 45 to 50% of 1 RM are needed to increase dynamic muscular strength in previously untrained individuals.[53] This initial phase of lifting is characterized by improved motor learning and coordination.[54] Thus, heavy loads are not required to increase strength at this level of training. However, greater loading is needed as one progresses to the novice, moderate, and advanced levels of training. Häkkinen et al.[48] reported that loads greater than 80% of 1 RM were needed to produce further neural adaptations during resistance exercise in advanced lifters. Neural adaptations are crucial to resistance training because they precede hypertrophy during intense training periods. For example, Ploutz[55] showed that less motor units are recruited for a given workload following resistance training when hypertrophy occurs. With enlarged muscle fibers, fewer motor units are needed to lift a specific load during weight training as greater force production accommodates an increase in muscle cross-sectional area (CSA).[56] In order to continually recruit these higher-threshold motor units, progressively heavier loads are needed. Maximizing strength and hypertrophy may only be accomplished when the maximal number of motor units are recruited. Thus, heavy loading in more experienced lifters is needed to recruit the high-threshold motor units that are not typically involved in light-to-moderate lifting.

There exists an inverse relationship between the amount of weight lifted and the number of repetitions performed. Several studies have indicated that training with loads corresponding to 1 to 6 RM were most conducive to increasing maximal dynamic strength.[57–59] This loading range appears to maximally recruit muscle fibers and is most specific to increasing dynamic 1 RM strength.[48] Although significant strength increases have been reported using loads corresponding to 8 to 12 RM,[5,60–62] this load range appears most effective for increasing muscular hypertrophy,[63] particularly when one-minute rest periods are used.[44,64] The magnitude of hypertrophy associated with both loading ranges is unclear. Considering that both stimulate muscle growth, it may be that the volume associated with 8 to 12 repetitions has a greater overall effect on protein synthesis.[65] Lighter loads, 12 to 15 RM and lighter, have only had small effects on maximal strength in previously untrained individuals,[66] but have been shown to be very effective for increasing local muscular endurance.[67] Although training with high loads and low repetitions, 1 to 6 RM, is most specific for increasing maximal strength, it appears that optimal strength training requires the systematic use of various loading strategies.[12] Therefore, periodized training in which great load variation is included appears most effective for long-term improvements in muscular fitness.

Training to increase muscular power requires two general loading strategies because both force and time components are relevant to maximizing power. First, moderate-to-heavy loads are required to recruit the high-threshold fast-twitch motor units needed for strength increases. However, as depicted by the force–velocity curve, with greater loading comes a decrease in lifting velocity such that performing heavy resistance training only, 1 to 6 repetitions with greater than 85% of 1 RM, would increase force production, but this does not maximize power due to the time component of a slow lifting velocity. Thus, the second strategy is to incorporate light-to-moderate loads performed at explosive lifting velocity. Wilson et al.[68] reported that 30% of 1 RM was the optimal loading that produced the greatest power output during ballistic resistance training. With ballistic resistance exercise, the load is maximally accelerated either by jumping, such as jump squats, or by releasing the weight using specialized equipment. During nonballistic traditional weight training exercises performed at an explosive velocity, a study has shown that 40 to 60% of 1 RM may be most beneficial.[69] Therefore, training for maximal power requires various loading strategies performed at high velocity.

1.3.3   Volume

The volume of weight training is an important concept for progression. Training volume is a summation of the total number of repetitions performed during a workout session. It is dependent upon several variables including the loads used, the number of exercises selected, frequency, and muscle actions used. There is an inverse relationship between training volume and intensity as it pertains to performance increase while reducing the risk of overtraining. In general, high-volume (i.e., moderate-to-heavy load, 8 to 12 repetitions per exercise or greater, moderate-to-high number of sets) programs are most conducive to increasing lean body mass and local muscular endurance,[67,70] whereas low-volume (i.e., high load, low repetitions, moderate-to-high number of sets) programs involve high-intensity contractions synonymous with strength and power training.[48] Thus, the volume of resistance exercise has been shown to affect neural,[23,71] hypertrophic,[72,73] metabolic,[22,41] and hormonal[44,45,74,75] responses and adaptations to weight training.

Altering training volume can be accomplished by changing the number of exercises performed per session, changing the number of repetitions performed per set, or changing the number of sets per exercise. Total volume per workout session has received attention in the literature. Studies using 2,[76,77] 3,[20,62,78,79] 4 to 5,[33,34,79–82] and 6 or more[83,84] sets per exercise have all produced significant increases in muscular strength in both trained and untrained individuals. In direct comparison, studies have reported similar strength increases between 2 and 3 sets,[85] and 2 and 4 sets,[86] whereas 3 sets have been reported superior.[57] Thus, little or no differences have been reported between variation in set number within multiple-set weight training programs. It appears that other variables such as intensity, the number of exercises performed, rest periods, frequency, and training goals are important for determining the number of sets per workout and/or per exercise.

Another aspect of training volume that has received considerable attention is the comparison of single- and multiple-set weight training programs. It is important to note that not all exercises have to be performed for the same number of sets in a workout. Variation in set number may depend upon the exercise selected. However, for the majority of the referenced studies, one set per exercise performed for 8 to 12 RM at a slow velocity has been compared to both periodized and nonperiodized multiple-set programs. In untrained subjects, several studies have reported similar strength increases between single- and multiple-set programs,[87–92] whereas several studies reported multiple-set programs superior.[14,16,57,85,93] In resistance-trained subjects, multiple-set programs have been superior for strength,[5,15,20,94] power,[4,94] hypertrophy,[5] and high-intensity endurance[5,15] enhancement. To date, no study has shown single-set training superior to multiple-set training in either trained or untrained individuals. It appears that both programs are effective for increasing strength in untrained subjects during short-term training periods such as 6 to 12 weeks. However, long-term studies support the contention that a higher volume of training is needed for further improvement. Recently, Marx et al.[17] had previously untrained women train for 6 months using either low-volume, single-set training or periodized, multiple-set training. Both training groups significantly increased muscular strength during the first 3 months. However, only the periodized multiple-set group showed continued improvement over the 6-month period. Thus, the need for variation is critical for continued improvement. The key factor may be the use of "periodization" of training volume rather than number of sets, which represents only one factor in a volume and intensity periodization model.

Considering the number of variables involved in resistance training, comparing single- and multiple-set protocols may be an oversimplification. For example, several of the aforementioned studies compared programs of different set number regardless of differences in intensity, exercise selection, and repetition speed. In addition, the use of untrained subjects during short-term training periods has also raised criticism,[94] because untrained subjects have been reported to respond favorably to most programs.[6,95] Part of this has evolved because of the popularity of a specific single-set program[96] in which researchers desired to compare this regimen to other protocols. Based upon the available data, it appears that previously untrained individuals may not be sensitive to training volume during the initial 6 to 12 weeks of training.

However, it also appears that greater volume is needed beyond this point in training to produce optimal improvements. In advanced lifters, further increases in volume may be counter-productive, but it appears that the correct manipulation of both volume and intensity produces optimal performance gains and avoids overtraining.[24,97]

1.3.4   Exercise Selection

The exercises chosen during weight training are very important as they relate to the adaptations desired and the need to be selected for specific training goals. It is generally recommended that exercises be chosen that stress all major muscle groups in order to maintain muscular balance. There are two basic types of exercises: single-joint and multiple-joint exercises. *Single-joint exercises* target one general muscle group or joint action. *Multiple-joint exercises* target more than one muscle group or involve multiple joint actions and interactions. There are two types of multiple-joint exercises: basic strength and Olympic lifts. Basic strength exercises involve mostly 2 to 3 joints; examples are the squat, bench press, and lat pulldown. The Olympic lifts are total body lifts that involve most major muscle groups; examples are the clean and jerk, snatch, and their variations.

There has been little research concerning the efficacy of performing different exercises on various assessments. Both single-[98–100] and multiple-joint exercises[5,9,23,24] have been effective for increasing muscular strength and hypertrophy of the targeted muscle groups. Exercises stressing multiple or large muscle groups have shown the greatest acute metabolic responses.[101–103] For example, exercises such as the squat, leg press, leg extension, and bent-over row have been shown to produce greater oxygen consumption than exercises such as the behind-the-neck press, bench press, and arm curl.[102,103] In addition, these exercises have shown greater acute hormonal response[104–107] and require greater recovery between training sessions.[108] Deadlifts,[106] squat jumps,[107] and Olympic lifts[105] have produced greater acute growth hormone (GH) and testosterone responses compared to exercises such as the bench press and seated press. Thus, the amount and size of the muscle mass used is important during the acute response.

It has been generally recommended that both single- and multiple-joint exercises be included in a training program. Multiple-joint exercises have generally been regarded as most effective for the increase of overall muscular strength and hypertrophy in trained individuals because they allow a great amount of weight to be lifted.[95] Furthermore, they allow enhanced intermuscular communication and coordination of force, producing elements vital to human performance. A recent study by Chilibeck et al.[109] has shown that in previously untrained women, multiple-joint exercises require a longer initial neural adaptation phase compared to single-joint exercises due to the complexity of movement and joint actions involved. Thus, single-joint exercises are accompanied by a short neural phase and result in an earlier onset of hypertrophy in untrained individuals.[109] In addition, performing multiple-joint exercises may have greater impact on multiple-joint activities involved in daily living or in athletics.[1] Thus, multiple-joint exercises are important for strength, power, and hypertrophy training. Single-joint exercises are effective for increasing strength and hypertrophy and are commonly used in a variety of programs. Training goals may dictate what and how many exercises to include. In addition, the use of barbells, dumbbells, or machines, or altering grip/foot width, hand position, body position, or contraction pattern, such as unilateral, bilateral, or alternate, are also used to vary exercises during periodized resistance training.

1.3.5 Exercise Order

The sequence of exercises that are performed during a training session significantly affects performance and subsequent adaptation. Sequencing of exercises is based on training goals and is highly dependent on energy metabolism and fatigue. For strength training it is recommended that basic strength exercises such as the squat and bench press be performed initially during the workout. Training for enhanced speed and power entails performance of total-body explosive lifts such as the power clean and power snatch initially during the workout. Bodybuilding, or training for hypertrophy, entails performance of many exercises under various conditions where training through fatigue is paramount. Improper sequencing of exercises can compromise the lifter's ability to perform the desired number of repetitions with the desired load. Therefore, exercise order needs to correspond with specific training goals. A few general methods for sequencing exercises for both multiple or single muscle group training sessions have been suggested. Although there are some exceptions to these general guidelines, training goals such as increased strength, size, and power may be optimized when:

- Large muscle mass exercises are performed before smaller muscle mass exercises
- Agonist/antagonist exercises, those which train opposing muscle groups, are rotated for total-body sessions
- Upper and lower body exercises are rotated for total-body sessions
- Multi-joint exercises are performed before single-joint exercises
- Weak-point exercises are performed before strong exercises
- Total-body exercises such as Olympic lifts are performed before basic strength and single joint exercises
- When using split routines, training specific muscle groups, high-intensity exercises are performed before lower-intensity exercises

Research has shown that changing order significantly affects exercise performance. Sforzo and Touey[110] investigated the squat and bench press using different orders. Session 1 began with multi-joint exercises and ended with single-joint exercises (squat, leg extension, leg curl, bench press, shoulder press, and triceps pushdown). Session 2 was the reverse (leg curl, leg extension, squat, triceps pushdown, shoulder press, and bench press). Each exercise was performed for 4 sets of 8 RM with 2 minutes rest between sets and 3 minutes rest between exercises. Overall, there was a 75% decline in bench press performance and a 22% decline in squat performance when the reverse order was used. The results of this study demonstrated that either fewer repetitions with a specific workload are performed or significantly less weight is used when these exercises are performed in a fatigued state. Considering the importance of these exercises for increased size and strength, it is recommended that these exercises be performed early in the workout when fatigue is minimal.

1.3.6   Rest Periods

The amount of rest taken between sets, exercises, and/or repetitions significantly affects performance and subsequent adaptation.[111,112] Rest period length depends on training intensity, goals, fitness level, and targeted energy system utilization. In addition, other factors such as changing weights or exercises and equipment availability contribute to the length of the rest period. For example, strength/power training stresses the ATP–PC system predominately, while hypertrophy/strength (8 to 12 RM) affects mostly ATP–PC and glycolytic pathways with minor aerobic contributions (@ 20%). Endurance training (high repetition, short rest periods) increases the contribution of energy liberation from aerobic sources. In addition, an active rest period has been shown to improve performance of subsequent sets of the bench press.[113]

Research studies comparing weight training performance with various rest periods are few. The length of the rest period significantly increases the metabolic,[114,115] hormonal,[44,64] and cardiovascular[52] responses to an acute bout of resistance exercise, as well as performance of subsequent sets.[5] Larson and Potteiger[116] reported no significant difference in performance among 3 different rest period lengths (heart rate recovery method, 3 minutes, or 1:3 work/relief ratio) during 4 sets of squats at 85% of 10 RM. Kraemer[5] reported differences in performance with 3- vs. 1-minute rest periods. All lifters were able to perform 10 repetitions with 10 RM loads for 3 sets with 3-minute rest periods for the leg press and bench press. However, when rest periods were reduced to 1 minute, 10, 8, and 7 repetitions were performed, respectively.

When training for absolute strength or power, rest periods of at least 3 to 5 minutes are recommended. Robinson et al.[117] reported a 7% increase in squat performance after 5 weeks of training when 3-minute rest periods were used compared to only a 2% increase when 30-second rest periods were used. Pincivero et al.[118] reported significantly greater strength gains (5 to 8%) when 160-second rest intervals were used compared to 40 second. Strength and power performance is highly dependent on anaerobic energy metabolism, primarily the phosphagens. Studies show that the majority of phosphagen repletion occurs within 3 minutes.[119,120] In addition, sufficient removal of lactate and subsequent buffering of H^+ may require at least 4 minutes.[117] Therefore, performance of maximal lifts requires maximal energy substrate availability prior to the set with minimal or no fatigue.

Stressing the glycolytic and ATP–PC energy systems may enhance training for hypertrophy, thus less rest between sets appears to be effective. Rest periods of 1 to 2 minutes for basic strength exercises are commonly used. Considering that heavy resistance exercise has been effective for increasing hypertrophy,[48] maximal hypertrophy may be attained through the combination of strength and hypertrophy training. Thus, periodization of volume and intensity may be most beneficial.

Training for muscular endurance implies the individual: (1) performs several repetitions (or long-duration sets), (2) trains to and beyond the point of fatigue, and (3) minimizes recovery between sets (i.e., training in a semi-fatigued state). Therefore, high repetitions and shorter rest periods (30 to 90 seconds or less) for endurance training appear to be most effective.[66]

The amount of rest taken between repetitions has only been partially investigated. Rooney et al.[121] had subjects train using 6 to 10 consecutive high-intensity repetitions or 6 to 10 repetitions separated by 30-second rest periods and reported significantly greater strength improvement with consecutive repetitions (56%) than with extended rest between repetitions (41%). These findings demonstrate that fatigue may contribute to the strength training stimulus.

1.3.7 Frequency

The number of training sessions performed during a specific period (i.e., 1 week) may affect subsequent training adaptations. Frequency also includes the number of times certain exercises or muscle groups are trained per week. It depends on several factors such as volume and intensity, exercise selection, level of conditioning and/or training status, recovery ability, nutrition, and goals. Training with heavy loads increases the recuperation time needed prior to subsequent sessions, especially for multi-joint exercises involving similar muscle groups.[108] The use of extremely heavy loads, especially when heavy eccentric training is performed, may require 72 hours of recovery, whereas large and moderate loads may require less recovery time (48 and 24 hours, respectively).[65] In addition, reduced frequency is adequate during maintenance training. Training 1 to 2 days per week is adequate for mass, power, and strength retention.[108] However, this appears effective for short-term training, mostly because in long-term maintenance training, reduced frequency and volume may lead to detraining.

Numerous resistance training studies have used frequencies of 2 to 3 alternating days per week in untrained subjects.[33,34,70,122] This has been shown to be a very effective initial frequency.[78] Graves et al.[123] reported 3 days/week superior to 2 days/week during the initial 10 weeks of training. These workouts typically stress the total body. In addition, two studies have shown higher frequencies as superior. Hunter[124] reported 4 days superior to 3 for increasing bench press strength and endurance. Gilliam[125] reported 3 to 5 days superior to 1 to 2 days of training per week for improving 1 RM bench press, with 5 RM producing the greatest increase. The progression from beginning to novice status does not necessitate a change in frequency, but may be more dependent upon alterations in other acute variables such as exercise selection, volume, and intensity. However, it is common to see novice lifters train 3 to 4 days/week. Increasing training frequency allows for greater specialization such as greater exercise selection per muscle group and/or volume in accordance with more specific goals. Thus, an upper/lower body split or muscle group split routine is common.[1] Similar improvements in performance have been observed between upper/lower workouts and total-body workouts.[126] In addition, it is recommended that similar muscle groups or selected exercises not be performed on consecutive days to allow adequate recovery and to minimize the risk of overtraining.

Frequency for advanced or elite athletes may vary considerably, depending on intensity, volume, and goals. One study demonstrated that football players who trained 4 to 5 days/week achieved better results than those who self-selected frequencies of 3 and 6 days/week.[127] Weightlifters and body builders typically use high-frequency training, at least 4 to 6 sessions per week. Double-split routines, or two training sessions per day, are common[65,128] during preparatory training phases, which may result in 8 to 12 training sessions per week. Frequencies as high as 18 sessions per week have been reported in Bulgarian weight lifters.[65] The rationale for this high-frequency training is that frequent short sessions followed by periods of recovery, supplementation, and food intake allow for high-intensity training via maximal energy utilization and reduced fatigue during exercise performance.[1,108] Häkkinen and Kallinen[129] reported greater increases in muscle CSA and strength when training volume was divided into 2 sessions per day as opposed to 1 in female athletes. In addition, exercises such as total-body lifts performed by Olympic lifters require technique mastery which may increase total training volume and frequency. Elite power lifters typically train with frequencies of 4 to 6 sessions per week.[1] It should be noted that training at these high frequencies would result in overtraining in most individuals. However, the superior conditioning of these athletes combined with other factors, which may possibly include anabolic drug use, enables the successful use of high-frequency programs.

1.3.8 Repetition Speed

The contraction velocity used to perform dynamic muscle actions affects the adaptations to resistance training. Repetition speed depends on training loads, fatigue, and goals. In addition, repetition speed has been shown to significantly affect neural,[28,50] hypertrophic,[83,122] and metabolic[102] adaptations to weight training.

Force production and contraction velocity directly interact during exercise performance. Generally, force production is greatest at slower velocities and lowest during high-velocity isokinetic movements.[1] This relationship is graphically represented as a force–velocity curve. The implications for the force–velocity curve demonstrate that training at a slow-to-moderate velocity is effective for increasing strength, and training with high velocity is effective for power/speed enhancement. This is generally the case for isokinetic exercise. However, dynamic resistance exercise poses a different type of stimulus, as speed is not controlled, in which attempting to control movement velocity limits force production and strength development.[130,131]

Generally, moderate-to-rapid velocities are most effective for enhanced muscular performance (number of repetitions performed, work and power output, volume), whereas slow velocity is effective for increasing local muscular endurance and isometric strength for a specific number of repetitions. LaChance and Hortobagyi[132] reported significantly greater average power, work, and total number of repetitions performed using a self-selected, rapid velocity compared to 2:2, or 2:4 (2-second positive, 4-second negative) cadence. Thus, improving set performance, the number of repetitions, or load may be best accomplished with use of moderate-to-fast velocities.

Studies that have used isokinetic resistance exercise have shown strength increases specific to the training velocity with some spillover above (as great as 210°/second) and below (as great as 180°/second) the training velocity, mostly at moderate and fast velocities but not at very slow velocities (i.e., 30°/second).[1] Several researchers have trained subjects at 30°/second,[25] 36°/second,[133] 60°/second,[122,134] 100°/second,[135] 108°/second,[133] 120°/second,[83,136] 179°/second,[134] 240°/second,[137] 300°/second[122,134] and reported significant increases in muscular strength. However, it appears that training at moderate velocity (180 to 240°/second) produced the greatest strength increases across all testing velocities.[134] Therefore, isokinetic training is most beneficial when training velocity is goal specific. Otherwise, training at fast, moderate, and slow velocities may produce the greatest strength increases across all testing velocities.[1]

During conventional weight training, free weights and machines, both fast and moderate contraction velocities can increase local muscular endurance depending on the number of repetitions performed and rest between sets. However, slow-velocity training, 3:3 ratio and slower, places continual tension on the muscles for an extended period of time with less generated momentum, thus making it most conducive to increasing local muscular endurance. However, significant reductions in RM loads are observed with slow contraction velocities. Keogh et al.[130] reported that concentric force production was significantly lower for slow velocity (5:5 ratio) lifting compared to traditional (moderate) velocity (771 vs. 1167 N) with a corresponding lower IEMG observed for the slow velocity. These data indicate that motor unit recruitment may be limited when attempting to slow contraction velocity. In addition, the lighter loads required for very slow velocities of training may not provide an optimal stimulus for strength enhancement. Thus, slow training velocities during dynamic resistance exercise may not maximize increases in muscular strength.

Moderate velocities, the velocities most typically used during resistance training, are effective for increasing muscular strength at *all* velocities,[1] whereas training with fast velocities appears most effective for enhancing muscular power and speed.[138] However, for hypertrophy training it appears that fast velocities are not as effective for inducing muscle growth compared to slow or moderate velocities.[50] In addition, high-velocity training imposes less metabolic demand in exercises such as the leg extension, squat, row, and curl compared to slow and moderate velocities.[102]

One limitation to performing high-velocity repetitions with free weights is the deceleration phase. The deceleration phase is that point near the end of the concentric phase in which bar velocity decreases prior to completion of the repetition. The length of this phase depends upon the load used and the average velocity. For example, the load may be decelerated for approximately 24% of the concentric phase, which may increase to 52% or greater when lighter loads are used.[139] Thus, power increases may be most specific only to the initial segment of the ROM as power/speed development throughout the full ROM is limited because the load cannot be maximally accelerated throughout and safely released.[140] A new piece of equipment, the *Plyometric Power System*, has been developed which allows the lifter to safely release the weight using a computerized braking mechanism, thus allowing maximal power output without deceleration.[141] This piece of equipment is beneficial for both upper and lower body ballistic training.

Another popular technique used for both strength and power training is *compensatory acceleration*.[140,142] Compensatory acceleration requires the lifter to accelerate the load maximally throughout the ROM, regardless of momentum, during the concentric action, thus striving to increase bar velocity to maximal levels. A major advantage is that this technique can be used with heavy loads such that there are small deceleration phases and is quite effective, especially for multi-joint exercises.[81] Hunter and Culpepper[143] and Jones et al.[131] reported significant strength and power increases throughout the ROM when compensatory acceleration was used, with the increases greater than that observed for traditional slow-to-moderate velocity concentric actions.[131]

1.4   Summary

Success in weight training depends on the proper manipulation of the acute program variables in accordance with specific training needs and goals. Factors such as the exercises selected and their order, muscle actions involved, intensity, volume, movement velocity, rest periods, and training frequency are all important for program design and affect the body's physiological adaptations to weight training. Perhaps the three most important concepts for long-term progression during weight training are specificity, progressive overload, and variation. The gradual increase in program intensity is necessary to elicit further positive adaptations. In addition, the systematic variation of the training stimulus (periodization) is mandatory for long-term improvements in muscular fitness. In addition to the design of weight training programs, which include optimal periods of rest and recovery, proper nutritional intake is of equal importance for optimal athletic performance. This information is provided in the remaining chapters of this book.

References

1. Fleck, S. J. and Kraemer, W. J., *Designing Resistance Training Programs, 2nd ed.*, Human Kinetics, Champaign, IL, 1997.
2. Mookerjee, S. and Ratamess N. A., Comparison of strength differences and joint action durations between full and partial range-of-motion bench press exercise, *J. Strength Cond. Res.*, 13, 76, 1999.
3. Baker, D., Wilson, G., and Carlyon, R., Generality versus specificity: a comparison of dynamic and isometric measures of strength and speed-strength, *Eur. J. Appl. Physiol.*, 68, 350, 1994.
4. Matveyev, L., *Fundamentals of Sports Training*, Progress, Moscow, 1981.
5. Kraemer, W. J., A series of studies — the physiological basis for strength training in American football: fact over philosophy, *J. Strength Cond. Res.*, 11, 131, 1997.
6. Häkkinen, K., Factors influencing trainability of muscular strength during short term and prolonged training, *NSCA J.*, 7, 32, 1985.
7. Kibler, W. B. and Chandler, T. J., Sport-specific conditioning, *Amer. J. Sports Med.*, 22, 424, 1994.
8. Dolezal, B. A. and Potteiger, J. A., Concurrent resistance and endurance training influence basal metabolic rate in nondieting individuals, *J. Appl. Physiol.*, 85: 695, 1998.
9. Stone, M. H., O'Bryant, H., and Garhammer, J., A hypothetical model for strength training, *J. Sports Med.*, 21, 342, 1981.
10. Fees, M., Decker, T., Snyder-Mackler, L., and Axe, M. J., Upper extremity weight-training modifications for the injured athlete: a clinical perspective, *Amer. J. Sports Med.*, 26, 732, 1998.

11. Gibala, M. J., MacDougall, J. D., and Sale, D. G., The effects of tapering on strength performance in trained athletes, *Int. J. Sports Med.*, 15, 492, 1994.
12. Fleck, S. J., Periodized strength training: a critical review, *J. Strength Cond. Res.*, 13, 82, 1999.
13. Baker, D., Wilson, G., and Carlyon, R., Periodization: the effect on strength of manipulating volume and intensity, *J. Strength Cond. Res.*, 8, 235, 1994.
14. Stowers, T., McMillan, J., Scala, D., Davis, V., Wilson, D., and Stone, M., The short-term effects of three different strength-power training modes, *NSCA J.*, 5, 24, 1983.
15. McGee, D., Jessee, T. C., Stone, M. H., and Blessing, D., Leg and hip endurance adaptations to three weight training programs, *J. Appl. Sports Sci. Res.*, 6, 92, 1992.
16. Sanborn, K., Boros, R., Hruaby, J., Schilling, B., O'Bryant, H., Johnson, R., Hoke, T., Stone, M., and Stone, M. H., Performance effects of weight training with multiple sets not to failure versus a single set to failure in women: a preliminary study, in *International Conference on Weightlifting and Strength Training*, Häkkinen, K., Ed., Funnerus Printing, Jyväskylä, Finland, 1998, 157.
17. Marx, J. O., Nindl, B. C., Ratamess, N. A., Gotshalk, L. A., Volek, J. S., Harman, F. S., Dohi, K., Bush, J. A., Fleck, S. J., Häkkinen, K., and Kraemer, W. J., The effects of single-set vs. periodized multiple-set resistance training on muscular performance and hormonal concentrations in women, *Med. & Sci. Sports & Exerc.*, in press. 2000.
18. O'Bryant, H. S., Byrd, R., and Stone, M. H., Cycle ergometer performance and maximum leg and hip strength adaptations to two different methods of weight-training, *J. Appl. Sport Sci. Res.*, 2, 27, 1988.
19. Herrick, A. B. and Stone, W. J., The effects of periodization versus progressive resistance exercise on upper and lower body strength in women, *J. Strength Cond. Res.*, 10, 72, 1996.
20. Kramer, J. B., Stone, M. H., O'Bryant, H. S., Conley, M. S., Johnson, R. L., Nieman, D. C., Honeycutt, D. R., and Hoke, T. P., Effects of single vs. multiple sets of weight training: impact of volume, intensity, and variation, *J. Strength Cond. Res.*, 11, 143, 1997.
21. Schiotz, M. K., Potteiger, J. A., Huntsinger, P. G., and Denmark, D. C., The short-term effects of periodized and constant-intensity training on body composition, strength, and performance, *J. Strength Cond. Res.*, 12, 173, 1998.
22. Willoughby, D. S., Training volume equated: a comparison of periodized and progressive resistance weight training programs, *J. Hum. Move. Stud.*, 21, 233, 1991.
23. Häkkinen, K., Pakarinen, A., Alen, M., Kauhanen, H., and Komi, P. V., Relationships between training volume, physical performance capacity, and serum hormone concentrations during prolonged training in elite weight lifters, *Int. J. Sports Med.*, 8 (suppl.), 61, 1987.
24. Häkkinen, K., Pakarinen, A., Alen, M., Kauhanen, H., and Komi, P. V., Neuromuscular and hormonal adaptations in athletes to strength training in two years, *J. Appl. Physiol.*, 65, 2406, 1988.
25. Knapik, J. J., Mawdsley, R. H., and Ramos, M. U., Angular specificity and test mode specificity of isometric and isokinetic strength training, *J. Ortho. Sports Phys. Ther.*, 5, 58, 1983.
26. McDonagh, M. J. N. and Davies, C. T. M., Adaptive response of mammalian skeletal muscle to exercise with high loads, *Eur. J. Appl. Physiol.*, 52, 139, 1984.

27. Komi, P. V., Kaneko, M., and Aura, O., EMG activity of leg extensor muscles with special reference to mechanical efficiency in concentric and eccentric exercise, *Int. J. Sports Med.*, 8, 22(supp.), 1987.

28. Eloranta, V. and Komi, P. V., Function of the quadriceps femoris muscle under maximal concentric and eccentric contraction, *Electromyo. Clin. Neurophysiol.*, 20, 159, 1980.

29. Bonde-Peterson, F., Knuttgen, H. G., and Henriksson, J., Muscle metabolism during exercise with concentric and eccentric contractions, *J. Appl. Physiol.*, 33, 792, 1972.

30. Evans, W. J., Patton, J. F., Fisher, E. C., and Knuttgen, H. G., Muscle metabolism during high intensity eccentric exercise, in *Biochemistry of Exercise*, Human Kinetics, Champaign, IL, 1983, 225.

31. Hather, B. M., Tesch, P., Buchanan, P., and Dudley, G. A., Influence of eccentric actions on skeletal muscle adaptations to resistance training, *Acta Physiol. Scand.*, 143, 177, 1991.

32. Ebbeling, C. B. and Clarkson, P. M., Exercise-induced muscle damage and adaptation, *Sports Med.*, 7, 207, 1989.

33. Dudley, G. A., Tesch, P. A., Miller, B. J., and Buchanan, M. D., Importance of eccentric actions in performance adaptations to resistance training, *Aviat. Space Envir. Med.*, 62, 543, 1991.

34. Dudley, G. A., Tesch, P. A., Harris, R. T., Golden, C. L., and Buchanan, P., Influence of eccentric actions on the metabolic cost of resistance exercise. *Aviat. Space Envir. Med.*, 62, 678, 1991.

35. Hettinger, R. and Muller, E., Muskelleistung und muskeltraining, *Arbeits Physiol.*, 15, 111,

36. Bandy, W. D. and Hanten, W. P., Changes in torque and electromyographic activity of the quadriceps femoris muscles following isometric training., *Phys. Ther.*, 73, 455, 1993.

37. Rarick, L. G. and Larsen, G. L., The effects of variations in the intensity and frequency of isometric muscular effort on the development of static muscular strength in pre-pubescent males, *Int. Zeitschrift fur Angewandte Physiol. einschliesslich Arbeitsphysiol.*, 18, 13, 1959.

38. Atha, J., Strengthening muscle, *Exerc. Sports Sci. Rev.*, 9, 1, 1981.

39. Always, S. E., Grumbt, W. H., Gonyea, W. J., and Stray-Gundersen, J., Contrasts in muscle and myofibers of elite male and female bodybuilders, *J. Appl. Physiol.*, 67, 24, 1989.

40. Jackson, A., Jackson, T., Hnatek, J., and West, J., Strength development: using functional isometrics in an isotonic strength training program, *Res. Q. Exerc. Sport*, 56, 234, 1985.

41. Collins, M. A., Cureton, K. J., Hill, D. W., and Ray, C. A., Relation of plasma volume change to intensity of weight lifting, *Med. Sci. Sports Exerc.*, 21, 178, 1989.

42. Dudley, G. A., Metabolic consequences of resistive-type exercise, *Med. Sci. Sports Exerc.*, 20(suppl.), S158, 1988.

43. Willoughby, D. S., Chilek, D. R., Schiller, D. A., and Coast, J. R., The metabolic effects of three different free weight parallel squatting intensities *J. Hum. Move. Stud.*, 21, 53, 1991.

44. Kraemer, W. J., Marchitelli, L., Gordon, S. E., Harman, E., Dziados, J. E., Mello, R., Frykman, P., McCurry, D., and Fleck, S. J., Hormonal and growth factor responses to heavy resistance exercise protocols, *J. Appl. Physiol.*, 69, 1442, 1990.

45. Kraemer, W. J., Fry, A. C., Warren, B. J., Stone, M. H., Fleck, S. J., Kearney, J. T., Conroy, B. P., Maresh, C. M., Weseman, C. A., Triplett, N. T., and Gordon, S. E., Acute hormonal responses in elite junior weightlifters, *Int. J. Sports Med.*, 13, 103, 1992.

46. Craig, B. W. and Kang, H., Growth hormone release following single versus multiple sets of back squats: total work versus power, *J. Strength Cond. Res.*, 8, 270, 1994.

47. Komi, P. V. and Viitasalo, J. H. T., Signal characteristics of EMG at different levels of muscle tension, *Acta Physiol. Scand.*, 96, 267, 1976.

48. Häkkinen, K., Alen, M., and Komi, P. V., Changes in isometric force- and relaxation-time, electromyographic and muscle fibre characteristics of human skeletal muscle during strength training and detraining, *Acta Physiol. Scand.*, 125, 573, 1985.

49. Sale, D. G., Neural adaptations to strength training, in *Strength and Power in Sport*, Komi, P. V., (Ed.), Blackwell Scientific Publications, Boston, 1992, 249.

50. Häkkinen, K., Komi, P. V., and Alen, M., Effect of explosive type strength training on isometric force-and relaxation-time, electromyographic and muscle fibre characteristics of leg extensor muscles, *Acta Physiol. Scand.*, 125, 587, 1985.

51. Fleck, S. J., Cardiovascular adaptations to resistance training, *Med. Sci. Sports Exerc.*, 20, S146, 1988.

52. Fleck, S. J., Pattany, P. M., Stone, M. H., Kraemer, W. J., Thrush, J., and Wong, K., Magnetic resonance imaging determination of left ventricular mass: junior Olympic weightlifters, *Med. Sci. Sports Exerc.*, 25, 522, 1993.

53. Wathen, D., Load assignment, in *Essentials of Strength Training and Conditioning*, Baechle, T. (Ed.), Human Kinetics, Champaign, IL, 1994, 435.

54. Rutherford, O. M. and Jones, D. A., The role of learning and coordination in strength training, *Eur. J. Appl. Physiol.*, 55, 10, 1986.

55. Ploutz, L. L., Tesch, P. A., Biro, R. C. L., and Dudley, G. A., Effect of resistance training on muscle use during exercise, *J. Appl. Physiol.*, 76, 1675, 1994.

56. Ikai, M. and Fukunaga, T., A study on training effect on strength per unit cross-sectional area of muscle by means of ultrasonic measurement, *Int. Zeitschrift fur Angewandte Physiol.*, 28, 173, 1970.

57. Berger, R. A., Optimum repetitions for the development of strength, *Res. Q.*, 33, 334, 1962.

58. O'Shea, P., Effects of selected weight training programs on the development of strength and muscle hypertrophy, *Res. Q.*, 37, 95, 1966.

59. Weiss, L. W., Coney, H. D., and Clark, F. C., Differential functional adaptations to short-term low-, moderate-, and high-repetition weight training, *J. Strength Cond. Res.*, 13, 236, 1999.

60. DeLorme, T. L. and Watkins, A. L., Techniques of progressive resistance exercise, *Arch. Phys. Med.*, 29, 263, 1948.

61. MacDougall, J. D., Ward, G. R., Sale, D. G., and Sutton, J. R., Biochemical adaptation of human skeletal muscle to heavy resistance training and immobilization, *J. Appl. Physiol.*, 43, 700, 1977.

62. Staron, R. S., Karapondo, D. L., Kraemer, W. J., Fry, A. C., Gordon, S. E., Falkel, J. E., Hagerman, F. C., and Hikida, R. S., Skeletal muscle adaptations during early phase of heavy-resistance training in men and women, *J. Appl. Physiol.*, 76, 1247, 1994.

63. Kraemer, W. J., Fleck, S. J., and Evans, W. J., Strength and power training: physiological mechanisms of adaptation, in *Exercise and Sport Science Reviews, Vol. 24*, Holloszy, J. O. (Ed.), Williams and Wilkins, Philadelphia, 1996, 363.

64. Kraemer, W. J., Gordon, S. E., Fleck, S. J., Marchitelli, L. J., Mello, R., Dziados, J. E., Friedl, K., Harman, E., Maresh, C., and Fry, A. C., Endogenous anabolic hormonal and growth factor responses to heavy resistance exercise in males and females, *Int. J. Sports Med.*, 12, 228, 1991.

65. Zatsiorsky, V., *Science and Practice of Strength Training*, Human Kinetics, Champaign, IL, 1995.

66. Anderson, T. and Kearney, J. T., Effects of three resistance training programs on muscular strength and absolute and relative endurance, *Res. Q. Exerc. Sport*, 53, 1, 1982.

67. Stone, W. J. and Coulter, S. P., Strength/endurance effects from three resistance training protocols with women, *J. Strength Cond. Res.*, 8, 231, 1994.

68. Wilson, G. J., Newton, R. U., Murphy, A. J., and Humphries, B. J., The optimal training load for the development of dynamic athletic performance, *Med. Sci. Sports Exerc.*, 25, 1279, 1993.

69. Newton, R. U., Kraemer, W. J., and Häkkinen, K., Effects of ballistic training on preseason preparation of elite volleyball players, *Med. Sci. Sports Exerc.*, 31(2), 323, 1999.

70. Hickson, R. C., Hidaka, K., and Foster, C., Skeletal muscle fiber type, resistance training, and strength-related performance, *Med. Sci. Sports Exerc.*, 26, 593, 1994.

71. Häkkinen, K., Pakarinen, A., Alen, M., Kauhanen, H., and Komi, P. V., Daily hormonal and neuromuscular responses to intensive strength training in 1 week, *Int. J. Sports Med.*, 9, 422, 1988.

72. Dons, B., Bollerup, K., Bonde-Petersen, F., and Hancke, S., The effect of weightlifting exercise related to muscle fiber composition and muscle cross-sectional area in humans., *Eur. J. Appl. Physiol.*, 40, 95, 1979.

73. Tesch, P. A., Komi, P. V., and Häkkinen, K., Enzymatic adaptations consequent to long-term strength training, *Int. J. Sports Med.*, 8(Suppl.), 66, 1987.

74. Kraemer, W. J., Fleck, S. J., Dziados, J. E., Harman, E. A., Marchitelli, L. J., Gordon, S. E., Mello, R., Frykman, P. N., Koziris, L. P., and Triplett, N. T., Changes in hormonal concentrations after different heavy-resistance exercise protocols in women, *J. Appl. Physiol.*, 75, 594, 1993.

75. Potteiger, J. A., Judge, L. W., Cerny, J. A., and Potteiger, V. M., Effects of altering training volume and intensity on body mass, performance, and hormonal concentrations in weight-event athletes, *J. Strength Cond. Res.*, 9, 55, 1995.

76. Mayhew, J. L. and Gross, P. M., Body composition changes in young women with high resistance training, *Res. Q.*, 45, 433, 1974.

77. Dudley, G. A. and Djamil, R., Incompatibility of endurance- and strength-training modes of exercise, *J. Appl. Physiol.*, 59, 1446, 1985.

78. Berger, R. A., Effect of varied weight training programs on strength, *Res. Q.*, 33, 168, 1962.

79. Staron, R. S., Malicky, E. S., Leonardi, M. J., Falkel, J. E., Hagerman, F. C., and Dudley, G. A., Muscle hypertrophy and fast fiber type conversions in heavy resistance-trained women, *Eur. J. Appl. Physiol.*, 60, 71, 1989.

80. McMorris, R. O. and Elkins, E. C., A study of production and evaluation of muscular hypertrophy, *Arch. Phys. Med. Rehab.*, 35, 420, 1954.

81. Jones, D. A. and Rutherford, O. M., Human muscle strength training: the effects of three different regimes and the nature of the resultant changes, *J. Physiol.*, 391, 1, 1987.

82. Hortobagyi, T., Barrier, J., Beard, D., Braspenninex, J., Koens, P., DeVita, P., Dempsey, L., and Lambert, J., Greater initial adaptations to submaximal muscle lengthening than maximal shortening, *J. Appl. Physiol.*, 1677, 1996.

83. Housh, D. J., Housh, T. J., Johnson, G. O., and Chu, W. K., Hypertrophic response to unilateral concentric isokinetic resistance training, *J. Appl. Physiol.*, 7, 65, 1992.

84. Sale, D. G., Jacobs, I., MacDougall, J. D., and Garner, S., Comparisons of two regimens of concurrent strength and endurance training, *Med. Sci. Sports Exerc.*, 22, 348, 1990.

85. Capen, E. K., Study of four programs of heavy resistance exercises for development of muscular strength, *Res. Q.*, 27, 132, 1956.

86. Ostrowski, K. J., Wilson, G. J., Weatherby, R., Murphy, P. W., and Lyttle, A. D., The effect of weight training volume on hormonal output and muscular size and function, *J. Strength Cond. Res.*, 11, 148, 1997.

87. Reid, C. M., Yeater, R. A., and Ullrich, I. H., Weight training and strength, cardiorespiratory functioning and body composition of men, *Brit. J. Sports Med.*, 21, 40, 1987.

88. Coleman, A. E., Nautilus vs. universal gym strength training in adult males, *Amer. Correct. Ther. J.*, 31, 103, 1977.

89. Jacobson, B. H., A comparison of two progressive weight training techniques on knee extensor strength, *Ath. Train.*, 21, 315, 1986.

90. Silvester, L. J., Stiggins, C., McGown, C., and Bryce, G. R., The effect of variable resistance and free-weight training programs on strength and vertical jump, *NSCA J.*, 3, 30, 1982.

91. Messier, S. P. and Dill, M. E., Alterations in strength and maximal oxygen uptake consequent to Nautilus circuit weight training, *Res. Q. Exerc. Sport*, 56, 345, 1985.

92. Starkey, D. B., Pollock, M. L., Ishida, Y., Welsch, M. A., Brechue, W. F., Graves, J. E., and Feigenbaum, M. S., Effect of resistance training volume on strength and muscle thickness, *Med. Sci. Sports Exerc.*, 28, 1311, 1996.

93. Stone, M. H., Johnson, R. L., and Carter, D. R., A short term comparison of two different methods of resistance training on leg strength and power, *Ath. Train.*, 158, 1979.

94. Kraemer, W. J., Ratamess, N., Fry, A. C., Triplett-McBride, T., Koziris, L. P., Bauer, J. A., Lynch, J. M., and Fleck, S. J., Influence of resistance training volume and periodization on physiological and performance adaptations in college women tennis players, *Am. J. Sports Med.*, in press.

95. Stone, M. H., Plisk, S. S., Stone, M. E., Schilling, B. K., O'Bryant, H. S., and Pierce, K. C., Athletic performance development: volume load — 1 set vs. multiple sets, training velocity and training variation, *Strength & Cond.*, 20, 22, 1998.

96. Jones, A., The best kind of exercise, *Iron Man*, 32, 36, 1973.

97. Häkkinen, K., Komi, P. V., Alen, M., and Kauhanen, H., EMG, muscle fibre and force production characteristics during a 1 year training period in elite weightlifters, *Eur. J. Appl. Physiol.*, 56, 419, 1987.

98. O'Hagan, F. T., Sale, D. G., MacDougall, J. D., and Garner, S. H., Comparative effectiveness of accommodating and weight resistance training modes, *Med. Sci. Sports Exerc.*, 27, 1210, 1995.

99. Willoughby, D. S. and Simpson, S., Supplemental EMS and dynamic weight training: effects on knee extensor strength and vertical jump of female college track & field athletes, *J. Strength Cond. Res.*, 12, 131, 1998.

100. Colliander, E. B. and Tesch, P. A., Effects of eccentric and concentric muscle actions in resistance training, *Acta Physiol. Scand.*, 140, 31, 1990.

101. Scala, D., McMillan, J., Blessing, D., Rozenek, R., and Stone, M., Metabolic cost of a preparatory phase of training in weight lifting: a practical observation, *J. Appl. Sports Sci. Res.*, 1, 48, 1987.

102. Ballor, D. L., Becque, M. D., and Katch, V. L., Metabolic responses during hydraulic resistance exercise, *Med. Sci. Sports Exerc.*, 19, 363, 1987.

103. Tesch, P. A., Short- and long-term histochemical and biochemical adaptations in muscle, in *Strength and Power in Sports*, Komi, P. V. (Ed.), Blackwell Scientific Publications, Boston, 1992, 239.

104. Kraemer, W. J., Hormonal mechanisms related to the expression of muscular strength and power, in *Strength and Power in Sports*, Komi, P. V. (Ed.), Blackwell Scientific Publications, Boston, 1992, 64.

105. Kraemer, W. J., Endocrine responses and adaptations to strength training, in *Strength and Power in Sports*, Komi, P. V. (Ed.), Blackwell Scientific Publications, Boston, 1992, 291.

106. Fahey, T. D., Rolph, R., Moungmee, P., Nagel, J., and Mortara, S., Serum testosterone, body composition, and strength of young adults, *Med. Sci. Sports*, 8, 31, 1976.

107. Volek, J. S., Boetes, M., Bush, J. A., Putukian, M., Sebastianelli, W. J., and Kraemer, W. J., Response of testosterone and cortisol concentrations to high-intensity resistance exercise following creatine supplementation, *J. Strength Cond. Res.*, 11, 182, 1997.

108. Wathen, D., Exercise selection, in *Essentials of Strength Training and Conditioning*, Baechle, T. (Ed.), Human Kinetics, Champaign, IL, 1994, 416.

109. Chilibeck, P. D., Calder, A. W., Sale, D. G., and Webber, C. E., A comparison of strength and muscle mass increases during resistance training in young women, *Eur. J. Appl. Physiol.*, 77, 170, 1998.

110. Sforzo, G. A. and Touey, P. R., Manipulating exercise order affects muscular performance during a resistance exercise training session, *J. Strength Cond. Res.*, 10, 20, 1996.

111. Kraemer, W. J., Noble, B. J., Clark, M. J., and Culver, B. W., Physiologic responses to heavy-resistance exercise with very short rest periods, *Int. J. Sports Med.*, 8, 247, 1987.

112. Kraemer, W. J., Endocrine responses to resistance exercise, *Med. Sci. Sports Exerc.*, 20, S152, 1988.

113. Hannie, P. Q., Hunter, G. R., Kekes-Szabo, T., Nicholson, C., and Harrison, P. C., The effects of recovery on force production, blood lactate, and work performed during bench press exercise, *J. Strength Cond. Res.*, 9, 8, 1995.

114. Kraemer, W. J., Neuroendocrine responses to resistance exercise, in *Essentials of Strength Training and Conditioning*, Baechle, T. (Ed.), Human Kinetics, Champaign, IL, 1994, 86.

115. Kraemer, W. J., General adaptations to resistance and endurance training programs, in *Essentials of Strength Training and Conditioning*, Baechle, T. (Ed.), Human Kinetics, Champaign, IL, 1994, 127.

116. Larson, G. D. and Potteiger, J. A., A comparison of three different rest intervals between multiple squat bouts, *J. Strength Cond. Res.*, 11, 115, 1997.

117. Robinson, J. M., Stone, M. H., Johnson, R. L., Penland, C. M., Warren, B. J., and Lewis, R. D., Effects of different weight training exercise/rest intervals on strength, power, and high intensity exercise endurance, *J. Strength Cond. Res.*, 9, 216, 1995.

118. Pincivero, D. M., Lephart, S. M., and Karunakara, R. G., Effects of rest interval on isokinetic strength and functional performance after short term high intensity training, *Br. J. Sports Med.*, 31, 229, 1997.

119. Fleck, S. J., Bridging the gap: interval training physiological basis, *NSCA J.*, 5, 40, 57, 1983.

120. Volek, J. S. and Kraemer, W. J., Creatine supplementation: its effect on human muscular performance and body composition, *J. Strength Cond. Res.*, 10, 200, 1996.

121. Rooney, K. J., Herbert, R. D., and Balwave, R. J., Fatigue contributes to the strength training stimulus, *Med. Sci. Sports Exerc.*, 26, 1160, 1994.

122. Coyle, E. F., Feiring, D. C., Rotkis, T. C., Cote, R. W., Roby, F. B., Lee, W., and Wilmore, J. H., Specificity of power improvements through slow and fast isokinetic training, *J. Appl. Physiol.*, 51, 1437, 1981.

123. Graves, J. E., Pollock, M. L., Jones, A. E., Colvin, A. B., and Leggett, S. H., Specificity of limited range of motion variable resistance training, *Med. Sci. Sports Exerc.*, 21, 84, 1989.

124. Hunter, G. R., Changes in body composition, body build and performance associated with different weight training frequencies in males and females, *NSCA J.*, 7, 26, 1985.

125. Gilliam, G. M., Effects of frequency of weight training on muscle strength enhancement, *J. Sports Med.*, 21, 432, 1981.

126. Calder, A. W., Chilibeck, P. D., Webber, C. E., and Sale, D. G., Comparison of whole and split weight training routines in young women, *Can. J. Appl. Physiol.*, 19, 185, 1994.

127. Hoffman, J. R., Kraemer, W. J., Fry, A. C., Deschenes, M., and Kemp, M., The effects of self-selection for frequency of training in a winter conditioning program for football, *J. Appl. Sport Sci. Res.*, 4, 76, 1990.

128. Häkkinen, K., Pakarinen, A., Alen, M., Kauhanen, H., and Komi, P. V., Neuromuscular and hormonal responses in elite athletes to two successive strength training sessions in one day, *Eur. J. Appl. Physiol.*, 57, 133, 1988.

129. Häkkinen, K. and Kallinen, M., Distribution of strength training volume into one or two daily sessions and neuromuscular adaptations in female athletes, *Electromyo. Clin. Neurophysiol.*, 34, 117, 1994.

130. Keogh, J. W. L., Wilson, G. J., and Weatherby, R. P., A cross-sectional comparison of different resistance training techniques in the bench press, *J. Strength Cond. Res.*, 13, 247, 1999.

131. Jones, K., Hunter, G., Fleisig, G., Escamilla, R., and Lemak, L., The effects of compensatory acceleration on upper-body strength and power in collegiate football players, *J. Strength Cond. Res.*, 13, 99, 1999.

132. LaChance, P. F. and Hortobagyi, T., Influence of cadence on muscular performance during push-up and pull-up exercises, *J. Strength Cond. Res.*, 8, 76, 1994.

133. Moffroid, M. and Whipple, R. H., Specificity of speed of exercise, *Phys. Ther.*, 50, 1692, 1970.
134. Kanehisa, H. and Miyashita, M., Specificity of velocity in strength training, *Eur. J. Appl. Physiol.*, 52, 104, 1983.
135. Tomberline, J. P., Basford, J. R., Schwen, E. E., Orte, P. A., Scott, S. G., Laughman, R. K., and Ilstrup, D. M., Comparative study of isokinetic eccentric and concentric quadriceps training, *J. Ortho. Sports Phys. Ther.*, 14, 31, 1991.
136. Narici, M. V., Roi, G. S., Landoni, L., Minetti, A. E., and Cerretelli, P., Changes in force, cross-sectional area and neural activation during strength training and detraining of the human quadriceps, *Eur. J. Appl. Physiol.*, 59, 310, 1989.
137. Ewing, J. L., Wolfe, D. R., Rogers, M. A., Amundson, M. L., and Stull, G. A., Effects of velocity of isokinetic training on strength, power, and quadriceps muscle fibre characteristics, *Eur. J. Appl. Physiol.*, 61, 159, 1990.
138. Morrissey, M. C., Harman, E. A., Frykman, P. N., and Han, K. H., Early phase differential effects of slow and fast barbell squat training, *Am. J. Sports Med.*, 26, 221, 1998.
139. Elliott, B. C., Wilson, G. J., and Kerr, G. K., A biomechanical analysis of the sticking region in the bench press, *Med. Sci. Sports Exerc.*, 21, 450, 1989.
140. Wilson, G. J., Strength and power in sport, in *Applied Anatomy and Biomechanics in Sport*, Blackwell Scientific Publications, Boston, 1994, 110.
141. Newton, R. U., Kraemer, W. J., Häkkinen, W. J., Humphries, B. J., and Murphy, A. J., Kinematics, kinetics, and muscle activation during explosive upper body movements: implications for power development, *J. Appl. Biomech.*, 12, 31, 1996.
142. Hatfield, F. C., *Power: A Scientific Approach*, Contemporary Books, Inc., Chicago, 1989.
143. Hunter, G. R. and Culpepper, M. I., Joint angle specificity of fixed mass versus hydraulic resistance knee flexion training, *J. Strength Cond. Res.*, 9, 13, 1995.
144. Bell, G., Syrotuik, D., Socha, T., Maclean, I., and Quinney, H. A., Effect of strength training and concurrent strength and endurance training on strength, testosterone, and cortisol, *J. Strength Cond. Res.*, 11(1), 57, 1997.

2

General Nutritional Considerations for Strength Athletes

Jeff S. Volek

CONTENTS

0-8493-8198-3/01/$0.00+$.50
© 2001 by CRC Press LLC

2.1 Introduction

Strength training is no longer limited to only bodybuilders and power lifters. Athletes participating in almost every sport incorporate resistance training into their overall training program. Expectations from a resistance training program differ somewhat from athlete to athlete; however, increased muscular strength and power and lean body mass are general goals of most programs. The structural and metabolic demands of resistance training are intense, and continued gains depend heavily on recovery from successive workouts. Adequate nutrition is essential for optimal recovery between workouts and maximal adaptations to a training program. There are many factors that contribute to individual nutrient requirements, such as genetics, training goals, phase of training, and training status. However, data from the scientific literature can be extremely useful in planning a general diet that can serve as a template for strength athletes.

In a discussion of nutrition for strength athletes, it is important to first identify mechanisms by which diet can enhance performance of individual resistance exercise workouts. This will help to clarify exactly what we are trying to influence with nutrition and will also help to evaluate the efficacy of a particular dietary strategy. Diet can influence the storage, mobilization, and utilization of nutrients. For example, a high-carbohydrate diet increases storage of glycogen and increases the oxidation of carbohydrate over fat. Second, dietary intake can influence important recovery processes that are required to maximize physiological adaptations over a training cycle. For example, adequate protein is required to meet the demands of increased protein synthesis. Third, dietary intake can influence the concentrations of hormones, which in turn regulate nearly every physiological process in the body. Anabolic hormones like testosterone, growth hormone, insulin, and insulin-like growth factor I are extremely important in mediating many of the positive adaptations to resistance training such as muscle growth. Hormones also influence the relative proportion of carbohydrate and fat utilization at rest and during exercise.

Central to understanding how nutrition can influence performance is a basic understanding of energy metabolism and the metabolic demands of resistance training. An overview of protein, carbohydrate, and fat will follow, emphasizing the classification and sources of each macronutrient. Research on protein requirements for strength athletes and carbohydrate supplementation before, during, and after resistance exercise will be presented. The role of fat in the diet and other nutritional concerns for strength athletes will be discussed.

2.2   Metabolic Demands of Resistance Training

In general, resistance exercise requires high contraction frequency and high power or force outputs of specific muscles such that fatigue (a decline in force/power output or inability to complete a repetition) occurs rapidly. High-intensity exercise of this nature cannot be performed continuously for extended periods due to selective muscle fiber type depletion of energy substrates (phosphocreatine and glycogen) and/or accumulation of metabolic products (lactate, H^+, ammonia). However, a large number of repetitions can be accomplished when performed intermittently. Typically, multiple repetitions are performed continuously, which constitutes a single set. The rest period between sets can vary and influences metabolic and hormonal responses. Multiple sets are usually performed for different exercises targeting various muscle groups. The metabolic demands of resistance exercise will vary to some degree depending on the configuration of these acute program variables but are much different compared to prolonged continuous endurance exercise.

The final energy currency in the body is ATP, and high-intensity exercise, especially resistance exercise, requires high rates of ATP turnover. Since storage of ATP is minimal, metabolic pathways exist that rapidly generate the required ATP necessary to perform resistance exercise. Immediate generation of ATP occurs anaerobically (without oxygen) via the high-energy phosphate compound phosphocreatine, which is rapidly dephosphorylated to reform ATP at the onset of high-intensity exercise. Glycolysis, the breakdown of glucose into pyruvate, is also simultaneously activated at the onset of exercise and contributes to the formation of ATP anaerobically. Glucose is derived from the breakdown of glycogen which occurs at the onset of intense exercise. After only approximately 10 to 15 seconds phosphocreatine stores are depleted and glycolysis becomes the primary energy system to generate ATP. During high-intensity exercise, or high repetition sets of resistance exercise with short rest periods, lactate accumulation and the rising H^+ concentration ultimately lead to fatigue. If exercise continues at a low intensity, ATP resynthesis occurs primarily at the expense of oxidation of carbohydrates (plasma glucose or muscle glycogen) and fats (intramuscular triglycerides or plasma fatty acids). During rest or periods of low-intensity activity, such as recovery periods between sets of resistance exercises, phosphocreatine is resynthesized, and lactate is cleared from the muscle so that subsequent sets can be performed at maximal intensity.

Compared to endurance exercise there are relatively few studies examining energy metabolism during resistance exercise. One of the few studies designed to examine muscle metabolism during resistance exercise was performed in a group of bodybuilders who completed a very intense workout consisting of 5 sets each of front and back squats, leg press, and knee extensions.[1] Muscle biopsies were obtained prior to and about 30 seconds after the workout session in order to measure energy substrates. There was a small decline in muscle ATP concentrations and an almost 50% depletion in phosphocreatine. The resynthesis of phosphocreatine during recovery is an oxygen-dependent process with a half-life of approximately 30 seconds.[2] Thus, depletion of phosphocreatine was probably greater considering the fact that the biopsy in this study was obtained 30 seconds after the exercise workout. It can be concluded that phosphagen metabolism is very important for resistance exercise, which probably explains why creatine supplementation is beneficial for resistance exercise.[3] In these same subjects, muscle glycogen was depleted by about one third.[4] Surprising was the nearly one third reduction in muscle triglyceride stores observed in these athletes. It is generally thought that lipids contribute little to ATP production during exercise intensities greater than 70 to 80% of VO_2max. These data challenge that notion and suggest that triglycerides are an important energy source during resistance exercise. In fact, triglyceride utilization played a more important role than glycogen breakdown in some subjects. Interestingly, the depletion of muscle triglycerides was related to the resting pre-exercise muscle triglyceride concentration. Those subjects with higher pre-exercise triglycerides demonstrated the greatest depletion in triglyceride stores. Thus, if muscle triglycerides are available, they will probably be used for energy and may spare muscle glycogen. This is the only study that has measured muscle triglycerides in response to resistance exercise.

Other studies have examined glycogen depletion and resynthesis in response to resistance exercise. Robergs et al.[5] studied glycogen depletion patterns in response to a low- and high-intensity knee extension protocol performed at 30% and 70% of one-repetition maximum. Repetitions were adjusted so that an equal amount of work was performed during both knee extension protocols. Glycogen depletion was about 30% and was similar for both exercise intensities. Glycogen resynthesis slowly increased toward resting values over 2 hours post-exercise. Other studies have demonstrated a similar depletion in muscle glycogen of about 30% in response to resistance exercise.[6,7]

An overview of energy metabolism during a bout of resistance exercise is shown in Figure 2.1. The few studies examining muscle metabolism during resistance exercise indicate a large reliance on phosphocreatine in addition to muscle glycogen and triglyceride stores. The relative contribution from these sources may depend on availability, especially in the case of triglyceride stores. Thus, from a nutritional standpoint it would be advantageous to optimize the use of phosphocreatine (creatine supplementation) because this is the most powerful energy system in terms of ATP provision. Since glycogen and perhaps even triglycerides contribute significantly to the provision of energy during resistance exercise, replenishing these energy stores should be an important component of an overall dietary strategy for strength athletes.

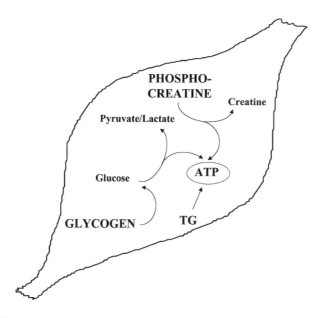

FIGURE 2.1

Skeletal muscle energy substrates utilized to synthesize ATP during resistance exercise. Phosphocreatine is an immediate energy buffer that supplies ATP anaerobically via the creatine kinase reaction. Breakdown of muscle glycogen into glucose is further metabolized in anaerobic glycolysis into lactate, with concomitant production of ATP. There is some indication that triglycerides might be an important energy source for ATP during resistance exercise. Triglycerides must first be hydrolyzed into fatty acids that must enter the mitochondria to be further metabolized aerobically via β-oxidation, the Kreb's cycle, and the electron transport chain.

2.3 Protein

Dietary protein contains 4 kcal per gram energy and has functions related to structural (collagen of bone and skin), regulatory (peptide hormones), contractile (actin and myosin filaments), transport (hemoglobin), catalytic (enzymatic), and energetic (gluconeogenic) roles. Proteins and their component parts, amino acids, are essential dietary nutrients to sustain life and serve as the building blocks for synthesis of proteins into skeletal muscle. While our bodies have the capacity to synthesize certain amino acids (nonessential or dispensable amino acids), others must be obtained from the diet and are called essential or indispensable amino acids (Table 2.1). Under certain physiological and pathological conditions, synthesis of nonessential amino acids may be insufficient and may become conditionally essential. All amino acids are important, not just the essential amino acids. For protein synthesis to take place, all amino acids must be available and present. Individual requirements for amino acids have not been determined. Rather, dietary recommendations are for protein, which contains amino acids. Rich sources of protein include meat (beef, chicken, turkey, fish), dairy (eggs, milk, cheese), and nuts/seeds.

TABLE 2.1

Classification of Amino Acids

Nutritionally Essential	Conditionally Essential	Nutritionally Nonessential
Isoleucine	Arginine	Aspartic acid
Leucine	Cysteine	Asparagine
Lysine	Glutamine	Glutamic acid
Methionine	Glycine	Alanine
Phenylalanine	Histidine	Serine
Threonine	Proline	
Tryptophan	Taurine	
Valine	Tyrosine	

2.3.1   Types of Protein

Not all protein foods are of equal nutritional value. Depending on the presence and ratio of amino acids in a particular protein food, it may be classified as high-quality, intermediate-quality, or low-quality. High-quality or complete proteins contain all the essential amino acids; intermediate-quality proteins are lacking in one of the essential amino acids; and low-quality proteins are lacking in more than one essential amino acid (Table 2.2). Adequate essential amino acid intake can be achieved by complementing lower-quality protein sources that lack different essential amino acids.

TABLE 2.2

Quality of Different Protein Sources

High-Quality	Milk	
	Eggs	Animal Sources
	Meat (beef, chicken, fish)	
Intermediate-Quality	Nuts/seeds	
	Rice	
	Soy	
	Potatoes	
	Oats	Plant Sources
Low-Quality	Peas	
	Cornmeal	
	White flour	
	Gelatin	

2.3.2 Protein Requirements for Strength Athletes

In order to promote increases in muscle size (hypertrophy) and increases in strength it is an absolute requirement that athletes be in a positive nitrogen status. Nitrogen status is determined by measuring dietary nitrogen intake (protein is 16% nitrogen) and subtracting nitrogen loss (urine, sweat, feces). A question debated for over 100 years is whether large quantities of dietary protein are necessary to optimize protein synthesis and enhance muscular hypertrophy and strength. The current recommended daily allowance (RDA) for protein is 0.8 grams per kilogram body weight. The RDA for protein was derived from both short- and long-term nitrogen balance studies from subjects whose lifestyles were essentially sedentary.

Resistance training is a powerful stimulus to increase the rate of amino acid incorporation into muscle proteins.[8] In recent years, evidence has accumulated indicating that protein in excess of the current RDA is necessary to maintain nitrogen balance and optimize muscle development. Based on nitrogen balance and metabolic tracer studies examining the optimal protein requirement for strength and power athletes, protein intake should be about 1.7 to 1.8 g/kg/day.[9] Consuming protein at levels >2 g/kg/day will cause an increase in amino acid oxidation without increasing whole-body protein synthesis.[10] Other dietary factors may also affect protein requirements. Total energy intake as well as the composition of the diet can alter protein metabolism. If insufficient calories are consumed, protein intakes that would normally promote a positive nitrogen balance can induce a negative nitrogen status.[11] Further, if dietary carbohydrates are reduced, glycogen stores may become depleted more quickly and enhance the utilization of protein as a fuel source.[12] Thus, under conditions of inadequate energy consumption and/or low carbohydrate intake protein requirements may be further increased. The negative health concerns associated with increasing protein intake to these levels are unsubstantiated. Protein intakes up to 2 g/kg/day can be easily and safely consumed in a typical Western diet.

The source and quality of protein may also impact adaptations to resistance training. Consuming higher-quality protein, meat in particular, may augment gains in strength and increases in lean body mass and muscle fiber hypertrophy compared to a vegetarian diet lacking meat.[13] A possible explanation for the greater adaptations observed with consumption of meat is higher testosterone concentrations. Testosterone is a steroid hormone secreted from the Leydig cells of the testes that has both anabolic and anticatabolic effects upon muscle tissue. A vegetarian or meatless diet results in lower circulating concentrations of testosterone compared to a mixed Western or a high-meat diet.[14–17] Raben et al.[18] reported a significant decrease in resting testosterone concentrations and an attenuation in the exercise-induced increase in testosterone in male endurance athletes who switched from a meat-rich diet to a lacto-ovo vegetarian diet. The diets contained equal percentages of calories derived from protein, carbohydrate, and fat, but the source of protein in the vegetarian diet was derived mainly from vegetable sources (83%), whereas the mixed diet contained significantly less vegetable protein (35%). The exact mechanism linking nutrition to testosterone is unknown, but it appears that including red meat in the diet is beneficial in terms of promoting an anabolic environment in the body.

2.3.3   Practical Guidelines

Based on several studies evaluating protein requirements for strength athletes, there is general agreement that the RDA is not adequate. An intake ranging from 1.5 to 2.0 g/kg/day should maintain a positive nitrogen balance in strength athletes. This is equivalent to 112 to 150 grams of protein for a 75-kg (165 lbs) athlete or about 450 to 600 kcal of protein per day. These levels can be easily achieved by consuming a wide variety of protein sources from lean meats (beef, chicken, fish), eggs, cheese, cottage cheese, yogurt, milk, and nuts and seeds.

2.4   Carbohydrate

Dietary carbohydrates contain 4 kcal per gram energy and function primarily as an energy substrate. Rich sources of carbohydrates include breads, pastas, rice, beans, cereals, fruits and fruit juices, and vegetables.

2.4.1   Types of Carbohydrate

Structurally, carbohydrates can be classified as monosaccharides (one sugar), disaccharides (two sugars), or polysaccharides (many sugars). The primary dietary monosaccharides, disaccharides, and polysaccharides are shown in Table 2.3. Monosaccharides and disaccharides are collectively referred to as "simple" carbohydrates, and polysaccharides as "complex" carbohydrates. This classification system is based on chemical structure and does not reflect any physiological or metabolic effect of the carbohydrate. A more useful classification system based on a metabolic outcome is the glycemic index (GI).

2.4.2   Glycemic Index (GI)

The GI provides a method to classify foods based on their acute glycemic impact.[19] The GI of a food is based on a standard food (usually glucose or white bread), which is given an arbitrary value of 100. The GI of a food is calculated by integrating the 2-hour glycemic-response curve after ingestion of the test food containing 50 g of available carbohydrate. Foods that are digested quickly and appear in the bloodstream rapidly have a high GI, and

TABLE 2.3

Structural Classification of Carbohydrates

Monosaccharides "Simple Carbohydrates"

Glucose
Fructose
Galactose

Disaccharides "Simple Carbohydrates"

Sucrose (glucose + fructose)
Lactose (glucose + galactose)
Maltose (glucose + glucose)

Polysaccharides "Complex Carbohydrates"

Starch
Cellulose

foods that are more resistant to digestion and appear in the bloodstream at a slower rate have a low GI. Foods with a high GI cause blood sugar and insulin concentrations to rise faster than low GI foods. There is no obvious correlation between the prevalent chemical classification system of simple or complex carbohydrates and the GI of a food. For example, complex carbohydrates such as white bread and potatoes have a high GI, whereas the simple carbohydrate fructose has a low GI. The main determinant of the GI and the metabolic effect of a food is the rate at which it is digested.[20] Factors that influence the digestion of foods and thus the GI include type of sugar (fructose is lower than sucrose or glucose), nature of the starch (amylose is lower than amylopectin), fiber content, portion size, degree of processing, protein and fat in the food, and food preparation method. Table 2.4 lists several foods and their corresponding GI.

2.4.3   Carbohydrates Before and During Resistance Exercise

Nearly all of the literature pertaining to consumption of foods and fluids prior to and during exercise has been based on the performance of endurance athletes. Carbohydrate consumed prior to and/or during endurance exercise can provide an energy source late in exercise when glycogen concentrations in muscle and liver have become depleted, and subsequently delay fatigue and enhance performance.[22] As reviewed above, resistance exercise depletes muscle glycogen, especially in Type II or fast-twitch muscle fibers. Thus, carbohydrates may enhance resistance training workouts if glycogen depletion limits performance. Specific Type II muscle fiber glycogen depletion may limit performance if a high volume of work is performed or if multiple workouts are performed in a single day. At least one recent study

TABLE 2.4

Glycemic Index (GI) of Various Foods

Bakery Products		Fruits		Dairy Foods	
Angel food cake	95	Apple	52		
Sponge cake	66	Apple juice	58	Ice cream	87
Croissant	96	Banana	76	Ice cream (low-fat)	71
Doughnut (cake type)	108	Cherries	32	Milk (whole)	39
Muffin (bran)	85	Fruit cocktail	79	Milk (skim)	46
Waffles	109	Grapefruit	36	Yogurt	20
		Grapefruit juice	69		
Breads		Grapes	62	**Snack Foods**	
		Orange	62		
Bagel	103	Orange juice	74	Oatmeal cookies	79
Hamburger bun	87	Pear	47	Vanilla wafers	110
Kaiser rolls	104	Pineapple	94	Rice cakes	117
Wheat bread	99	Plum	34	Jelly beans	114
		Raisins	91	Chocolate	70
Cereals		Watermelon	103	Popcorn	79
				Corn chips	105
All-Bran	60	**Legumes**		Potato chips	77
Cheerios	106			Peanuts	21
Corn flakes	119	Baked beans	69		
Oat bran	78	Chickpeas	47	**Sugars**	
Puffed wheat	105	Kidney beans	42		
Rice Krispies	117	Lentils	41	Honey	104
Shredded wheat	99	Lima beans	46	Fructose	32
		Pinto beans	55	Glucose	138
Cereal Grains/Pasta		Split peas	45	Sucrose	92
				Lactose	65
Barley	36	**Vegetables**		Maltose	150
White rice	81				
Brown rice	79	Carrots	101	**Soups**	
Instant rice	128	Potato (baked)	121		
Rye	48	Sweet potato	77	Lentil	63
Wheat	59	Peas	68	Split pea	86
Linguine	65	Corn	78	Tomato	54
Spaghetti	59				

GI values from Foster-Powell and Miller.[21]

reported a beneficial effect of carbohydrate supplementation on resistance exercise performance.[23]

Haff et al.[23] examined the effects of carbohydrate supplementation or placebo on the ability to perform multiple sets of squat exercise during a second training session of a single day. A glycogen-depleting resistance exercise session (15 sets of various squat exercises) was performed in the morning, and then 4 hours later subjects were required to squat to exhaustion. The squat protocol consisted of sets of 10 repetitions at 55% of one-repetition maximum with 3 minutes recovery between sets. The carbohydrate supplement was a 20% maltodextrin and dextrose solution, which yielded 0.3 grams per kilogram body weight. The supplement was provided before the morning workout, throughout the 4-hour recovery period, and during the squat-to-exhaustion test. Compared to placebo, carbohydrate supplementation significantly improved the number of sets (18.7 vs. 11.3), number of repetitions (199 vs. 131), and duration (78 vs. 46 min). The results indicate that carbohydrate supplementation may be beneficial for athletes who perform more than one training session per day.

The value of carbohydrate supplementation for single resistance training sessions is questionable. If resistance training proceeds beyond approximately 1 hour, glycogen depletion may limit performance, and therefore carbohydrate supplementation would be hypothesized to improve muscular strength and muscular endurance. Although no data exist, carbohydrate supplementation before and during exercise may enhance glycogen resynthesis during the recovery period between multiple sets of resistance exercise.

2.4.4 Carbohydrates After Resistance Exercise

In the scientific literature, ingestion of carbohydrates immediately after resistance exercise has been evaluated based on two outcomes. First, carbohydrates consumed after a workout can enhance the rate of glycogen resynthesis, which may be important for athletes performing 2 training sessions per day or 1 long session. Second, carbohydrate supplementation after a bout of resistance exercise has been shown to alter exercise-induced hormonal responses, which may positively impact recovery by influencing glycogen resynthesis and protein metabolism.

2.4.4.1 Glycogen Resynthesis

Dietary factors may influence muscle glycogen resynthesis by increasing the supply of substrate to muscle, thereby enhancing uptake, and by affecting hormones such as insulin, which may activate important steps involved in glycogen resynthesis (glycogen synthase). One dietary strategy to increase glycogen resynthesis is to simply increase carbohydrate intake during recovery. Only a few studies have examined the influence of carbohydrates provided after a bout of resistance exercise.

Using a leg extension protocol, Pascoe et al.[7] examined the influence of post-resistance exercise carbohydrate supplementation on muscle glycogen resynthesis. Subjects in this study received either a carbohydrate solution (1.5 g/kg body weight) or water immediately and 1 hour post-exercise. Muscle biopsies were obtained at 0, 2, and 6 hours after exercise to measure muscle glycogen. Muscle glycogen was depleted by about 30% immediately after exercise during both conditions. The rate of glycogen resynthesis was significantly greater during the initial 2 hours of recovery with carbohydrate ingestion. After 6 hours, glycogen was restored to 91% of pre-exercise with carbohydrate and 75% of pre-exercise with water.

Roy and Tarnopolosky[6] examined the influence of a carbohydrate or a mixed drink containing carbohydrate, protein, and fat on muscle glycogen resynthesis after resistance exercise. In all trials there was a similar degree of glycogen depletion of about 30%. The rate of glycogen resynthesis was significantly greater for carbohydrate and mixed trials compared to placebo. However, there was no difference between drinks. Thus, protein and fat do not interfere with glycogen resynthesis and may help in other processes such as supplying needed amino acids for incorporation into muscle proteins or enhancing the hormonal environment. These studies examined muscle glycogen resynthesis in response to carbohydrate supplementation provided during the immediate post-exercise period. An important question is how much carbohydrate is needed during the entire period between successive bouts of resistance exercise on different days.

Although theirs was not a resistance exercise study, MacDougall et al.[24] had subjects perform high-intensity exhaustive cycle ergometry to deplete glycogen levels and then had them consume either a mixed diet (3100 kcals) or a mixed diet plus an additional 2500 kcal of carbohydrate during the 24-hour period following exercise. Muscle glycogen was depleted to 28% of pre-exercise values immediately after exercise, which was similar to other resistance exercise studies; depleted levels returned to resting levels after 24 hours of recovery. There was no difference in glycogen resynthesis rate between dietary conditions, indicating that consumption of higher than normal amounts of carbohydrate cannot accelerate the rate of glycogen resynthesis.

The data presented support a role for carbohydrate supplementation immediately post-exercise if rapid resynthesis of glycogen is desired, such as when multiple training sessions or competitions are performed in the same day. Combining protein and fat with the carbohydrate after exercise will probably not hinder[25] and may even enhance[26] glycogen resynthesis because of the greater rise in insulin associated with ingestion of protein–carbohydrate mixtures compared to carbohydrate alone.

2.4.4.2 Hormonal Responses

The endocrine system plays an important regulatory role in many important physiological processes related to energy metabolism and recovery from exercise. An acute bout of resistance exercise results in increased concentrations of growth hormone, testosterone, epinephrine, and cortisol immediately post-exercise.[27] Certain aspects of the resistance exercise bout will influence the magnitude of these hormonal responses, such as muscle mass involved, rest periods between sets, and number of repetitions.[28] Nutrition, in particular post-exercise meals, can alter hormonal responses to exercise.[29,30]

Our laboratory recently examined the influence of a liquid carbohydrate–protein supplement on the acute hormonal responses to heavy resistance exercise workouts performed on 3 consecutive days.[29] Nine healthy resistance-trained men consumed either a high-calorie liquid protein–carbohydrate supplement consisting of 33% protein (predigested casein and albumin) and 67% carbohydrate (glucose polymers, glucose, crystalline fructose, and xylitol) or placebo for 1 week in a double-blind, balanced, crossover design separated by a 7-day washout period. On the last 3 days of each treatment, subjects performed resistance exercise workouts having consumed the supplement 2 hours before and immediately after the workout. Blood samples were obtained at rest, and at 0, 15, 30, 45, and 60 minutes post-exercise. On exercise days, subjects drank 1/2 serving 2 hours prior to their workout and 1/2 serving after the immediate post-exercise blood draw. The remaining two servings were consumed later in the evening. Each full serving of the supplement provided 7.9 kcal·kg^{-1}·day^{-1}, 1.3 g carbohydrate·kg^{-1}·day^{-1}, and 0.7 g protein·kg^{-1}·day^{-1} (between 525 and 825 kcal per serving). The lactate response declined over the 3 days and was significantly lower during supplementation on Days 2 and 3. The growth hormone response to exercise on Day 1 during supplementation was significantly greater than placebo. There were no differences in the cortisol response to exercise between treatments. Glucose was elevated above rest by 30 minutes post-exercise during supplementation and remained stable during placebo. Insulin declined slightly below resting immediately post-exercise and increased >500% above pre-exercise by 45 minutes post-exercise during supplementation, whereas insulin was unchanged during placebo. Insulin-like growth factor-I (IGF-I) did not increase with exercise but was significantly higher during supplementation on Days 2 and 3. These data indicate that protein–carbohydrate supplementation before and after training can alter the metabolic and hormonal responses to consecutive days of heavy resistance exercise training.

Two other studies have examined the effects of ingesting a dietary supplement comprised of protein and carbohydrate on the hormonal responses to resistance exercise. Chandler et al.[30] showed that insulin and growth hormone concentrations during recovery from a high-intensity resistance training session were higher and testosterone lower when subjects consumed a protein–carbohydrate supplement immediately and 2 hours following the workout. Fahey et al.[31] showed that insulin concentrations were higher at the end of exercise when subjects consumed a protein–carbohydrate supplement 30 minutes prior to and intermittently during a 2-hour weight training session. These studies indicate that carbohydrate and protein consumed prior to, during, and after resistance exercise alter the typical hormonal responses.

2.4.5 Practical Guidelines

Pre-exercise carbohydrate may be beneficial if multiple training sessions are performed in a single day or if one long, intense workout (at least greater than 1 hour) is performed. Pre-exercise carbohydrate will probably not enhance strength performance in shorter workouts because glycogen depletion is probably not a limiting factor in performance. The immediate post-exercise meal should be consumed as soon as possible following the activity, preferably within 1 hour after exercise, to take advantage of the increased rate of glycogen resynthesis and possibly to augment anabolic hormone concentrations. Although the effects of different post-exercise GI carbohydrates have not been investigated after resistance exercise, based on data from endurance exercise it may be beneficial to consume a high-GI carbohydrate after exercise because glycogen resynthesis is faster compared to consumption of a low-GI food.[32] A quality source of protein should also be consumed with the immediate post-exercise meal to ensure all amino acids are available to meet the increased demands of protein synthesis following a bout of resistance exercise.[8] The rest of the meals consumed until the pre-event meal the following day should be comprised of low-to-moderate GI foods, which will keep blood glucose and insulin concentrations more stable without compromising glycogen resynthesis. Over 24 hours the diet should provide approximately 6 to 8 g carbohydrate per kilogram body weight or about 450 to 600 g (1800 to 2400 kcal) per day for a 75-kg athlete. The majority of carbohydrates consumed throughout the day should have a low-to-moderate-GI, thereby preventing surges in blood glucose and insulin. This will enhance energy levels, decrease hunger, promote oxidation of lipid over carbohydrate, and minimize the potential to store excess calories as triglycerides in adipose tissue. A wide variety of unprocessed foods including whole grains, legumes, fruits, and vegetables should be chosen.

2.5 Fat

Dietary fatty acids contain hydrocarbon chains ranging in length from 4 to 20 carbons. Three fatty acids are esterfied with a single glycerol molecule to form triglyceride, the storage form of fat in the body. Compared to carbohydrates, fats are an efficient storage form of energy in the body because they are stored anhydrous (without water) and they contain 9 kcal per gram, over twice the energy per gram as carbohydrate or protein. Based on the degree of saturation, fatty acids may be classified as saturated (no double bonds), polyunsaturated (more than one double bond), and monounsaturated (one double bond). There are two dietary essential polyunsaturated fatty acids, α-linoleic and γ-linolenic acids.

2.5.1 Types of Fat

Saturated fatty acids (SFA) obtained in the diet contain different lengths of hydrocarbon chains; the most common SFA are between 12 and 18 carbons in length. There are no double bonds between the carbons in SFA. The fats associated with animal products (beef, chicken, dairy products) are predominately saturated. Additionally, SFA are usually solid at room temperature.

Unlike SFA, polyunsaturated fatty acids (PUFA) contain two or more double bonds in their hydrocarbon chain. Depending on where the double bonds are located, PUFA may be classified as either n-3 or n-6 series. For example, an n-6 PUFA has the first double bond beginning at the 6th carbon, and an n-3 PUFA has the first double bond beginning at the 3rd carbon. The most common dietary PUFA from the n-6 series is linoleic acid (18:2n-6), and it is also one of the dietary essential fatty acids. Fish oils (or marine oils), which have received considerable attention in the literature recently due to their potent triglyceride-lowering effects,[33] are an example of an n-3 PUFA. Generally, PUFA are the predominant fat in foods derived from plants including most oils, nuts, and seeds. They are usually liquid at room temperature.

Monounsaturated fatty acids (MUFA) contain a single double bond in their hydrocarbon chain; the most common dietary MUFA is oleic acid (18:1n-9). Similar to PUFA, MUFA are usually found in plant-derived foods and are particularly high in olive and canola oils and macadamia nuts.

Trans fatty acids are a type of unsaturated fat that occurs in relatively small amounts in natural foods. However, during the processing of unsaturated oils and other fats such as margarine, the configuration of the double bonds can be switched from the more common *cis* to the *trans* isomer. This occurs during the hydrogenation process to make butter and margarine more solid. Trans fatty acids not only increase LDL cholesterol, but they also decrease HDL cholesterol;[34] hence, they increase the risk for cardiovascular disease.

Cholesterol is a waxy substance that occurs naturally in all parts of our bodies and is manufactured internally; thus, it is not an essential dietary nutrient. Cholesterol is a type of lipid that has a chemical structure similar to many steroids; in fact cholesterol is the precursor to many hormones such as estrogen, progesterone, testosterone, and cortisol. Dietary cholesterol is only present in foods of animal origin such as meats and dairy products, not plant oils. Cholesterol is also involved in producing bile acids, which help in the digestion of dietary fat. In general, our bodies produce cholesterol based on body requirements and the mechanism is under negative feedback control. If dietary intake is low, cholesterol biosynthesis is increased. When dietary cholesterol intake is high, cholesterol biosynthesis is down-regulated.

2.5.2 Role of Fat for Strength Athletes

Compared to carbohydrate and protein, there is less information about the role of fat in the diet of athletes. Fat in an athlete's diet is important for several reasons and should not be avoided. Dietary lipids may be hypothesized to be very important in terms of promoting lipid oxidation and thereby conserving glucose for other tissues,[35] replenishing muscle triglyceride stores after high-intensity exercise,[36] enhancing immune function,[37] and improving the hormonal environment for optimal recovery.[18,38] A low-fat, high-carbohydrate diet promotes oxidation of carbohydrate over fat, which may be a metabolic disadvantage for weight control, cardiovascular health, and exercise performance.

Dietary nutrients, in particular fat, have been shown to affect testosterone. Individuals consuming a diet containing about 20% fat compared to a diet containing 40% fat have significantly lower concentrations of testosterone.[14–17] The specific type or quality of macronutrient may also impact testosterone, independent of a change in diet composition. Volek et al.[38] reported significant positive correlations between dietary fat, specifically saturated and monounsaturated fatty acids, and resting testosterone concentrations in a group of young resistance-trained men. The potential reduction in testosterone on a low-fat diet may have a negative impact on physiological adaptations, especially if the decline in testosterone was substantial.

Compared to muscle glycogen, there is very limited data available on the importance of intramuscular triglycerides for resistance exercise and the rate and regulation of resynthesis after strength exercises. One study did show significant depletion of muscle triglycerides in response to a bout of resistance exercise, especially in athletes with high triglyceride stores before the workout.[4] The enzyme lipoprotein lipase (LPL) has an important role in replenishment of muscle triglycerides.[39] Localization of LPL on the luminal surface of endothelial cells of capillaries allows the enzyme to hydrolyze plasma triglycerides in very-low-density lipoproteins (VLDLs) and chylomicrons and thus provide fatty acids for oxidation or incorporation into triglycerides within skeletal muscle. Exercise training[40] and a high-fat diet[41,42] increase, whereas a high-carbohydrate diet[41] decreases, LPL activity. Upregulation of LPL activity may be responsible for the lower plasma triglycerides in athletes[43] and persons on a higher-fat diet.[44] Kiens et al.[42] demonstrated that switching from a dietary fat intake of 43% to 54% of energy for 4 weeks was associated with an 80% increase in muscle LPL activity and a 57% increase in resting muscle triglyceride stores.

Only one study has examined the effects of diet on intramuscular triglyceride resynthesis after exercise and involved endurance activity. Consumption of a low-carbohydrate, high-fat (68% of energy) diet for 24 hours following a 120-minute cycling bout significantly increased muscle triglyceride stores above pre-exercise levels and to a greater extent than an isocaloric high-carbohydrate, low-fat (5% of energy) diet.[36] The significant increase in intramuscular triglycerides after 24 hours of a high-fat diet was probably mediated via stimulation of LPL activity induced by exercise and the high-fat nature of the diet. The need to provide dietary fat after exercise and the impact on performance is unknown.

2.5.3   Practical Guidelines

In addition to effects on performance and body composition, recommendations for dietary fat should also consider the potential impact on blood lipid profiles and therefore cardiovascular disease risk. A diet that emphasizes

PUFA and MUFA, especially fish oil, has definite advantages over a diet rich in SFA in terms of cardiovascular disease. When either PUFA or MUFA are substituted for carbohydrate in the diet, there are improvements in total cholesterol, LDL cholesterol, HDL cholesterol, and triglycerides.[45,46] These "healthy" fats should account for the majority of fat in an athlete's diet. The optimal amount of fat in the diet is controversial, and research in this area for strength athletes is not available. If fat is derived from unsaturated sources, extremely high intakes do not result in adverse blood lipid responses; in fact triglycerides are actually improved.[44] An intake of between 30 and 40% of total energy intake is probably a good place to start if the majority of these calories are from unsaturated sources, especially if weight gain is a goal of the resistance training program. Rich sources of PUFA are most vegetable oils, nuts and seeds, peanut butter, and fatty fish. Rich sources of MUFA are canola oil, olive oil, olives, macadamia nuts, and avocados.

2.6 Other Nutritional Concerns

2.6.1 Weight Gain/Weight Loss

If weight maintenance is desired, total energy intake should match energy expenditure. A stable body weight is strong evidence that adequate energy is being consumed. In order to increase lean body mass, energy intake must be greater than energy input. A moderate increase in caloric or energy intake (300 to 500 kcal/day), primarily from protein and unsaturated fat, while simultaneously decreasing aerobic training volume is recommended. If weight loss is a goal, caloric intake should be decreased by approximately 300 to 500 kcal/day. Protein intake may need to be increased in order to maintain a positive nitrogen balance. High glycemic index carbohydrates should be minimized to help keep insulin low and fatty acid mobilization and oxidation elevated. Resistance training workouts should be performed in addition to moderate amounts of aerobic exercise to enhance energy expenditure. Small frequent meals are recommended over large infrequent meals. More frequent meals allow for more complete absorption and fewer episodes of hypoglycemia in susceptible persons.

2.6.2 Dietary Supplements

Although nutrition is the cornerstone of a strength athlete's training program, dietary supplements may be useful as well. Once an athlete has obtained a sound nutritional program, there may be some advantage to using a daily multivitamin/mineral supplying levels at the RDA. Since strength training relies heavily on phosphocreatine as an energy source, creatine supplementation may provide a way to enhance the intensity of individual workouts[3,47,48] and the adaptations to a resistance training program.[49] Creatine supplementation is discussed in detail in Chapter 8.

2.7 Summary

For the athlete engaged in daily strenuous intermittent exercise sessions, optimal nutrition is an extremely important component of the training program. The optimal diet for an athlete involved in resistance exercise should contain adequate carbohydrate, protein, and fat to meet the energy and tissue remodeling needs imposed by the training. Incorporating creatine supplementation into the athlete's nutritional plan may also enhance the quality of training sessions and improve exercise performance. Consuming a diet with adequate protein, carbohydrate, and fat and incorporating the GI into the daily eating plan allows the athlete to take advantage of the physiological and hormonal responses elicited by ingestion of dietary nutrients. Protein requirements are the least controversial and should supply between 1.5 and 2.0 grams per kilogram body weight per day. For athletes training multiple times per day, there may be a relatively greater need for carbohydrate to replace glycogen. Incorporation of these nutritional strategies will strengthen the foundation on which athletes build their entire training paradigm. Experimentation is the only way to find the ideal ratio of macronutrients for each person. There is always an adaptation period that occurs with any dietary change. Thus, allow enough time to accurately assess the efficacy of a change in diet, preferably at least 2 to 3 weeks.

References

1. Tesch, P. A., Colliander, B., and Kaiser, P., Muscle metabolism during intense, heavy resistance exercise, *Eur. J. Appl. Physiol.*, 55, 363, 1986.
2. Harris, R. C., Edwards, R. H. T., Hultman, E., Nordesjö, L.-O., Nylind, B., and Sahlin, K., The time course of phosphocreatine resynthesis during recovery of the quadriceps muscle in man, *Eur. J. Physiol.*, 367, 137, 1976.
3. Volek, J. S., Kraemer, W. J., Bush, J. A., Boetes, M., Incledon, T., Clark, K. L., and Lynch, J. M., Creatine supplementation enhances muscular performance during high-intensity resistance exercise, *J. Am. Diet. Assoc.*, 97, 765, 1997.
4. Essen-Gustavsson, B. and Tesch, P. A., Glycogen and triglyceride utilization in relation to muscle metabolic characteristics in men performing heavy-resistance exercise, *Eur. J. Appl. Physiol.*, 61, 5, 1990.

5. Robergs, R. A., Pearson, D. R., Costill, D. L., Fink, W. J., Pascoe, D. D., Benedict, M. A., Lambert, C. P., and Zachweija, J. J., Muscle glycogenolysis during different intensities of weight-resistance exercise, *J. Appl. Physiol.,* 70, 1700, 1991.

6. Roy, B. D. and Tarnopolosky, M. A., Influence of differing macronutrient intakes on muscle glycogen resynthesis after resistance exercise, *J. Appl. Physiol.,* 72, 1854, 1998.

7. Pascoe, D. D., Costill, D. L., Fink, W. J., Robergs, R. A., and Zachwieja, J. J., Glycogen resynthesis in skeletal muscle following resistive exercise, *Med. Sci. Sports Exerc.,* 25, 349, 1993.

8. Chesley, A., MacDougall, J. D., Tarnopolosky, M. A., Atkinson, S. A., and Smith, K., Changes in human muscle protein synthesis after resistance exercise, *J. Appl. Physiol.,* 73, 1383, 1992.

9. Lemon, P. W. R., Is increased dietary protein necessary or beneficial for individuals with a physically active lifestyle? *Nutr. Rev.,* 54(suppl), S169, 1996.

10. Tarnopolsky, M. A., Atkinson, S. A., MacDougall, J. D., Chesley, A., Philips, S., and Schwartz, H. P., Evaluation of protein requirements for trained strength athletes, *J. Appl. Physiol.,* 73, 1986, 1992.

11. Walberg, J. L., Leidy, M. K., Sturgill, D. J., Hinkle, D. E., Ritchey, S. J., and Sebolt, D. R., Macronutrient content of a hypoenergy diet affects nitrogen retention and muscle function in weight lifters, *Int. J. Sports Med.,* 9, 261, 1988.

12. Lemon, P. W. R. and Mullin, J. P., Effect of initial muscle glycogen levels on protein catabolism during exercise, *J. Appl. Physiol.,* 48, 624, 1980.

13. Campbell, W. W., Barton, M. L., Cyr-Campbell, D., Davey, S. L., Beard, J. L., Parise, G., and Evans, W. J., Effects of omnivorous diet compared with a lactoovovegetarian diet on resistance-training-induced changes in body composition and skeletal muscle in older men, *Am. J. Clin. Nutr.,* 70, 1032, 1999.

14. Goldin, B. R., Woods, M. N., Spiegelman, D. L., Longcope, C., Morrill-LaBrode, A., Dwyer, J. T., Gualtieri, L. J., Hertzmark, E., and Gorbach, S. L., The effect of dietary fat and fiber on serum estrogen concentrations in premenopausal women under controlled dietary conditions, *Cancer,* 74, 1125, 1994.

15. Hämäläinen, E., Aldercreutz, H., Puska, P., and Pietinen, P., Diet and serum sex hormones in healthy men, *J. Steroid Biochem.,* 20, 459, 1984.

16. Ingram, D. M., Bennett, F. C., Wilcox, D., and de Klerk, N., Effect of low-fat diet on female sex hormone levels, *J. Natl. Cancer Inst.,* 79, 1225, 1987.

17. Reed, M. J., Cheng, R. W., Simmonds, M., Richmond, W., and James, V. H. T., Dietary lipids: an additional regulator of plasma levels of sex hormone binding globulin, *J. Clin. Endocrin. Metab.,* 64, 1083, 1987.

18. Raben, A., Kiens, B., Ritchter, E. A., Rasmussen, L. B., Svenstrup, B., Micic, S., and Bennett, P., Serum sex hormones and endurance performance after a lactoovo vegetarian and a mixed diet, *Med. Sci. Sports Exerc.,* 24, 1290, 1992.

19. Jenkins, D. J. A., Wolever, T. M. S., Taylor, R. H., Baker, H., Fielden, H., Baldwin, J. M., Bowling, A. C., Newman, H. C., Jenkins, A. L., and Goff, D. V., Glycemic index of foods: a physiological basis for carbohydrate exchange, *Am. J. Clin. Nutr.,* 34, 362, 1981.

20. Wolever, T. M. S., Jenkins, D. J. A., Jenkins, A. L., and Josse, R. G., The glycemic index: methodology and clinical implications, *Am. J. Clin. Nutr.,* 54, 846, 1991.

21. Foster-Powell, K. and Miller, J. B., International tables of glycemic index, *Am. J. Clin. Nutr.,* 62, 871S, 1995.

22. Coyle, E. F., Hagberg, J. M., Hurley, B. F., Martin, W. H., Ehsani, A. A., and Holloszy, J. O., Carbohydrate feeding during prolonged endurance exercise can delay fatigue, *J. Appl. Physiol.*, 55, 230, 1983.

23. Haff, G. G., Stone, M. H., Warren, B. J., Keith, R., Johnson, R. L., Nieman, D. C., Williams, F., and Kirksey, B., The effect of carbohydrate supplementation on multiple sessions and bouts of resistance exercise, *J. Strength Cond. Res.*, 13, 111, 1999.

24. MacDougall, J. D., Ward, G. R., Sale, D. G., and Sutton, J. R., Muscle glycogen resynthesis after high-intensity intermittent exercise, *J. Appl. Physiol.*, 42, 129, 1977.

25. Burke, L. M., Collier, G. R., Beasley, S. K., Davis, P. G., Fricker, P. A., Heeley, P., Walder, K., and Hargreaves, M., Effect of coingestion of fat and protein with carbohydrate feedings on muscle glycogen storage, *J. Appl. Physiol.*, 78, 2187, 1995.

26. Zawadzki, K. M., Yaspelkis III, B. B., and Ivy, J. L., Carbohydrate-protein complex increases the rate of muscle glycogen storage after exercise, *J. Appl. Physiol.*, 72, 1854, 1992.

27. Kraemer, W. J., Marchitelli, L. J., Gordon, S. E., Harman, E., Dziados, J. E., Mello, R., Frykman, P., McCurry, K., and Fleck, S. J., Hormonal and growth factor responses to heavy-resistance exercise protocols, *J. Appl. Physiol.*, 69, 1442, 1990.

28. Kraemer, W. J., Endocrine responses to resistance exercise, *Med. Sci. Sports Exerc.*, 20(suppl), S152, 1988.

29. Kraemer, W. J., Volek, J. S., Bush, J. A., Putukian, M., and Sebastianelli, W. J., Hormonal responses to consecutive days of heavy-resistance exercise with or without nutritional supplementation, *J. Appl. Physiol.*, 85, 1544, 1998.

30. Chandler, R. M., Byrne, H. K., Patterson, J. G., and Ivy, J. L., Dietary supplements affect the anabolic hormones after weight-training exercise, *J. Appl. Physiol.*, 76, 839, 1994.

31. Fahey, T. D., Hoffman, K., Colvin, W., and Lauten, G., The effects of intermittent liquid meal feeding on selected hormones and substrates during intense weight training, *Int. J. Sports Nutr.*, 3, 67, 1993.

32. Burke, L. M., Collier, G. R., and Hargreaves, M., Muscle glycogen storage after prolonged exercise: effect of the glycemic index of carbohydrate feedings, *J. Appl. Physiol.*, 75, 1019, 1993.

33. Harris, W. S., n-3 Fatty acids and serum lipoproteins: human studies., *Am. J. Clin. Nutr.*, 65(suppl), 1645S, 1997.

34. Mensink, R. P. and Katan, M. B., Trans monounsaturated fatty acids in nutrition and their impact on serum lipoprotein levels in man, *Prog. Lipid Res.*, 32, 111, 1993.

35. Phinney, S. D., Bistrian, B. R., Evans, W. J., Gervino, E., and Blackburn, G. L., The human metabolic response to chronic ketosis without caloric restriction: preservation of submaximal exercise capacity with reduced carbohydrate oxidation, *Metabolism*, 32, 769, 1983.

36. Starling, R. D., Trappe, T. A., Parcell, A. C., Kerr, C. G., Fink, W. J., and Costill, D. L., Effects of diet on muscle triglyceride and endurance performance, *J. Appl. Physiol.*, 82, 1185, 1997.

37. Venkatraman, J. T., Rowland, J. A., Denardin, E., Horvath, P. J., and Pendergast, D., Influence of the level of dietary lipid intake and maximal exercise on the immune status in runners, *Med. Sci. Sports Exerc.*, 29, 333, 1997.

38. Volek, J. S., Boetes, M., Bush, J. A., Incledon, T., and Kraemer, W. J., Testosterone and cortisol in relationship to dietary nutrients and heavy resistance exercise, *J. Appl. Physiol.*, 82, 49, 1997.

39. Oscai, L. B., Essig, D. A., and Palmer, W. K., Lipase regulation of muscle triglyceride hydrolysis, *J. Appl. Physiol.*, 69, 1571, 1990.

40. Nikkila, E. A., Taskinen, M.-R., Rehunen, S., and Harkonen, M., Lipoprotein lipase activity in adipose tissue and skeletal muscle of runners: relation to serum lipoproteins, *Metabolism*, 27, 1661, 1978.

41. Jacobs, I., Lithell, H., and Karlsson, J., Dietary effects on glycogen and lipoprotein lipase activity in skeletal muscle in man, *Acta Physiol. Scand.*, 115, 85, 1982.

42. Kiens, B., Essen-Gustavsson, B., Gad, P., and Lithell, H., Lipoprotein lipase activity and intramuscular triglyceride stores after long-term high-fat and high-carbohydrate diets in physically trained men, *Clin. Physiol.*, 7, 1, 1987.

43. Haskell, W. L., The influence of exercise on the concentrations of triglyceride and cholesterol in human plasma, in *Exercise and Sport Science Reviews, Vol. 12*, Terjung, R. L. (Ed.), Collamore Press, Lexington, MA, 1984, 205-244.

44. Volek, J. S., Gómez, A. L., and Kraemer, W. J., Fasting lipoprotein and post-prandial triacylglycerol responses to a low-carbohydrate diet supplemented with n-3 fatty acids, *J. Am. Coll. Nutr.*, 19, 383, 2000.

45. Katan, M. J., Zock, P. L., and Mensink, R. P., Dietary oils, serum lipoproteins, and coronary heart disease, *Am. J. Clin. Nutr.*, 61(suppl), 1368S, 1995.

46. Kris-Etherton, P. M. and Yu, S., Individual fatty acid effects on plasma lipids and lipoproteins: human studies, *Am. J. Clin. Nutr.*, 65(suppl), 1628S, 1997.

47. Volek, J. S. and Kraemer, W. J., Creatine supplementation: its effect on human muscular performance and body composition, *J. Strength Cond. Res.*, 10, 198, 1996.

48. Volek, J. S., Kraemer, W. J., Bush, J. A., Boetes, M., Incledon, T., Clark, K. L., and Lynch, J. M., Creatine supplementation enhances muscular performance during high-intensity resistance exercise, *J. Am. Diet. Assoc.*, 97, 765, 1997.

49. Volek, J. S., Duncan, N. D., Mazzetti, S. A., Putukian, M., Staron, R., Putukian, M., Gómez, A. L., Pearson, D. R., Fink, W. J., and Kraemer, W. J., Performance and muscle fiber adaptations to creatine supplementation and heavy resistance training, *Med. Sci. Sports Exerc.*, 31, 1147, 1999.

3

Energy Yielding Nutrients for the Resistive-Trained Athlete

Jacobo O. Morales

CONTENTS

3.1 Introduction

In order to support ongoing bodily processes, such as active transport mechanisms, endocrine secretions, anabolism, and circulation, the human body requires a continuous supply of potential energy. The latter, obtained from the foods we consume, is ultimately converted into a usable energy form (ATP) as a result of the process known as bioenergetics. Once ATP is synthesized, this high-energy phosphate can provide usable chemical energy for mechanical work or other noncontractile functions. Because ATP is an intermediate in a cell's energy exchange process, this phosphagen can be thought of as a molecule for capturing and transferring G (free energy).

The uninterrupted need for ATP regeneration is pronounced whenever the body's physiology deviates from homeostasis, as during physical exercise. Thus, whenever humans sustain a run, swim, or engage in a resistive-type workout, the phosphorylation of adenosine diphosphate, ADP, must be positively modulated in order to meet the heightened contractile demands of the exercising muscles. The resulting increase in energy exchange within the working muscle fiber cells depletes the body's potential energy stores, as exercise mechanical work is only possible through the conversion of stored chemical potential energy into the former. Consequently, those who engage in regular physical exercise must make sure to balance their energy output with adequate dietary energy input in order to carry out normal tissue growth, repair, and maintenance.

Energy intake by an athletically inclined population is required not only for replenishing purposes but also to support any required (anabolic) processes conducive to exercise adaptations. For example, people undergoing endurance-type training will convert food into energy to be used for replication of mitochondrial protein, myoglobin, and capillary beds, as well as replete catabolized protein when amino acids are required as an auxiliary fuel source. Those dedicated to resistive-type training will need replication of myofibrillar protein in order to support the anabolic stimulus known to accompany chronic resistive exercise.

The purpose of this chapter is to discuss the energy demands of those who rely primarily on resistive training as the conditioning modality to enhance athletic performance. Examples of such individuals include track and field throwers, Olympic weightlifters, bodybuilders, and powerlifters. Focus will be placed on the energy-yielding nutrients (carbohydrates, proteins, and fats), and consideration will be given to nutrient demands based on: (a) reliance during training or participation, and (b) nutrient requirements for adaptations.

3.2   Metabolic Profile of a Resistive Training Bout

In order to appreciate the nature of the nutrient blend during physical exercise, the metabolic profile of the specific exercise must be identified. For example, during submaximal (steady-state) exercise (running, cycling at 40% VO_2max), ATP regeneration can be adequately achieved by oxidation of fat and carbohydrate stores.[1] However, when this exercise is performed at high intensity (non-steady state), the relatively slow activation and rate of energy delivery through oxidative phosphorylation cannot fully meet the energy requirements of muscle actions.[1] Given these circumstances, anaerobic energy delivery becomes the fundamental mechanism to support ongoing muscle actions. Although the above statements have been classically used to address the metabolic characteristics of rhythmic, uninterrupted exercise, during a typical resistive training session, reliance on the latter is also applicable. That is, weight training is an activity in which the ATP/CP system (alactic anaerobic) as well as glycolysis (lactic anaerobic) are likely to support the required ATP resynthesis—the reason being that they have faster rates of caloric yield (kcal·min^{-1}) when compared to those of the oxidative pathways. For instance, according to Brooks et al.,[2] the maximal *power* (kcal·min^{-1}) for the immediate energy sources (ATP and CP) is ≈ 36, whereas the nonoxidative (anaerobic glycolysis) value is 16. For the oxidative energy source (substrate = glycogen) the rate is 10.[2] The difference observed within the anaerobic systems in terms of rate of ATP resynthesis suggests that the rapid utilization of CP may buffer the momentary lag in energy provision from glycolysis.[1] This point exemplifies the critical importance of CP at the onset of, for example, a set of supine bench presses. Without substantial hydrolysis of CP at this time, the probability for force output to be quickly impaired is very likely. Nevertheless, the expeditious rates of ATP synthesis provided by the anaerobic energy systems are probably required when resistive training is done for athletic conditioning purposes. During conditioning, performers must produce very high muscular forces in a ballistic fashion during workouts that may exceed 60 minutes. In order for these voluntary efforts to be carried out, the myosin cross-bridges require a continuous and fast exposure to ATP, which can only be brought about by a fast-yielding pathway with ample substrate to operate.

3.2.1 Reliance on Carbohydrates

Although depleted high-energy phosphates (ATP, CP) may be replenished between sets of weight training exercises, during high-intensity lifting, anaerobic glycolysis may eventually become the primary means of regenerating ATP. During structured, serious training, continuous recruitment of muscle may prevent the full repletion of the limited ATP and CP stores, thus *forcing* reliance on the anaerobic degradation of carbohydrates. Therefore, as the exercise bout duration increases, the contribution of glycolysis to ATP regeneration rises, as CP regeneration remains incomplete. This observation is supported by a large body of evidence suggesting that muscle glycogen rather than phosphocreatine or stored ATP is the predominant fuel for high-intensity exercise of short duration[3–5] including resistance training.[6] A sustained reliance on glycolysis will have implications (to be discussed later) regarding the importance of adequate glycogen intake and stores for successful performance during training.

3.2.2 Reliance on Fats

While the energy density of simple fats (triglycerides) is higher than that of carbohydrates (9 kcal·g^{-1} for palmitic acid vs. 4 kcal·g^{-1} for glucose), fats are used to a lesser extent as fuel during resistive training.[7] A fundamental reason to explain this observation is that the individual fatty acid (FA) constituents can only be degraded through mitochondrial respiration. Since resistive exercise has traditionally been labeled as *anaerobic* in nature, the use of FAs as a significant substrate is arguable. Also, while FAs provide more ATP per molecule than glucose (129 from palmitate vs. 38 from glucose), in order to produce the equivalent amount of ATP, the complete oxidation of FAs requires more oxygen (and thus, more time) than the oxidation of carbohydrates. For example, to completely degrade one molecule of 6-C glucose through oxidative phosphorylation only 6 molecules of oxygen must be expended; for 16-C palmitic acid, 23 molecules of oxygen are consumed. Given that fats can only be metabolized aerobically, and that during their oxidation a lower extent of ATP is produced per unit of time, it may be concluded that significant reliance on FAs as a substrate during mostly anaerobic, fast ATP-demanding tasks is unlikely and perhaps, illogical.

Consider also the various steps that must be taken in order to oxidize lipids during exercise. For the sake of simplicity, use of extramuscular triglycerides will be considered. First, peripheral lipolysis must be stimulated in order to promote the breakdown of stored triglycerides and the subsequent mobilization into circulation of the released FAs. Once in the bloodstream, FAs must be carried to the target tissue, exercising skeletal muscle, and then transported across the capillary–muscle interface. Within the sarcoplasm, FAs must be activated and translocated across the mitochondrial membrane. Inside the organelle, the pathways of β-oxidation and the TCA cycle will completely oxidize the substrate, and the resulting reduction of electron carriers (FADH$_2$, NADH) will promote ATP synthesis via oxidative phosphorylation.

The first stage in this process, the mobilization of lipids, plays a key role in the subsequent regulation of FA utilization.[7] During an intense weightlifting session, the resulting increase in blood lactate concentration, and accompanying hydrogen ion accumulation, is likely to inhibit lipolysis and promote the esterification of FAs to triglycerides.[8] This will certainly compromise the supply of FAs to blood and the muscle cells and their contribution as a fuel during this kind of exercise. Second, lipolysis within peripheral triglyceride stores (adipocytes) is a process that requires upregulation of the enzyme HSL (hormone sensitive lipase). This enzymatic modulation occurs through the cyclic AMP second messenger mechanism, activated by blood epinephrine, or by norepinephrine released by local sympathetic nerve endings. Due to the non-continuous nature of resistive training, peripheral, and perhaps intramuscular, lipolysis may be insufficiently upregulated to result in enhanced blood FA supply. Since the flux of FAs from blood into muscle depends on the blood FA concentration, their extent of mitochondrial oxidation may also be affected in response to limited blood, and eventually, intramuscular accumulation.

3.2.3　Reliance on Proteins

Although the main function of dietary protein is its contribution of amino acids to various anabolic processes, protein is also catabolized for energy.[9] In well-nourished individuals at rest, protein metabolism contributes between 2 and 5% of the body's total energy requirement. During exercise, much of the information regarding protein metabolism has been derived from nitrogen balance[10–12] and urinary excretion measurements.[13–16] These methods, however, do not provide information about the effects of exercise upon the rates and regulation of amino acid oxidation/protein synthesis during and after exercise.[17] In order to address this concern, stable isotope (primarily, L-[1-^{13}C]) traced studies performed on experimental animals and, more recently in humans, demonstrate that the oxidation of particular amino acids, including essential amino acids such as leucine, is increased in proportion to the increase in VO_2 during prolonged submaximal exercise.[18] However, the contribution of amino acids in supplying fuel to any appreciable extent is relatively small (approximately 5 to 15% during aerobic activity)[18,19] as long as the dietary energy supply is adequate.[20]

The quantitative importance of protein metabolism during resistive exercises has only recently been investigated. Tarnopolsky et al.[17] utilized continuous L-[1-^{13}C] leucine infusion during a typical 60-minute resistive training session that consisted of 9 exercises: 3 sets of 10 repetitions of each exercise at 70% of one repetition maximum (1 RM). The authors observed no change in whole-body leucine oxidation during the exercise or for 2 hours of recovery. As suggested by Lemon,[21] these results are likely due to the fact that strength exercise is so intense that a major portion of the necessary energy must be derived via anaerobic metabolism rather than via oxidative pathways. Although studies replicating these findings are needed, these data support the conclusion of Astrand and Rodahl[20] that, at least with strength/power exercise, protein/amino acids contribute very little to exercise fuel.[22]

3.3　The Role of Carbohydrates for Resistive-Type Athletes

Although a decrease in blood glucose is not normally associated with a resistance training session,[23–25] a significant decrease in muscle glycogen has been reported after resistance exercise[24,26–28] and other forms of high-intensity intermittent exercise.[4,5,29] For example, MacDougall[24] et al. have reported a 25% reduction in muscle glycogen after 3 sets of biceps curls to failure, while Tesch et al.,[26] found a 26% reduction in glycogen stores of the vastus lateralis after a multiple-bout resistance exercise session. In a follow-up investigation, Tesch et al.,[27] showed glycogen decrements in the same muscle of up to 40% over 3 exercise bouts performed at 30, 45, and 60% 1 RM, respectively (5 sets of 10 knee extensions). These results are supported by the earlier work of

Robergs et al.,[28] who demonstrated that 6 sets of leg extensions performed at
70 and 35% of 1 RM decreases muscle glycogen by 39 and 38%, respectively.
Clearly, these investigations demonstrate that muscle glycogen is an important fuel source during weight training activities.[30] If muscle glycogen levels
become limiting, the potential ergogenic effect of a high-carbohydrate training diet may only be derived from an increase in the storage of muscle
glycogen prior to the start of the next training bout. With a bigger fuel
compartment, the performer may be able to withstand longer, more intense
sessions, and thus, achieve a better training effect. This may be the reason
why it is common practice for athletes involved in resistive-training programs to ingest carbohydrate beverages with the intent of enhancing their
performance.[31]

3.3.1   Carbohydrate Supplementation and Exercise Performance

Although the importance of muscle glycogen as an energy source during
endurance exercise is well documented,[32–36] published research on the effect of
carbohydrate ingestion on the performance of resistance-training exercise is
very limited. One of the first studies addressing this question was done by
Lambert et al.[31] In their investigation male subjects were fed either a placebo
or a 10% glucose polymer beverage (1 g·kg^{-1}) immediately before and also
between the 5th, 10th, and 15th sets of a weight training session. The subjects
performed repeated sets of 10 repetitions with 3 minutes of recovery separat-
ing the sets. Subjects tended to do more total repetitions (149 vs. 129, P = .056)
and more total sets (17.1 vs. 14.4, P = .067) when they consumed the carbohydrate beverage than when they drank the placebo. Their results suggested that
glucose polymer ingestion tends to increase performance during multiple-
bout (approximately 15 sets) resistance exercise.

A study by Haff et al.[30] had subjects participate in a double-blind protocol
in which a carbohydrate supplement (0.3 g·kg^{-1}) or placebo (P) was ingested
during a morning session, a 4-hour recovery period, and an afternoon session
with sets of squats performed to exhaustion. Performance measured in number of sets, repetitions, and duration was statistically different between the
carbohydrate and the P group. The authors concluded that carbohydrate
supplementation enhances the performance of multiple sets to exhaustion
during the second workout of a given day.

Recent research by Conley[37] as cited by Haff et al.[30] has indicated that carbohydrate supplementation before and during weight training does not significantly improve performance when executing sets of squats to failure.
Conley[37] suggested that the shorter duration of his workout (35 minutes) may
have accounted for the lack of performance increase from carbohydrate
ingestion since glycolysis may become a limiting factor when the substrate is
lacking. Apparently, under the current experimental conditions, 35 minutes
was not enough time to induce significant depletion of on-site glycogen
stores. In the investigations where carbohydrate feeding seemed to have

played a role in performance,[30,31] workout durations were 77 and 56 minutes, respectively.

3.3.2 Carbohydrate Restriction and Exercise Performance

As opposed to supplementation, Leveritt and Abernethy[38] investigated the effect of a carbohydrate restriction program (CRP) on squat (3 sets at 80% 1 RM until failure) and isokinetic knee extensions (5 sets of 5 repetitions) performance. The CRP consisted of 60 minutes of cycling at 75% peak cycling VO$_2$ (PVO$_2$) followed by four 1-minute bouts at 100% PVO$_2$, followed by 2 days of reduced carbohydrate intake (1.2 ± 0.5 g·kg^{-1}·d^{-1}). Subjects performed the exercises under no experimental intervention and after the 2-day CRP. Squat repetitions were significantly reduced after the CRP; however, isokinetic torque measures were not significantly different from the control measurements at any of the five contractile speeds tested (1.05, 2.09, 3.14, 4.19, and 5.24 rads·s^{-1}). The authors explained such results based on the intensity and duration associated with each exercise modality. In contrast to the relatively short duration of the isokinetic exercise (periods of 3 to 15 seconds), the squat exercise involved 3 bouts of near maximal muscular contraction lasting approximately 30 seconds each. The capacity of anaerobic pathways to support ATP regeneration during maximal exercise implies that glycogen metabolism would be much greater during the longer-lasting squat exercise. The authors concluded that the CRP may have compromised squat performance due to lack of substrate available for anaerobic glycolysis.[38]

It should be noted that the mechanism underlying the resulting shift in performance (or lack of[37]) in response to carbohydrate supplementation[30,31] and/or restriction[38] is not clear because intramuscular glycogen was not measured in these investigations. Thus, whether muscle function paralleled changes in muscle carbohydrate storage cannot be answered by the reviewed literature. Also, protocol differences and methods employed have combined to make estimations of *potential* glycogen depletion difficult when attempting to compare these studies[30,31,37,38] among themselves, or with those just documenting depletion in response to exercise.[24,26-28] Moreover, none of the above supplementation studies have assessed lifting performance during a *real-life*, complete weight training session. Appreciation of the significant differences in training volume (sets × reps), intensity (% RM), rest intervals, etc., employed by the athletes this chapter deals with, raises the question of a carry-over effect of present results to the weight room.

Additional research investigating the effect of carbohydrate restriction on strength performance is equivocal and may be because this effect is dependent on the type of strength tests used.[38] For example, an investigation by Grisdale et al.[39] had subjects perform a one-leg ergometry exercise to deplete muscle glycogen stores in that leg. Even though a high-carbohydrate diet replaced muscle glycogen within 24 hours, the ability of the previously depleted leg to sustain repeated 25-second intervals of isometric concentrations at 50% maximal effort (90-second rest intervals) remained impaired relative to the leg that was not glycogen depleted. Thus, results showed that the residual adverse effect of prior exercise on performance of high-intensity efforts 24 hours later was not caused by inadequate glycogen availability during the second exercise task. While the previous authors tested isometrically, a study by Symons and Jacobs[40] showed that neither electrically evoked muscle force production nor maximal isokinetic strength and endurance was marred by several days of a low-carbohydrate diet (meals contained 8 to18% carbohydrate), when muscle glycogen was reduced by 36%. Until more consistent experimental designs are developed and tried, the association between carbohydrate restriction and resistive performance will remain elusive.

3.3.3   Carbohydrate Requirements of Resistive-Trained Populations

There is sufficient evidence to show that carbohydrate consumption immediately before and during endurance exercise can prolong exercise duration[41-43] and increase work output[44-46] for a given duration. Although the previous review addressed carbohydrate supplementation (or restriction) during resistive activity, the fact remains that for this kind of exercise, the ergogenic efficacy of pre-exercise muscle glycogen stores and carbohydrate consumption is less clear.[47] In addition to a lack of investigations, protocol differences and methods employed make interpretation of the various results difficult. However, as mentioned above, there is ample evidence pointing to the fact that skeletal muscle glycogen loss is evoked by resistive exercise[24,26-28] implying that carbohydrate availability may become a limiting factor during such exercise. Like endurance athletes, those relying on resistance exercise to improve performance may experience significant glycogen loss in the weight room. The questions now become: (a) how much is needed for day-to-day replenishment of muscle glycogen, and (b) what is the best way to achieve this goal?

3.3.4   Optimizing Glycogen Recovery After Exercise

Given the importance of muscle glycogen in prolonged endurance performance,[48] several reviews have addressed the optimal dietary regimen for replenishment following exhaustive exercise.[49-51] This information has led to methods of achieving glycogen *supercompensation*[52] in order to achieve an ergogenic effect from glycogen storage overload. These regimens have proven effective in increasing glycogen stores to high values consistent with good endurance exercise performance.[48,52] For the strength-trained athlete, however, the concern is how to replenish muscle glycogen following intense weight lifting in order to have ample substrate for upcoming training sessions.

After exercise that is of sufficient intensity and duration to deplete the muscle glycogen stores, the activity of glycogen synthase is increased.[53] This enzyme is rate-limiting in the glycogenesis pathway and its activity is upregulated when muscle glycogen levels are low.[47] Given this association, a low post-exercise glycogen concentration can catalyze the rapid restoration of glycogen only if adequate substrate is available. This availability is possible only if glucose transport across the plasma membrane is facilitated. It happens that following a bout of heavy exercise, the membrane's permeability for glucose is increased due to the insulin-like effects of muscle contraction. Recognition that contractions induce GLUT-4 translocation through a separate, insulin-independent mechanism,[54] together with the activation of glycogen synthase, allows for an initial rapid, insulin-independent resynthesis of muscle glycogen following exercise. The increased permeability for glucose induced by a contraction-signaling pathway reverses rapidly in the absence of insulin.[53] This is compensated by a marked increase in the muscle's sensitivity to insulin, which remains elevated for a long time, perhaps until glycogen supercompensation has occurred.[55,56]

Regardless of the increase in glycogen synthase activity, the muscle cell's permeability to glucose, and the muscle's sensitivity to insulin, full repletion of glycogen following a bout of intense exercise is not possible in the absence of carbohydrate feeding after exercise. The latter probably stimulates glycogenesis by increasing plasma insulin and glucose concentrations. Unless sufficient carbohydrate is ingested, a day-to-day glycogen depletion–repletion balance may not be obtained between resistive training bouts, nor will efforts to supercompensate stores[53] be successful.

The time period between cessation of a training bout and the consumption of a carbohydrate supplement will significantly influence the rate of muscle glycogen resynthesis.[57] A carbohydrate supplement in excess of 1 g·kg^{-1} body weight needs to be taken immediately after exercise and should be repeated every 2 hours for 6 hours.[48,58] When supplements are administered in this fashion, a high rate of resynthesis (5 to 6 $\mu\text{mol·g}^{-1}$ wet weight·h^{-1})[57–59] is maintained for approximately 2 hours before decline begins as the blood glucose and insulin levels do the same.[57] Nevertheless, this protocol seems to maximize glycogen rate of storage for up to 6 hours after exercise.

Increasing the amount of carbohydrate consumption above 1.0 to 1.5 g·kg^{-1} body weight appears to provide no additional benefit, and may have the adverse effect of causing nausea and diarrhea.[53] Also, glucose or its polymers are more advantageous than those composed primarily of fructose. However, endurance athletes should also ingest some fructose because it may be better than glucose for replenishing liver glycogen.[60,61] As reviewed by Coyle and Coggan,[62] numerous studies have reported that consumption of liquid or solid carbohydrates *during* exercise can improve endurance performance. When compared to carbohydrate consumed for glycogen replenishing purposes immediately *after* exercise, similar results have been obtained. Nonetheless, liquid supplements are recommended because they are easier to digest and less filling, and provide a source of fluid for rehydration.[53]

Finally, athletes should realize that if they are achieving the dietary goal of 58% of calories from carbohydrates they might already be consuming what is needed to replace muscle glycogen on a day-to-day basis. For example, if an athlete requires 4000 kcal per day for caloric balance (energy intake) and 58% is derived from carbohydrates, then 2320 kcal (0.58 × 4000), or 580 grams of carbohydrate, will be consumed. This quantity is consistent with what is needed to restore muscle glycogen to normal levels 24 hours after strenuous exercise (500 to 700 grams).[60,61,63]

3.4   The Role of Protein for Resistive-Type Athletes

Increased physical training appears to increase the protein needs of participants regardless of the nature of the exercise (resistive vs. endurance) when this need is contrasted with that of sedentary counterparts.[64] Previous investigations[65,66] have suggested that in order to maintain nitrogen balance, highly trained endurance athletes should exceed the current protein RDA of 0.8 gm/kg BW per day. If endurance athletes require more dietary protein/amino acids, the most probable causes for the increased need would be to cover the loss of amino acids oxidized during exercise[22] and to provide additional raw materials to replace any exercise-induced muscle damage, especially when the exercise has a large eccentric component.[67] For the strength/power athlete, the most probable cause for the increased need would be to provide supplemental raw materials to enhance muscle protein synthesis.[22] While protein breakdown generally increases only modestly with exercise, muscle protein synthesis rises markedly following both endurance and resistive-type exercise.[9] Thus, increasing the availability of amino acids from increased dietary protein could promote an accelerated rate of muscle protein synthesis if this practice is done in combination with chronic resistive exercise. In essence, a bigger amino acid supply may support the anabolic stimulus known to accompany chronic resistive exercise. Although probably not as important, protein supplementation may also cover the increased amino acid loss as a consequence of amino acid oxidation during exercise.[22]

3.4.1   Protein Supplementation and Exercise Performance

For many years athletes have taken amino acid supplements in an attempt to increase muscle mass, strength, and ultimately performance. These supplements have been highly touted as safe and effective alternatives to anabolic steroids for building muscle mass.[68] Given the tremendous pressure to excel in competition, numerous studies have evaluated the specific benefits of protein and/or amino acid supplementation on strength, body composition, and also on measures of human growth hormone (GH) activity.[64] Recent claims suggest that amino acid supplements, particularly arginine, stimulate the release of GH. Once released, this hormone can induce a number of effects on the body including growth of tissues and organs through enhanced protein synthesis.[68] Thus, the stimulation of GH by arginine may have an anabolic effect on muscular development. However, results of published studies have failed to establish a definite conclusion regarding the effects of this hormone because control of all the variables known to affect blood levels of GH is extremely difficult. For example, release of GH from the anterior pituitary occurs in a pulsatile nature which varies greatly throughout a 24-hour period due to the influence of various provocative stimuli. The latter include factors such as diet composition, body fatness, age, and exercise.[64] Not to be over-looked is the potential change in the hormone's response to exercise as the participant adapts to it.[69] Finally, while intravenous infusion of arginine has been demonstrated to induce secretion of GH,[70,71] oral administration may not sufficiently elevate plasma arginine levels to facilitate this response.[68] Given the array and complexity of issues related to evaluating the effects of GH, it is understandable that the results reported in the literature to date provide no consistent information.[64]

3.4.1.1 Amino Acid Supplementation and Muscle Function

Walber-Rankin et al.[72] found no evidence of arginine supplementation (0.1 g·kg^{-1}·body weight^{-1} administered twice daily) affecting the amount of lean or fat tissue lost during a hypocaloric diet combined with a weightlifting program. The authors saw no effect of supplement consumption on blood arginine or GH whether the subjects were in energy balance or energy deficit. Additionally, results of this investigation showed that neither body composition nor muscle function (tests of isokinetic peak torque) were altered by the amino acid supplement. Contrary to the above investigation, Elam et al.[73] reported significant improvement in total strength performance and lean body mass in a group of men taking an arginine/ornithine supplement (2 g each ornithine and arginine daily) compared to those taking a placebo after 5 weeks of strength training. However, these results are difficult to interpret since no baseline measurements (body composition, strength parameters) were made and nonexercised control groups were not used. Thus the strength changes due to the resistive-training program with supplement or placebo cannot be determined or compared.[72] Gater et al.[68] reported significant improvements in 1 RM measurements (bench press, squat, deadlift) over a 10-week period of resistive training. Nonetheless, no significant effects were noted for arginine/lysine supplementation (132 mg·kg^{-1}). Results by Hawkins et al.[74] did not support any value of oral arginine supplementation (1.0 g arginine·kg^{-1}·day^{-1}) in a group of 13 experienced male weight lifters. Subjects were divided into experimental and placebo groups during a 10-day low-calorie diet period. Following such period, postassessment of muscle function (isokinetic peak torque and endurance) revealed no effect for the type of supplement.

3.4.1.2 *Amino Acid Supplementation and Growth Hormone Levels*

Since a primary objective of amino acid supplementation is to induce the release of GH, and hopefully to promote anabolism of myofibrillar protein content of skeletal muscle, a number of studies have examined the effect of oral amino acid supplements on GH release. For example, an investigation by Fry et al.[75] examined the effect of high-volume Olympic weightlifting and amino acid supplementation on GH levels. The subjects in question were 28 elite junior weightlifters participating in a national training camp. The supplementation doses were as follows: 2.4 g amino acids prior to daily meals (3 doses per day) and 2.1 g of branched-chain amino acids along with L-glutamine and L-carnitine prior to each workout. Statistical analyses did not reveal a significant change on resting or post-exercise GH levels. The study presented above by Gater et al.[68] also failed to show GH release in response to arginine supplementation. Apparently, the supplementation dose (132 mg/kg BW) used in that study was insufficient to stimulate GH release as indicated by unchanging levels of its messenger, insulin-like growth factor-1 (IGF-1).[68] Data from Lambert et al.[76] and Fogelholm et al.[77] also showed failure of commercial amino acid supplements on GH blood concentration in male bodybuilders and weightlifters, respectively. As stated above, it seems that rigorous control of the variables known to affect GH levels makes it very difficult to design studies aimed to assess the biological effects of this hormone on muscle mass and, more important, the performance of resistive-trained athletes. The problem is exacerbated when such factors as diet, type of training, or % fat are combined within an experimental design or differ in combination and/or manipulation among experiments. For example, Isidori et al.[78] found that an orally administered supplement of arginine with lysine (1.2 mg each) significantly increased GH levels. However, when each amino acid was administered by itself, GH levels did not show an increase. These results suggest that the effects of amino acids on GH release may not be due to specific amino acids but to specific combinations.[64]

3.4.2 Protein Requirements of Resistive-Trained Populations

The very high protein intakes and the prevalence of amino acid supplementation common to strength athletes[79–81] indicates that athletes readily accept the link between muscular development and increased dietary protein[22] without scientific verification. Although there are some recent scientific data consistent with this idea, the issue of exercise effect on protein need is extremely complex, but there continues to be no consensus among sport nutritionists.[21] Lemon attributes the existing controversy, in part to the limitations of the measurement techniques used (complete or partial nitrogen balance and radio/stable isotopic metabolic tracers) and the established tradition that exercise has minimal effects on protein metabolism.[22] Butterfield[82] has also criticized many nitrogen balance studies of athletes because researchers failed to provide adequate energy intake, calories,[82] or they did not allow for an adequate period of adjustment to the diet and training regimen.[64]

Regardless of confounding arguments, several investigations attest to the fact that the current protein RDA (0.8 g·kg⁻¹·day⁻¹) is inadequate for persons participating in intense resistive exercise. For example, Tarnopolsky et al.[11] estimated that in order for strength athletes to achieve nitrogen balance, the protein intake should be 1.4 g·kg⁻¹·day⁻¹ compared to 0.89 g·kg⁻¹·day⁻¹ for sedentary controls. The authors estimated that protein intake for persons engaged in resistive training should be 1.76 g·kg⁻¹·day⁻¹, which is more than twice the RDA for men.[64] This RDA is higher than the 1.2 g·kg⁻¹·day⁻¹ previously reported by the same group.[65] Subsequently, whole-body protein synthesis was elevated when athletes participating in a resistive-training program increased their protein intake from 0.86 to 1.4 g·kg⁻¹·day⁻¹. This increment in protein synthesis was not associated with an increase in amino acid oxidation. Further increases in protein intake to 2.4 g·kg⁻¹·day⁻¹ resulted in no additional increments in whole-body protein synthesis but induced an increase in amino acid oxidation, indicating a protein overload at such value. Amino acid oxidation also increased in sedentary controls who had protein intakes of 1.4 and 2.4 g·kg⁻¹·day⁻¹. This suggests that at a protein intake of 1.4 g·kg⁻¹·day⁻¹, the amino acids consumed in excess of needs were removed from the body via oxidation in the sedentary subjects but were used to support an enhanced protein synthesis rate in the strength group.[21] With time, the latter should lead to increases in muscle mass, and potentially strength, if there is simultaneous inclusion of an adequate resistive training stimulus.

Walberg et al.[12] provided two groups of bodybuilders with different protein intakes (0.8 vs. 1.6 g·kg⁻¹·day⁻¹) and hypoenergy diets (18 kcal/kg) for a 7-day period. Throughout this period the diet higher in protein was consistently associated with a positive nitrogen balance, whereas the lower intake produced values that were generally negative.

Similar to Walberg et al.,[12] Lemon et al.[10] compared protein intakes of 2.62 vs. 0.99 g·kg⁻¹·day⁻¹ in novice bodybuilders during the first month of training. Based on nitrogen balance data and linear regression methodology, these investigators concluded that the protein requirement was 1.5 g·kg⁻¹·day⁻¹ and the recommended allowance (requirement + 2 SD) should be 1.7 g·kg⁻¹·day⁻¹. This last value is consistent with that obtained by Tarnopolsky et al.[11] (1.76 g·kg⁻¹·day⁻¹) for strength athletes.

Fern et al.[83] compared protein intakes in bodybuilders assigned to either 3.3 vs. 1.3 g·kg⁻¹·day⁻¹. Results showed significantly greater gains in body mass over 4 weeks of training at the higher protein intake. Metabolic tracer data indicated that protein synthesis increased with training regardless of diet; however, with the higher protein intake the increase in synthesis was fivefold greater. This observation is of considerable importance because it appears to be the first documentation that a protein intake of approximately four times the RDA, in combination with strength training, can promote greater muscle size gains than the same training with a diet containing adequate protein.[22] Unfortunately, amino acid oxidation also increased 150% on the higher intake, which suggested that the optimum protein intake was also exceeded.[21]

3.5 Recommendations

The fact that glycogen seems to be an important fuel source during weight training exercises,[24,26–28] may explain why it is common practice for athletes involved in resistive-training programs to ingest carbohydrate beverages with the intent of enhancing their performance.[31] However, support for the use of carbohydrate supplements for the latter purpose remains elusive, as the ergogenic efficacy of enhanced pre-exercise muscle glycogen stores and carbohydrate consumption is less clear.[47] Nevertheless, the trend of the current literature points to a carbohydrate intake above that of a normal diet for athletes involved in high-volume, high-intensity lifting. This recommendation may benefit athletes currently engaged in this type of training routine, as these variables (volume and intensity) are primary determinants of carbohydrate use during exercise.[84] For athletes who perform prolonged and intense resistance exercise, carbohydrate feeding may prevent acute glycogen loss, allowing them to maintain a given exercise intensity for a longer period of time.[31] This is likely to promote a better training stimulus along with increased performance. Those involved in rigorous training should consume sufficient carbohydrate to limit overtraining decrements due to chronic glycogen depletion.[27]

If resistive athletes decide to adopt a carbohydrate supplementation regimen, attention should be paid to the time period between cessation of a training bout and the consumption of the supplement. In order to stimulate a high rate of glycogen resynthesis, a carbohydrate supplement (liquid or solid) in excess of 1 g·kg^{-1} body weight (not to exceed 1.5 g·kg^{-1} body weight) needs to be taken immediately after exercise[57] and should be repeated every 2 hours for 6 hours.[48,58] Finally, resistance-trained athletes should realize that if they are achieving the dietary goal of 58% of calories from carbohydrates they might already be consuming what is needed to replace muscle glycogen on a day-to-day basis.

There is evidence to support that athletes engaged in resistance training appear to benefit from increased protein intakes over the RDA during periods of resistive training. The increases in lean body mass as well as its maintenance may be achieved with regular training provided that the dietary intakes of protein and energy are adequate to meet protein requirements.[64] However, of critical importance is the observation from tracer studies[11,83] that the efficacy of dietary protein appears to plateau somewhere between 1.4 and $2.4 \text{ g·kg}^{-1}\text{day}^{-1}$.[22] This is consistent with the recent nitrogen balance data[10–12] which suggests that the protein intake of strength/power athletes should be about 1.7 to 1.8 g·kg^{-1}·day^{-1} (225% of the current RDA). However, the issue of exercise effect on protein need is extremely complex, and there is still no absolute consensus.[21] Additionally, investigations supporting extremely high protein diets[83] customarily consumed by strength/power athletes are very limited. Thus, at this time there is no good evidence that such high protein intakes (>2 g kg^{-1}·day^{-1}) are either necessary or beneficial.

It appears that the increased protein needs can be met via appropriate food selection without consuming expensive protein supplements.[21] Results of previous investigations have failed to establish a definite conclusion regarding the use of oral protein/amino acid supplements by individuals involved in resistive training[72] because these products do not seem to have an effect on blood arginine,[72] GH,[68,72,75–77] or muscular performance.[68,72,74] The variability in GH responsiveness may be explained by the difficulty in controlling the known stimuli (diet composition, body fatness, age, and exercise) affecting the release of this hormone. This presents a challenge in designing studies attempting to clarify the interrelationships among those influencing variables and muscular performance.

References

1. Hultman, E. and Greenhaff, P. L., Carbohydrate metabolism in exercise, in *Nutrition in Sports*, Maughan, R. J. (Ed.), Blackwell Science, Oxford, 2000, chap. 6.
2. Brooks, G. A., Fahey, T. D., White, T. P., and Baldwin, K. M., *Exercise Physiology, Human Bioenergetics and its Applications*, 3rd ed., Mayfield Publishing Company, Mountain View, CA, 2000, chap. 3.
3. Cheetham, M. E., Boobis, L. H., Brooks, S., and Williams, C., Human muscle metabolism during sprint running, *J. Appl. Physiol.*, 61, 54, 1986.
4. McCartney, N., Spriet, L. L., Heigenhauser, G. J. F., Kowalchik, J. M., Sutton, J. R., and Jones, N. L., Muscle power and metabolism in maximal intermittent exercise, *J. Appl. Physiol.*, 60, 1164, 1986.
5. Spriet, L. L., Lindinger, M. I., McKelvie, R. S., Heigenhauser, G. J. F., and Jones, N. L., Muscle glycogenolysis and H$^+$ concentration during maximal intermittent cycling, *J. Appl. Physiol.*, 66, 8, 1989.
6. MacDougall, J. D., Ray, S., McCartney, N., Sale, D., Lee, P., and Garner, S., Substrate utilization during weightlifting, *Med. Sci. Sports Exerc.*, 20, S66, 1988.
7. Hawley, J. A., Jeukendrup, A. E., and Brouns, F., Fat metabolism during exercise, in *Nutrition in Sports*, Maughan, R. J. (Ed.), Blackwell Science, Oxford, 2000, chap. 13.
8. Brooks, G. A., Fahey, T. D., White, T. P., and Baldwin, K. M., *Exercise Physiology, Human Bioenergetics and Its Applications*, 3rd ed., Mayfield Publishing Company, Mountain View, CA, 2000, chap. 7.
9. McArdle, W. D., Katch, F. I., and Katch, V. L., *Exercise Physiology: Energy, Nutrition, and Human Performance*, 4th ed., Williams and Wilkins, Philadelphia, PA, 1996, chap. 1.

10. Lemon, P. W. R., Tarnopolsky, M. A., MacDougall, J. D., and Atkinson, S. A., Protein requirements and muscle mass/strength changes during intensive training in novice bodybuilders, *J. Appl. Physiol.*, 73, 767, 1992.

11. Tarnopolsky, M. A., Atkinson, S. A., MacDougall, J. D., Chesley, A., Phillips, S., and Schwarcz, H. P., Evaluation of protein requirements for trained strength athletes, *J. Appl. Physiol.*, 73, 1986, 1992.

12. Walberg, J. L., Leidy, M. K., Sturgill, D. J., Hinkle, D. E., Ritchey, S. J., and Sebolt, D. R., Macronutrient content of a hypoenergy diet affects nitrogen retention and muscle function in weightlifters, *Int. J. Sports Med.*, 9, 261, 1988.

13. Hickson, J. F., Wolinsky, I., Rodriguez, J. P., Pivarnik, J. M., Kent, M. C., and Shier, N. W., Failure of weight training to affect urinary indices of protein metabolism in men, *Med. Sci. Sports Exerc.*, 18, 563, 1986.

14. Marable, N. L., Hickson, J. K., Korslund, M. K., Herbert, G., Desjardins, R. F., and Thye, F. W., Urinary nitrogen excretion as influenced by a muscle-building exercise program and protein variation, *Nutr. Rep. Int.*, 19, 795, 1979.

15. Mole, P. and Johnson, R. E., Disclosure by dietary modification of an exercise-induced protein catabolism in man, *J. Appl. Physiol.*, 31, 185, 1971.

16. Chesley, A., MacDougall, J. D., Tarnopolsky, M. A., Atkinson, S. A., and Smith, K., Changes in human muscle protein synthesis after resistance training, *J. Appl. Physiol.*, 73, 1383, 1992.

17. Tarnopolsky, M. A., Atkinson, S. A., MacDougall, J. D., Senor, B. B., Lemon, P. W. R., and Schwarcz, H., Whole body leucine metabolism during and after resistance exercise in fed humans, *Med. Sci. Sports Exerc.*, 23, 326, 1991.

18. Brooks, G. A., Fahey, T. D., White, T. P., and Baldwin, K. M., *Exercise Physiology, Human Bioenergetics and Its Applications*, 3rd ed., Mayfield Publishing Company, Mountain View, CA, 2000, chap. 28.

19. Jackson, C. G. R., Overview of human bioenergetics and nutrition, in *Energy-Yielding Macronutrients and Energy Metabolism in Sports Nutrition*, Driskel, J. A. and Wolinsky, I. (Eds.), CRC Press, Boca Raton, 2000, chap. 2.

20. Astrand, P-O. and Rodahl, K., *Textbook of Work Physiology*, 3rd ed., McGraw-Hill, New York, 1986.

21. Lemon, P. W. R., Effects of exercise on protein metabolism, in *Nutrition in Sports*, Maughan, R. J. (Ed.), Blackwell Science, Oxford, 2000, chap. 10.

22. Lemon, P. W. R., Do athletes need more dietary protein and amino acids?, *Int. J. Sports Nut.*, 5, 1995.

23. Keul, J., Haralambie., J., Bruder, M., and Gottstein, H. J., The effect of weight lifting exercise on heart rate and metabolism in experienced lifters, *Med. Sci. Sports Exerc.*, 10, 13, 1978.

24. MacDougall, J. D., Ray, S., McCartney, N., Sale, D., Lee, P., and Gardner, S., Substrate utilization during weightlifting, *Med. Sci. Sports Exerc.*, 20, S66, 1988.

25. Peters, H. P. F., Van Schelven, W. F., Versappen, P. A., De Boer, R. W., Bol, E., Erich, W. B. M., Van Der Togt, C. R., and De Vries, W. R., Exercise performance as a function of semi-solid and liquid carbohydrate feedings during prolonged exercise, *Int. J. Sports Med.*, 16, 105, 1995.

26. Tesch. P. A., Colliander, E. B., and Kaiser, P., Muscle metabolism during intense, heavy resistance exercise, *Eur. J. Appl. Physiol.*, 55, 362, 1986.

27. Tesch, P. A., Ploutz-Snyder, L. L., Ystrom, L., Castro, M. J., and Dudley, G. A., Skeletal muscle glycogen loss evoked by resistance exercise, *J. Strength and Cond. Res.*, 12, 67, 1998.

28. Robergs, R. A., Pearson, D. R., Costill, D. L., Fink, W. J., Pascoe, D. D., Benedict, M. A., Lambert, C. P., and Zachweija, J. J., Muscle glycogenolysis during differing intensities of weight-resistance exercise, *J. Appl. Physiol.*, 70, 1700, 1991.

29. Hermansen, L. and Vaage, O., Lactate disappearance and glycogen synthesis in human muscle after maximal exercise, *Am. J. Physiol.*, 233, E422, 1977.

30. Haff, G. G., Stone, M. H., Warren, B. J., Keith, R., Johnson, R. L., Nieman, D. C., Williams, F., and Kirksey, K. B., The effect of carbohydrate supplementation on multiple sessions and bouts of resistance exercise, *J. Strength Cond. Res.*, 13, 111, 1999.

31. Lambert, C. P., Flynn, M. G., Boone, J. B., Michaud, T. J., and Rodriguez-Zayas, J., Effects of carbohydrate feeding on multiple-bout resistance exercise, *J. Appl. Sport Sci. Res.*, 5, 192, 1991.

32. Coggan, A. R. and Coyle, E. F., Effect of carbohydrate feedings during high-intensity exercise, *J. Appl. Physiol.*, 65, 1703, 1988.

33. Coyle, E. F., Coggan, A. R., Hemmert, M. K., and Ivy, J. L., Muscle glycogen utilization during prolonged strenuous exercise when fed carbohydrate, *J. Appl. Physiol.*, 61, 165, 1986.

34. Doyle, J. A., Sherman, W. M., and Strauss, R. L., Effects of eccentric and concentric exercise on muscle glycogen replenishment, *J. Appl. Physiol.*, 74, 1848, 1993.

35. Hargreaves, M. and Briggs, C. A., Effect of carbohydrate ingestion on exercise metabolism, *J. Appl. Physiol.*, 65, 1553, 1988.

36. Wright, D. A., Sherman, W. M., and Dernbach, A. R., Carbohydrate feedings before, during, or in combination improve cycling endurance performance, *J. Appl. Physiol.*, 71, 1082, 1991.

37. Conley, M. S., The effects of carbohydrate ingestion on multiple sets of resistance exercise, Master's Thesis, Appalachian State University, Boone, NC, 1993.

38. Leveritt, M. and Abernethy, P. J., Effects of carbohydrate restriction on strength performance, *J. Strength Cond. Res.*, 13, 52, 1999.

39. Grisdale, R. K., Jacobs, I., and Cafarelli, E., Relative effects of glycogen depletion and previous exercise on muscle force and endurance capacity, *J. Appl. Physiol.*, 69, 1276, 1990.

40. Symons, J. D. and Jacobs, I., High-intensity exercise performance is not impaired by low intramuscular glycogen, *Med. Sci. Sports Exerc.* 21, 550, 1989.

41. Coyle, E. F., Hagberg, J. M., Hurley, B. F., Martin, W. H., Ehsani, A. A., and Holloszy, J. O., Carbohydrate feeding during prolonged strenuous exercise can delay fatigue, *J. Appl. Physiol.*, 55, 230, 1983.

42. Fielding, R. A., Costill, D. L., Fink, W. J., King, D. S., Hargreaves, M., and Kovaleski, J. E., Effect of carbohydrate feeding frequencies and dosage on muscle glycogen use during exercise, *Med. Sci. Sports Exerc.* 17, 472, 1985.

43. Yaspelkis, B. B., Patterson, J. G., Anderla, P. A., Ding, Z., and Ivy, J. L., Carbohydrate supplementation spares muscle glycogen during variable-intensity exercise, *J. Appl. Physiol.*, 75, 1477, 1993.

44. Coggan, A. R. and Coyle, E. F., Reversal of fatigue during prolonged exercise by carbohydrate infusion or ingestion, *J. Appl. Physiol.*, 63, 2388, 1987.

45. Hargreaves, M., Costill, D. L., Coggan, A. R., Fink, W. J., and Nishibata, I., Effect of carbohydrate feedings on muscle glycogen utilization and exercise performance, *Med. Sci. Sports Exerc.* 16, 219, 1984.

46. Neufer, P. D., Costill, D. L., Flynn, M. G., Kirwan, J. P., Mitchell, J. B., and Houmard, J., Improvements in exercise performance: effects of carbohydrate feeding and diet, *J. Appl. Physiol.*, 62, 983, 1987.
47. Walberg-Rankin, J., Dietary carbohydrate as an ergogenic aid for prolonged and brief competitions in sport, *Int. J. Sport Nutr.*, 5, S13, 1995.
48. Powers, S. K. and Howley, E. T., *Exercise Physiology, Theory and Application to Fitness and Performance*, 3rd ed., Brown and Benchmark, Dubuque, IA, chap. 23.
49. Coyle, E. F. and Coyle, E., Carbohydrate that speed recovery from training, *Phys. Sportsmed.*, 21, 111, 1993.
50. Fallowfield, J. L. and Williams, C., Carbohydrate intake and recovery from prolonged exercise, *Int. J. Sport Nutr.*, 3, 150, 1993.
51. Robergs, R. S., Nutrition and exercise determinants of postexercise glycogen synthesis, *Int. J. Sport Nutr.*, 1, 307, 1991.
52. Sherman, W. M., Carbohydrates, muscle glycogen and muscle glycogen super-compensation, in *Ergogenic Aids in Sports*, Williams, M. H. (Ed.), Human Kinetics, Champaign, IL, 1983, chap. 1.
53. Ivy, J. L., Optimization of glycogen stores, in *Nutrition in Sports*, Maughan, R. J. (Ed.), Blackwell Science, Oxford, 2000, chap, 7.
54. Brooks, G. A., Fahey, T. D., White, T. P., and Baldwin, K. M., *Exercise Physiology, Human Bioenergetics and Its Applications*, 3rd ed., Mayfield Publishing Company, Mountain View, CA, 2000, chap. 9.
55. Cartee, G. D., Young, D. A., Sleeper, M. D., Zierath, J., Wallberg-Henriksson, H., and Holloszy, J. O., Prolonged increase in insulin-stimulated glucose transport in muscle after exercise, *Am. J. Physiol.*, 256, E494, 1989.
56. Garetto, L. P., Ritcher, E. A., Goodman, M. N., and Ruderman, N. B., Enhanced muscle glucose metabolism after exercise in the rat: the two phases, *Am. J. Physiol.*, 246, E471, 1984.
57. Ivy, J. L., Katz, A. L., Cutler, C. L., Sherman, W. M., and Coyle, E. F., Muscle glycogen synthesis after exercise: effect of time of carbohydrate ingestion, *J. Appl. Physiol.*, 64, 1480, 1988.
58. Blom, P. C. S., Hostmark, A. T., Vaage, O., Kardel, K. R., and Maehlum, S., Effect of different post-exercise sugar diets on the rate of muscle glycogen synthesis, *Med. Sci. Sports Exerc.* 19, 491, 1987.
59. Ivy, J. L., Lee, M. C., Brozinick, J. T., and Reed, M. J., Muscle glycogen storage after different amounts of carbohydrate ingestion, *J. Appl. Physiol.*, 65, 2018, 1988.
60. Friedman, J. E., Neufer, P. D., and Dohm, G. L., Regulation of glycogen synthesis following exercise: dietary considerations, *Sports Med.*, 11, 232, 1991.
61. Ivy, J. L., Muscle glycogen synthesis before and after exercise, *Sports Med.*, 11, 6, 1991.
62. Coyle, E. F. and Coggan, A. R., Effectiveness of carbohydrate feeding in delaying fatigue during prolonged exercise, *Sports Med.*, 1, 446, 1984.
63. Costill, D. L., The role of dietary carbohydrates in muscle glycogen resynthesis after strenuous running, *Am. J. Clin. Nutr.*, 34, 1831, 1981.
64. Bazzarre, T. L., Nutrition and strength, in *Nutrition in Exercise and Sport*, Wolinsky, I. (Ed.), CRC Press, Boca Raton, 1998, chap. 14.
65. Tarnopolsky, M. A., MacDougall, J. D., and Atkinson, S. A., Influence of protein intake and training status on nitrogen balance and lean body mass, *J. Appl. Physiol.*, 64, 187, 1988.

66. Murdoch, D. S., Bazzarre, T. L., Wu, S. L., Herr, D., and Snider, I. P., Nitrogen balance in highly trained athletes, *Med. Sci. Sports Exerc.*, 24, S178, 1992.

67. Evans, W. J. and Gannon, J. G., The metabolic effects of exercise-induced muscle damage, in *Exercise and Sports Sciences Reviews*, Holloszy, J. O. (Ed.), Williams and Wilkins, Baltimore, 1991.

68. Gater, D. R., Gater, D. A., Uribe, J. M., and Bunt, J. C., Impact of nutritional supplements and resistance training on body composition and insulin-like growth factor-1, *J. Appl. Sports Sci. Res.*, 6, 66, 1992.

69. Newsholme, E., The regulation of intracellular and intracellular fuel supply during sustained exercise, *Ann. NY Acad. Sci.*, 301, 81, 1977.

70. Eddy, R. L., Gilliland, P. F., Ibarra, J. D., McMurry, J. F., and Thompson, J. Q., Human growth hormone release: comparison of provocative test procedures, *Am. J. Med.*, 56, 179, 1974.

71. Penny, R., Blizzard, R. M., and Davis, W. T., Sequential study of arginine monochloride and normal saline as stimuli to growth hormone release, *Metab.*, 19, 165, 1970.

72. Walber-Rankin, J., Hawkins, C. E., Fild, D. S., and Seabolt, D. R., The effect of oral arginine during energy restriction in male weight trainers, *J. Strength Cond. Res.*, 8, 170, 1994.

73. Elam, R. P., Hardin, D. H., Sutton, R. A., and Hagen, L., Effects of arginine and ornithine on strength, lean body mass, and urinary hydroxyproline in adult males, *J. Sports Med. Phys. Fitness*, 29, 52, 1989.

74. Hawkins, C. E., Walber-Rankin, J., and Seabolt, D. R., Oral arginine does not affect body composition or muscle function in male weight lifters, *Med. Sci. Sports Exerc.*, 23, S15, 1991.

75. Fry, A. C., Kraemer, W. J., Stone, M. H., Warren B. J., Kearney, J. T., Maresh, C. M., Weseman, C. A., and Fleck, S. J., Endocrine and performance responses to high volume training and amino acid supplementation in elite junior weight lifters, *Int. J. Sport Nutr.*, 3, 306, 1993.

76. Lambert, M. I., Hefer, J. A., Millar, R. P., and Macfarlane, P. W., Failure of commercial oral amino acid supplements to increase serum growth hormone concentration in male bodybuilders, *Int. J. Sport Nutr.*, 3, 298, 1993.

77. Fogelholm, G. M., Naveri H. K., Kiilavuori, K. T. K., and Harkonen, M. H. A., Low-dose amino acid supplementation: no effects on serum human growth hormone and insulin in male weightlifters, *Int. J. Sport Nutr.*, 3, 290, 1993.

78. Isidori, A., Monaco, A. L., and Cappa, M., A study of growth hormone release in man after oral administration of amino acids, *Curr. Med. Res. Opin.*, 7, 475, 1981.

79. Hickson, J. F. and Wolinsky, I., Research directions in protein nutrition for athletes, in *Nutrition in Exercise and Sport*, 2nd ed., Wolinsky, I. and Hickson, J. F. (Eds.), CRC Press, Boca Raton, 1994.

80. Kleiner, S. M., Bazzarre, T. L., and Ainsworth, B. E., Nutritional status of nationally ranked elite bodybuilders, *Int. J. Sport Nutr.*, 4, 54, 1994.

81. Steen, S. N., Precontest strategy of a male bodybuilder, *Int. J. Sport Nutr.*, 1, 69, 1991.

82. Butterfield, G. E., Whole-body protein utilization in humans, *Med. Sci. Sports Exerc.*, 19, S157, 1987.

83. Fern, E. B., Bielinski, R. N., and Schutz, Y., Effects of exaggerated amino acid and protein supply in man, *Experientia*, 47, 168, 1991.

84. Gollnick, P. D., Armstrong, R. B., Sembrowich, W. L., Shepard, R. E., and Saltin, B., Glycogen depletion pattern in human skeletal muscle fibers after heavy exercise, *J. Appl. Physiol.*, 34, 615, 1973.

4

Vitamin and Mineral Considerations for Strength Training

Catherine G. Ratzin Jackson

CONTENTS

0-8493-8198-3/01/$0.00+$.50
© 2001 by CRC Press LLC

4.1   Energy Metabolism

In order to understand how best to meet dietary needs for vitamins and minerals in any type of activity, it is first important to determine whether the activity is primarily nonaerobic, anaerobic, aerobic, or combinations thereof. Many misconceptions about nutrition and exercise can be traced directly back to a poor understanding of energy metabolism. Not all dietary practices are appropriately used for all types of activities. It is now clear that the concept of specificity of nutritional practice, as has been recognized for some time in types of exercise, needs to be applied to nutrition as well.[1] It is further acknowledged that differences in dietary needs exist between women and men and that dietary practices should be specifically recommended to take this into account.[2]

In general, short-term and highly intense activities are nonaerobic and do not depend greatly on anything other than stores of ATP immediately available in the exercising muscle.[3] Dietary regimens adopted by the exerciser would therefore have little effect on energy availability. When exercise continues for 1 to 3 minutes, always considering that intensity will change time frames, an activity stresses the lactic acid system with a high reliance on carbohydrate stores for energy production. Should activity progress further to at least 5 minutes, the activity is characterized as aerobic metabolism and, while carbohydrate stores are necessary for the process to continue, the muscle can now use fat and protein for energy production. While the contributions of fat and carbohydrate are somewhat understood, the amount of energy delivery from protein is still not clear. It is thought that a person who exercises aerobically uses protein during exercise to a greater degree than one who exercises anaerobically. Strength training can generally be classified in the anaerobic spectrum of energy delivery. A thorough explanation of resistance training is found in Chapter 1.

4.2 Introduction to Vitamins and Minerals

4.2.1 General

The discovery of vitamins early in the 20th century marked the beginning of one of the most dynamic eras in the study of nutrition. However, it was soon apparent that controversies, which have continued to the present, had just begun. The first two vitamins were known to be "vital amines." It was then found that not all of these "vital" substances were amines, and it was also noted that there were different chemical structures within the general category of a particular "vitamin." This was only the beginning.

Vitamins are organic compounds which are classified as micronutrients because they are needed in very small amounts in comparison to the macronutrients carbohydrate, protein, fat, and water. They are essential to the diet and act, for the most part, as regulators of many different metabolic processes.[4] Vitamins are generally unrelated chemically and have widely varying physiological effects. Since most of the processes regulated by vitamins are found in energy delivery, it is easy to understand how the use of supplements can be thought to enhance athletic performance. However, describing a role of vitamins in metabolic processes is quite different from attributing ergogenic, or performance enhancing, effects to their use.

Minerals can be classified as macrominerals and microminerals.[5,6] While the definition of terms is sometimes problematic, the importance of minerals for normal metabolism and nutrition is significant. They interact to maintain body fluid electrolyte balance, maintain flow properties of body fluids, maintain integrity of teeth and bones, maintain normal cell activity, and they act as cofactors. Their uses are integral to normal physiologic functioning of the body, but the amounts needed are very small.

4.2.2 Vitamin and Mineral Supplement Industry

Currently in the United States, vitamins and minerals are certainly some of the most used and abused supplements, not only by athletes, but also by the general population. Among athletes, these supplements are particularly marketed to those who engage in weightlifting, bodybuilding, and any other sport or activity that can be characterized as resistance training. The individuals who weight train and bodybuild have been particularly targeted by the multibillion dollar supplement industry.[7] Great effort, along with a considerable amount of money, is spent on marketing and advertising vitamin and mineral supplements which promise shortcuts to good diet and hard work. It should be noted at this point that vitamins and minerals do not provide "energy" as it is measured in the scientific sense. However, the majority of marketing claims for benefits of supplements use the term.

There is no question that vitamin and mineral deficiencies will negatively affect performance and the activities of daily living. However, there is no evidence to suggest that athletes who consume adequate calories from a nutritionally balanced diet have deficiencies.[8] Studies have repeatedly shown that vitamin and mineral supplementation over long periods of time has no effect on any test of physical performance.[9,10]

Although rare, deficiencies may exist. The most common mineral deficiency in athletes is iron. Athletes who participate in resistance training where reductions in body weight are rapid and who place themselves on low energy or calorie intake diets may consider a modest level of vitamin/mineral supplement.[11] However, megadoses of vitamins and minerals along with the ingestion of other substances whose effects on the human body are unknown is unwarranted.

With little regulation from the federal government, as supplements are classified as "foods," thus circumventing the requirement of scientific proof of effects, manufacturers are free to claim almost anything they wish. The vast majority of performance claims are anecdotal with little or no scientific evidence to support effects or actual need for supplementation in healthy individuals. Additionally, although the individuals who strength train spend billions of dollars on supplements, the effects of these products in this particular population of athletes have rarely been studied. Far more information is available for those who participate regularly in endurance or aerobic activities.

Grunewald et al.[12] conducted a survey of 624 supplements targeted for bodybuilding athletes. Over 800 separate claims were made to suggest enhancement of athletic performance. Additional claims suggested improvement in mental function, sexual vigor, reduction of cancer risk, cholesterol levels, blood pressure control, and antioxidant effects. The majority of all claims were not supported by peer-reviewed research. The vitamin and mineral supplements were most commonly (57%) sold as "packs" for "multiple needs" of the athletes. The fact that none of the "needs" has been established scientifically was overlooked. Although the published literature generally does not support performance-enhancing, or ergogenic, effects of vitamin and mineral supplements, the claims continue to be made. The individuals purchasing the supplements are buying a dream more than a reality. The result is that strength-trained athletes have allowed themselves to be used as human guinea pigs in a monumental experiment, and they have personally paid billions of dollars for the privilege. A human subjects committee at any research institution in this country would never approve this type of experiment.

Another survey conducted by Philen et al.[13] focused on a much more serious problem than questionable performance claims. In advertisements in 12 magazines, 89 companies were identified that produced 311 products. Only 78% of the products listed ingredients. However, many of the ingredients that were listed have shown no effects in humans whatsoever, and these included such items as plant and insect steroids, substances known to induce cyanide poisoning, and hormones whose origins were unknown. Vitamin doses were frequently not given; in some instances they were many multiples of the RDA, to suggest that these were pharmacological or drug-like doses. Toxicological information could not be found for 139 ingredients. Many of the products contained unusual and unidentifiable ingredients; no one has any idea what effect these have on human metabolism. Considering the fact that individuals who strength train and bodybuild go to such great effort to improve the appearance of their bodies, it is unclear why they would consume huge quantities of substances whose internal effects on human physiology have not been identified. Again, the experiment is of enormous proportions, and the assumption of risk by athletes who allow themselves to be used as research subjects is clear. The advertising claims certainly support the goals and aspirations of the individuals who consume the supplements; however, the science does not.

4.2.3   Weight Gain and Weight Loss Practices

The most common strategy used to enhance weight gain and muscle growth by individuals who strength train, weightlift, and bodybuild is overfeeding.[14] Ironically, only 30 to 40% of this weight gain is typically fat-free mass, as most of the "bulk" gained is fat.[14] The energy intake of these individuals who try to "bulk up" tends to be high, between 4000 and 6000 kilocalories per day.[15,16] Therefore, it would be expected that nutrient intake would not be a problem. However, this is not the case. Overnutrition is frequently followed by severe dieting practices, particularly in the sport of competitive bodybuilding.[17] These dietary practices are followed by both males and females and span wide age ranges. Although the scientific literature is clear in showing that severe caloric restriction results in loss of lean body mass and muscle tissue, a commodity that bodybuilders spend a considerable amount of time enhancing, the facts have little effect on individual athlete's choices.

Energy or caloric intake needs to be adequate to meet not only the requirements for basal metabolism, which is the greatest need for calories and thus energy intake in the body, but activity must also be covered. While it is not known what the long-term effects are of severe weight loss for short periods of time over a lifespan, there are recommendations for safe weight loss regimens which should be followed (Appendix E). However, safe programs are seldom considered by resistance-trained athletes because such programs tend to be too slow; the athletes in these types of activities want the weight loss to be very rapid. There is an additional concern that these weight loss practices might impair normal growth in adolescents,[17,18] a group which increasingly participates in strength training and bodybuilding.

4.2.4   Dieting Risks and Vitamin and Mineral Deficiencies in Strength-Trained Females

Female athletes who bodybuild or strength train and who follow severe diet-ing practices aimed at weight loss are at particular risk. In general, the major-ity of women 19 to 50 years old in the United States show that they consume levels of iron, calcium, magnesium, zinc, vitamin B6, vitamin A, and folacin below the Recommended Dietary Allowance (RDA) even though 6 out of 10 women take supplements in addition to their normal diet.[19] Thus, it is clear that proper information about nutrition is needed more than the consump-tion of dietary supplements. It is recognized that intakes below the RDA do not necessarily indicate deficiency states. The RDAs are allowance levels for large population groups and are intentionally set slightly higher than known amounts to cover the needs of almost everyone within a specific category.[20] With respect to strength-trained athletes, vitamin and mineral supplements are very commonly used, but deficiencies can coexist with restricted food intake[21] and with inadequate knowledge about sound dietary practices. The reports of deficiencies appear to be specific to the groups investigated, but it is usually recognized that, as seen in the general population, female athletes of all types usually have low intakes of calcium, iron, and zinc.

Vitamin and mineral supplements are more commonly used by females who bodybuild and weight train than by men who participate in the same activities.[22] However, when nationally ranked elite bodybuilders had their nutritional status evaluated, even though all females supplemented their diets, they still failed to consume adequate amounts of vitamin D, calcium, zinc, copper, and chromium.[23] Their diets tended to be repetitive and monot-onous. It is clear that even with the use of vitamin and mineral supplements, adequate amounts of key nutrients may not be consumed and knowledge about proper nutrition is lacking.

4.2.5   Supplement Use

Of all of the practices followed by athletes who resistance train, the use of vitamin and mineral supplements is most acute in this group. Various studies have attempted to note the use of these substances; an extensive review by Bazzarre[24] has provided considerable insight. Anderson et al.[17] noted in-sea-son bodybuilder use of multivitamins (51%), vitamin C (46%), vitamin D (32%), B-complex vitamins (28%), calcium (33%), and potassium (30%). Oth-ers have noted vitamin and mineral supplement use in female competitive bodybuilders (100%[25]), female bodybuilders (100%,[23] 50%[26]), male body-builders (90%,[23] 63%,[27] 20%[26]) and male Olympic weightlifters (100%[28]). Weighted mean supplement consumption in decreasing level of prevalence was thus 100% for weightlifters and 69% for bodybuilders, the highest levels found in a 15-sport review.[29] Weightlifters state that food intake is not as important as the use of supplements.[28]

4.2.6   Information Sources for Strength-Trained Athletes

Resistance-trained athletes tend to get their information from friends, former competitors, health club staff members, magazines, books,[17,28] coaches,[30] trainers,[31] parents, and physicians.[32] Notably absent from all self-reported influences concerning vitamin and mineral supplementation are sport nutritionists, the only professional group with the appropriate knowledge and training to make recommendations, and exercise physiologists, the only professional group specializing in the study of human performance. Credible sources of information abound in the sport nutrition and exercise physiology literature. The reader is directed to several selected texts[33–38] and web sites (Appendix F).

4.2.7   Reasons for Supplement Use

Vitamin and mineral supplements are most often used as ergogenic aids, substances which are thought to enhance performance.[29] The scientific evidence thus far has overwhelmingly disputed this fact. It has been stated over and over again that there are no ergogenic effects of vitamin and mineral supplementation.[39–43] However, this repeated pronouncement has been virtually ignored by the individuals who strength train. Another reason resistance-trained athletes use vitamins and minerals is that they believe these substances supply energy[44] and build muscle. While vitamins are involved in energy metabolism, they do not supply energy, nor do they supply the materials that will build tissue. The use of vitamin and mineral supplementation by athletes to enhance performance, supply energy, and build muscle can be characterized as a modern-day myth of astronomical proportions.

4.3   Vitamins

4.3.1 Introduction

It has previously been stated that vitamins and minerals, in general, do not enhance performance. However, this has not stopped strength-trained athletes from being major consumers of these products. Herewith follows a listing of the vitamins and minerals thought to be involved in resistance-exercise performance. While the needs of those who exercise in an endurance mode have been studied, there is a general lack of information related to those who resistance train. It is certain that a chapter such as this will not dissuade athletes from supplementing with vitamins and minerals; however, the information is presented so the athlete may understand where pharmacological or drug dosages may exist and at what level toxicity may be anticipated

(Table 4.1). Very few recommendations have been made for resistance-trained athletes; included in Table 4.1 are recommendations for competitive strength-trained athletes from a single source.[45]

Many sources have clearly stated that healthy individuals should obtain their nutrient intakes from dietary sources and not from supplements.[46,47] It has also been stated that vitamin and mineral supplements do not enhance performance in individuals with adequate dietary intakes (Appendix F). Extensive literature reviews refute ergogenic claims while pointing to flawed research study design.[48,49] The potential exists that positive effects have been reported in humans who had deficiency states before the study.[48,49] However, many athletes, both recreational and competitive, still believe that performance is enhanced with supplements, and they continue to believe that it is imperative to consume them in large quantities. Therefore, information will be presented here on vitamins and minerals that are frequently included in supplements and which might be deficient in the diets of resistance-trained athletes. The information presented on individual vitamins and minerals has been adapted from numerous sources.[4,7,8,11,21,33–38,41,42] However, the reader is directed specifically to Reference 37, a sport nutrition source highly regarded for its in-depth information.

4.3.2 Fat-Soluble Vitamins

Fat-soluble vitamins are so named because their absorption and transport is associated with lipids. These vitamins are also stored in lipids within the body. The four currently recognized are vitamins A, D, E, and K.[4]

4.3.2.1 *Vitamin A*

Vitamin A is also known as retinol, an alcohol, and retinal, an aldehyde; the vitamin may be formed in the body by its precursor carotene (a carotenoid). There are numerous forms, which are chemically related. Functions within the body include maintaining proper vision, immune function, nervous function, bone integrity, growth, and skin integrity. Deficiency states in the United States are rare. Some signs and symptoms of inadequate stores include anorexia, immune deficiencies, growth difficulties, and night blindness. Toxic side effects of megadoses have been noted as hypervitaminosis A. The symptoms may include anorexia, skin conditions, hair loss, dizziness, muscle and bone pain, eye infections, headache, and damage to internal organs.

Since it is known that this vitamin may be used in synthesis of muscle proteins[50] and glycogen, it is speculated that aerobic exercise and muscle mass increase may be affected by supplementation. It has not, however, been shown that deficiency or enhanced intake affect endurance performance.[51] There is no evidence that supplementation has any beneficial effect on performance. It has been shown that bodybuilders may take 60,000 IU in the weeks just prior to competition,[52] although 50,000 IU has been listed as the

TABLE 4.1
Vitamins and Exercise

Vitamin	DRIs	Minimum Toxic Dose	Toxic Side Effects	Exercise Function	Marketing Claims	Competition Recommendations[45]
A	F-800 mg RE-RDA M-1000 mg RE-RDA	10 × the RDA	Bone and muscle pain, anorexia, organ damage, hair loss	Maintain vision, resist infection	Improve vision, improve immunity	2.8-3.8 mg
D	Adults-200 IU-AI 51-70y-400 IU-AI >70-600 IU-AI	Unclear-2000 IU/day if prolonged	Calcification of soft tissue, hypertension, anorexia, weakness, death	Bone growth and development	Build stronger bones	None
E	F-8 mg and M-10 mg α-tocopherol equiv. RDA	800 mg-3.2 g	Muscle weakness, fatigue, GI distress, double vision	Cell integrity, muscle metabolism	Increased endurance, improved performance	20-30 mg
K	F-60-65 mcg-RDA M-70-80 mcg-RDA	Natural Forms-no toxicity Synthetics-membrane destruction	Oxidation of membrane phospholipids; infants-anemia, jaundice	Normal blood clotting	Aids injury recovery	None
B_1 Thiamin	F-1.1 mg-RDA M-1.2 mg-RDA	Oral intake<500 mg no toxicity	Headache, weakness, interferes with other B absorption	Carbohydrate metabolism, nervous system function	Increased energy, endurance, performance; decreased fatigue	2.5-4.0 mg
B_2 Riboflavin	F-1.1 mg-RDA M-1.3 mg-RDA	None reported	None reported	Respiration and energy release	Increased energy, endurance, performance; decreased fatigue	4.0-5.5 mg
B_3 Niacin	F-14 mg-RDA M-16 mg-RDA	1g/day may produce side effects	Flushing @10 mg; liver injury, skin and GI problems	Respiration and energy release carbohydrate and fat metabolism	Increased energy, endurance, performance; decreased fatigue	20 mg

TABLE 4.1 (CONTINUED)

Vitamins and Exercise

Vitamin	DRIs	Minimum Toxic Dose	Toxic Side Effects	Exercise Function	Marketing Claims	Competition Recommendations[45]
B$_6$ Pyridoxine	1.3 mg DRI-RDA F>50y-1.5 mg M>50y-1.7 mg	Not clear; 500 mg/d associated with neurotoxicity	Degeneration in spinal cord, peripheral nerves; myelin loss	Protein and amino acid metabolism; RBC formation	Increased energy, endurance, performance; decreased fatigue	7–10 mg
B$_{12}$ Cobalamins	2.4 mcg-RDA >50y-increase	No clear toxicity	Allergy; liver damage	RBC development, maintains nervous tissue	Increased energy, endurance, performance; decreased fatigue	4–9 mcg
Biotin	30 mcg-AI	None reported	None reported	Amino acid metabolism, glycogen synthesis	Increased energy, endurance, performance; decreased fatigue	None
Folic Acid	400 mcg DFE	>0.4 mg = pharmacological dose, 5000 mcg masks B$_{12}$ deficiency	Insomnia, malaise, irritability, GI distress, zinc deficiency	Cell regulation, RBC formation	Increased energy, endurance, performance; decreased fatigue	None
Pantothenic Acid	5 mg-AI	None reported; 100 mg increases niacin excretion	GI distress and diarrhea	Energy metabolism	Increased energy, endurance, performance; decreased fatigue	None
C Ascorbic Acid	60 mg	Not clear; 2 g/d associated with diarrhea	May exacerbate existing conditions	Tissue repair, resistance to infection	Infection and illness protection, rapid injury recovery	175–200 mg

Legend: AI — Adequate Intakes[4], Competitor — Recommendations[4], Competitor — Recommendations made by Rogozkin[45], DFE — Dietary Folate Equivalents, DRIs — 1997-1998 Dietary Reference Intakes[4], Exercise Function and Marketing Claims — Adapted from Aronson[62], F — Female, g — gram, IU — International Units, M — Male, mcg — microgram, mg — milligram, Minimum Toxic Dose — Adapted from Groff and Gropper[4], RE — Retinol Equivalents[4], RDA — Recommended Dietary Allowances[20], Toxic Side Effects — Adapted from Aronson[62] and Groff and Gropper[4], y — years range for a minimum toxic dose (Table 4.1). Megadoses may produce toxic and undesirable effects.[36] Vitamin A intake is usually adequate in developed countries and frequently exceeds RDAs in athletes. It is suggested that no supplements of preformed vitamin A should be used to avoid toxicity. However, although no improvement in performance has been noted by supplementation, an intake of 1000 RE from animal food sources or fortified food products should "probably" be recommended to all strenuously exercising athletes.[53]

4.3.2.2　Vitamin D

Vitamin D represents a class of compounds, stored in body fat, which were shown to cure rickets. Functions within the body include interactions with a wide variety of cells and actions similar to hormones, but the most common association is with bone development, growth, and mineralization. Deficiencies include the development of rickets in children, bone abnormalities due to impaired calcium absorption in adults, muscle weakness, and muscle spasms. Exposure to natural sunlight prevents deficiencies for most individuals. The level of vitamin D intake associated with safety still remains unclear, while it is known that this vitamin interacts with calcium, phosphorus, vitamin K, and iron. Toxicity is noted with the development of kidney stones and calcification in soft tissue, hypertension, anorexia, nausea, renal failure, damage to the heart and lungs, damage to joints, and death.

Vitamin D helps maintain bone strength and mineralization through regulation of calcium and phosphate metabolism. It has been noted that female bodybuilders might completely exclude vitamin D from their diets due to their complete elimination of dairy products.[22] However, exposure to sunlight may ameliorate some effects of decreased intake. No improvement in performance has been noted by supplementation.[54]

4.3.2.3　Vitamin E

Vitamin E represents eight compounds, vitamers, whose richest sources are in plants. The most widely identified function of this vitamin is as an antioxidant which helps stabilize cell membranes. Deficiency states in humans are rare. Toxicity does not seem to be a problem unless there is a defect in the ability of the blood to coagulate. Large doses have occasionally been reported to cause fatigue, weakness, gastrointestinal upset, nausea, diarrhea, flatulence, and vision problems.

There is considerable interest in muscle damage associated with high levels of exercise, and it is attractive to speculate that antioxidants such as vitamin E will have cellular effects. It has been shown that vitamin E supplementation may affect the rate of repair of skeletal muscle damage in older subjects who train eccentrically.[55] Since toxicity is rare and vitamin E also has protective effects for the cardiovascular system, use is not precluded as a prophylactic measure. However, there are no known effects on the improvement of muscular strength, muscular endurance, or power. Nor has it been shown that supplementation of vitamin E will enhance performance or hasten exercise recovery.[56]

4.3.2.4 Vitamin K

Vitamin K is a coenzyme and represents several compounds found primarily in plants and synthesized in the human gut by bacteria. The most widely recognized function of this vitamin is as an aid to the normal clotting of blood. Deficiencies in normal adults are unlikely. When deficiencies do occur, they are often associated with antibiotic use. It is noted, however, that while deficiency may be rare, less than optimal intake in older adults may exacerbate atherosclerosis and osteoporosis. Toxicity is only noted in infants.

Recovery from injury would be supported by adequate amounts of vitamin K in the diet. However, there is no clear association between vitamin K and exercise; as a result there has been no research. Supplementation is completely unwarranted.[57]

4.3.2.5 General Statements about Fat-Soluble Vitamins

Vitamin and mineral supplements are generally safe unless large doses are consumed, and caution should be used in self-administered megadose therapy where the supplement achieves pharmacological status. Since vitamin and mineral supplements are more commonly used by females, some attention needs to be given to safety of their use. Fat-soluble vitamins are generally more toxic than water-soluble vitamins, and recent information indicates several concerns.[58-61] Two fat-soluble vitamins are associated with high dosage problems. Vitamin A intoxication has commonly been reported at levels of approximately 25,000 IU·d^{-1}. Some of the symptoms of toxicity include abdominal pain, anorexia, blurred vision, headache, drowsiness, muscle weakness, nausea, and vomiting. Vitamin E seems to have no side effects unless 300 IU·d^{-1} is exceeded. Symptoms of toxicity include nausea, fatigue, headache, elevation of serum lipids, and double vision; high intakes also interfere with vitamin K activity.[59]

4.3.3 Water-Soluble Vitamins

With the exception of vitamin C, water-soluble vitamins are members of the B complex. Their general functions fall into two broad categories: those that affect energy metabolism and those that affect the formation and function of blood. The vitamins categorized as energy related are thiamin (B_1), riboflavin (B_2), niacin (B_3), pantothenic acid, biotin, and vitamin B_6. The vitamins associated with blood and its function are folic acid, vitamin B_{12}, vitamin B_6, and pantothenic acid. Other functions of the aforementioned vitamins which are important for health are synthesis of sugars and electron transport substances (B_1), nerve and membrane conduction (B_1), synthesis of fatty acids (B_3), steroid hormone and cholesterol synthesis (B_3), synthesis of DNA precursors (B_3), oxidation of glutamate (B_3), synthesis of numerous compounds related to amino acid metabolism (B_6), metabolism of carbohydrate and fat (B_{12}), and DNA synthesis (folic acid).[4]

There have been no studies to date to support the notion that increased or megadoses of vitamins and minerals will have ergogenic or performance-enhancing effects on individuals with adequate vitamin and mineral intake. These recommendations have been published for quite some time.[62] Therefore, a detailed discussion of all of the water-soluble vitamins is not warranted. However, it has been noted through research that the dietary practices of some resistance-trained athletes may produce marginal deficiency states. Only those water-soluble vitamins will be considered here.

Bodybuilders frequently follow dietary regimens, usually associated with competition, which may lead to restriction in energy intake, and thus low levels of certain nutrients have been reported due to the quest for a very low fat diet. Repetitive diets with limited food choices characterize many precompetition diets.[26,63] Concomitantly, micronutrient intake may become inadequate. Low intakes were found for vitamins A,[23,64] D,[25,64] E,[25,64] C,[23,65] B_1,[64,65] B_6,[23] B_{12}[25] and folate,[23,25] generally in women. Generally speaking, male competitors in the same types of events have adequate energy intake, thus they tend to consume adequate amounts of micronutrients. It is known in other areas that females in general consume too little B_6.[19] The fact remains, however, that nutrient status is difficult to assess.[66] Since the fat-soluble vitamins have already been reviewed, the reader is directed to the previous section for this information.

4.3.3.1 Vitamin C

Vitamin C, ascorbic acid, is a strong chemical reducing agent that stimulates a number of enzymatic reactions involved in biosynthesis. It is known as a strong antioxidant against free radical compounds. Vitamin C also aids in non-heme iron absorption.[67]

Additional functions within the body include synthesis of collagen connective tissue, neurotransmitters, serotonin, carnitine, catecholamines, steroid hormones, conversion of cholesterol to bile acids, and others. Links have been established in the prevention of cardiovascular diseases, cancers, and cataracts. Reportedly there are exercise effects which include immune function stimulation,[68] fatigue and soreness reduction, and free radical damage protection.[69] The effects of exercise on the reduction of the vitamin C pool in the body is unknown.[70]

Deficiency states are characterized by abnormal bleeding of gums, capillaries, and joints, along with poor healing of wounds, fatigue, and abnormal psychological states. In the extreme, scurvy develops. Increased intake is frequently recommended for strenuous exercise. Megadoses of 1000 to 2000 mg can cause nausea, abdominal cramps, diarrhea, and other adverse symptoms.

Large doses are also linked with iron loading, decrease in B_{12} availability, and formation of urinary stones.

Effects of vitamin C would be more pronounced in endurance activities; however, reports of improvement of physical performance have been equivocal. They have ranged from improved performance to no effect at all. When methodological problems related to the studies are eliminated, it appears that vitamin C supplements have no effect on strength.[65,66] However, improved performance is to be expected in vitamin C-deficient individuals. It is known that some resistance-trained athletes, particularly bodybuilders,[23] may not have adequate intake, so their health would be improved by dietary changes or modest supplementation.

4.3.3.2 Vitamin B₁—Thiamin

Thiamin functions as a coenzyme crucial in carbohydrate metabolism.[4] Deficiency could impair aerobic metabolism at the cellular level along with the impairment of hemoglobin formation. Little research has been done with respect to thiamin effects on exercise. Although it has been recommended that there is a need for increased B_1 in those who exercise, the level recommended is low enough to be met by increased food intake.

Deficiency states produce muscle weakness, fast heart rates, anorexia, enlargement of the heart, and swelling of tissues. The most widely known syndrome associated with deficiency is beriberi. A particular form of deficiency is associated with excessive intake of alcohol. There seems to be little danger of toxicity associated with oral intakes of 500 mg/day. No studies link enhanced physical performance with elevated levels of thiamin intake.

4.3.3.3 Vitamin B₆

Vitamin B_6 is a series of compounds found primarily in muscle and integrated into the release of glucose from glycogen.[4] As a cofactor, it participates in numerous cellular reactions related to energy metabolism Theoretically, severe deficiency would impair energy release in the body along with hemoglobin synthesis.[67] Intake may stimulate growth hormone production. Results of performance enhancement with elevated intake are equivocal.

Deficiencies are rare but marginal deficiencies could exist in women and the elderly. Toxicity, although a limited problem, is characterized by neurological disorders and can be found at intakes exceeding 200 mg/day^{-1}. No evidence exists that elevated intake will improve resistance performance.[70] However, any deficiency in the B complex vitamins will impair performance.[73]

4.3.3.4 Vitamin B₁₂

Vitamin B_{12}, cobalamin, is involved with the formation and function of red blood cells.[4] Thus, all demands of oxidative metabolism are related to adequate B_{12} status. Much mythology, therefore, has surrounded B_{12} intake.

Aerobic capacity is only enhanced when frank deficiencies, as found in certain anemias, exist.[70] The widespread consumption of supplements and use of injections is completely unwarranted in most cases.

Since B_{12} is only found in animal products, vegetarians are constantly targets as possibly being at risk of low intake. However, most vegetarians are intelligent enough to know that sources exist in eggs, fermented cheeses, dry milk, milk, and milk products. Although toxic effects are not of great concern, no reports of enhanced performance in resistance-trained athletes who elevate their intakes have been reported.[73]

4.3.3.5   Folic Acid (Folate)

Folic acid, folate, is a coenzyme important in energy metabolism and in red blood cell formation.[4] While some have suggested that current recommendations have been seriously underestimated[74] and that all adults should consume supplements, the needs and potential deficiencies of athletes are unknown. It is known that overconsumption may mask pernicious anemia. There are no known studies assessing folic acid supplements on performance of any type.[70] Therefore, recommendations cannot be made.

4.3.3.6   Antioxidants

A current topic of interest to those who exercise is the effect of antioxidant vitamins on cellular repair and recovery.[75–78] While antioxidants are of primary concern to those who exercise aerobically and thus turn over high amounts of oxygen at the cellular level, contractions used in resistance training are also known to provoke muscle-damaging chemical reactions.[75] The antioxidants most commonly considered are vitamins C and E and beta carotene. However, many other nutrients, such as bioflavinoids, copper, cysteine, glutathione, lycopene, manganese, phytochemicals, selenium, and zinc, have antioxidant properties.

To date, the scientific studies have produced conflicting results and a lack of consensus among those who make recommendations for sport and exercise nutrition.[79] Antioxidants are not viewed as ergogenic aids but as supplements that may help ameliorate the negative effects of training and overtraining. Indiscriminate use is generally not justified, but a supplement whose constituents did not exceed 100% of the RDA for any particular nutrient would be acceptable to many sport nutritionists. An extensive review is available in Reference 80.

4.3.3.7   General Statements about Water-Soluble Vitamins

Water-soluble vitamins were thought to be very safe, but this has proved untrue in some cases. Pyridoxine (vitamin B_6) is neuroactive and produces symptoms of sensory neuropathy. The level shown to produce symptoms has consistently been reported lower and lower in the literature and the toxicity threshold for some individuals might be as low as 300 to 500 mg/day^{-1}. The controversy over vitamin C continues, but several of the widely reported effects have proved unfounded. Conditioned scurvy has not been substantiated; oxalate kidney stones have not been seen; and vitamin B$_{12}$ destruction was probably an artifact of the test used to measure vitamin C. Effects that have been substantiated include gastrointestinal distress (nausea, abdominal pain, diarrhea) with doses as low as 1000 mg, probably due to the acidity, not the vitamin itself; oxygen demand of tissue is increased, and problems may ensue if one ascends altitude; dental enamel may be eroded if chewable tablets are used daily; copper intake may be decreased; and, rarely, some individuals develop a rash showing delayed hypersensitivity allergy.[81]

4.4   Minerals

Mineral deficiencies and marginal intakes are more common than vitamin deficiencies.[63] In females and in males who live long enough, calcium is of perpetual concern. It is also known that females, in general, do not consume enough magnesium. Other minerals of concern, zinc and iron, are considered in Chapter 5 of this book. Therefore, only calcium and magnesium will be reviewed here.

4.4.1   Calcium

The most common mineral in the human body is calcium. An inevitable consequence of aging is loss of bone, with the end result being osteoporosis, a disorder of epidemic proportions in the United States costing at least $14 billion in health-care costs annually. Partly to blame may be the current trend of Americans who attempt to reduce caloric and cholesterol consumption by lowering their intake of dairy products, which contain the calcium that bones need. Women who bodybuild follow the at-risk dietary behaviors. The loss of calcium from the skeleton predisposes bone to fractures and compressions of the spine, leading to deformity. It is possible that the concern for reducing risk factors for cardiovascular disease may be increasing the risk for osteoporosis. We are just beginning to understand that the integrity of bone requires a complex integration of the hormones estrogen and testosterone, diet, and exercise and that focusing on one parameter at a time is too simplistic.

Bone mineral describes bone mass and is measured by the amount of calcium phosphate crystal present in bone.[82] Bone mineral density describes the amount of bone mineral found in a specific measured bone area.[82] A dynamic tissue, bone constantly adapts to the stresses placed on or removed from the skeleton, but the process is long and slow.

The highest bone density values are found in male weightlifters, thus suggesting that there is also an interaction of muscle mass which places stress on bone and forces it to adapt.[83] It was thought for some time that "weight bearing" exercise would be the best type of stimulus in the female to protect bone integrity, which is compromised by age, immobility, corticosteroid use, and premenopausal loss of the ability to produce estrogen. Heinrich and co-workers[84] found that weight training or resistance training may provide a good stimulus for increasing bone mineral content due to increased muscle weight. However, in general, the greatest bone densities are found in those who resistance train.

The interactions of exercise, hormones, diet, and bone density are complex. While it is not certain when the greatest bone mass is achieved, it is known that bone is gained during adolescence, plateaus perhaps in the third decade where it is somewhat stable (although decline has been observed) until approximately age 50, after which there is a gradual and progressive loss.[82] In females, this coincides with menopause, and the loss of bone density within the first 5 years after this event is dramatic.[85] Thus, if a line were drawn throughout a lifetime it would show progressive decline after the third decade, with the angle of decline modified by diet, exercise, and hormone balance. While much attention has been placed recently on understanding how to slow this loss, the fact remains that 75% of the variance may be hereditary and only 20% may be modifiable by activity or strength interventions.[82]

It has been shown that diet has a strong effect on bone status since stress fractures are more common in dancers with restrictive diets than in those whose diets are more liberal.[86] Exercise and load on the bone have a strong association, and Dalsky has written a thorough review.[87] The two factors may compete in resistance-trained athletes. It is known that excess calcium can create mineral imbalances. Zinc imbalance is an example.

In summary, it is known that bone density in males who resistance train is high. Bone status in females is probably most affected by female estrogen status. Diet and exercise are important. Therefore estrogen status should be maintained in females as long as possible; calcium intake should be high throughout their lifetimes; and females should adopt lifestyles that include exercise—the exact type, frequency, intensity, and duration of which is yet to be determined. Adults should consume between 1000–1500 mg calcium/day^{-1} and 400–600 IU/day^{-1} vitamin D.[88] The RDA is probably still too low in recommending 800 mg/day^{-1} for women 25 to 50; the RDA for 19- to 24-year-old women is 1200 mg/day^{-1}.[20] If hormone replacement therapy cannot or will not be considered, there are promising results from cyclic etidronate, alendronate, risedronate, estrogen receptor modulators, Tamoxifen, and salmon calcitonin.[88]

If both iron and calcium supplementation are chosen then it is important to coordinate their consumption. Calcium carbonate should be used, and both minerals should be consumed between meals. Calcium tends to inhibit non-heme iron absorption when both are consumed in the same meal, but the degree is unpredictable.[89] Attention should be paid to the use of alkaline-producing foods to ameliorate the effects of bone loss and help maintain bone mineral density.[90] If weight loss is also desired, as happens in bodybuilding, the athlete should follow the recommendations of the American College of Sports Medicine (Appendix F), which suggests that caloric deficit be matched equally with dietary caloric restriction and that weight loss be gradual.

4.4.2 Magnesium

Magnesium supplementation has been promoted as enhancing protein synthesis, growth, muscle contractility, and strength.[79] Research has been equivocal and has generally not supported these claims. Deficiency states will lead to impaired performance,[91] and it is known that Americans in general do not consume adequate amounts. Some studies have reported enhanced strength performance in untrained individuals with supplementation,[92] while results in other studies have been equivocal.[79,93,94] While there is no great concern about toxic effects, recommendations cannot be made until research is more conclusive.

4.5   Dietary Supplement Definition and Concerns

The difficulty in making appropriate choices for the nutritional support of exercise has been exacerbated by congressional legislation. In 1994 the Dietary Supplement Health and Education Act was passed by the U.S. Congress. Dietary supplements were defined as any product that contains a vitamin, mineral, amino acid, herb, or other botanical; or a concentrate, metabolite, constituent, extract, or combination of any of these ingredients. In real terms this means that herbs and plants that contain pharmaceutical agents or known drugs can be claimed by the manufacturer to be dietary supplements. Only federally recognized "dangerous" drugs are excluded. Thus, manufacturers have more freedom than ever to tout the efficacy of supplements to improve performance, the safety and purity of their product, and the "hint" of disease treatment without federal regulation, testing, or approval.[95] When people contact the Food and Drug Administration for help in assessing the manufacturer's claims, they are referred to the manufacturer for information. The manufacturers do not have to provide scientific evidence of their claims if they sell "dietary supplements."

It is certain that the deregulation of this industry will lead to and has already had disastrous consequences for the American public. The incidence of gastrointestinal and pulmonary cancers is associated with chromium use. Delayed development of cancer of the esophagus, a rare form of cancer whose incidence is rising, coincides in time with the popularity of herbals and megadose vitamins and minerals.[96] The more than 60 reported deaths linked to the use of the "natural" amphetamine, ephedra, attest to the fact that the concerns of sport nutritionists and exercise physiologists professional community are real. Since resistance-trained individuals are particular targets of "hyped" and "glitzy" campaigns, it is imperative to proceed with caution before they allow their bodies to become unregulated and unapproved experiments.

4.6   Summary and Recommendations

Many researchers in the field of sport and exercise nutrition suggest that athletes who strength train do not need to rely on vitamin and mineral supplements if they eat a good, well-balanced diet.[95,97-99] There is no research to support the concept that vitamin and mineral supplements help increase muscle mass.[99] Although it is unusual for athletes to have chronic vitamin and mineral deficiencies,[97] a deficiency should be properly diagnosed before supplements are self-prescribed. If it is known, by appropriate evaluation, that a diet is not well-balanced, a supplement that does not exceed 150% of any particular RDA is acceptable.[100] Therefore, the only support recommended for resistance-trained athletes is weight gainers, meal replacement products, and an occasional multivitamin/mineral supplement.[95,101]

The gain in muscle mass and muscle strength, so desired by those who resistance train, appears to depend on a well-nourished individual who participates in a well-designed program.[98] While good program design may be achievable with the contribution of Chapter 1 of this book, it is clear that those who resistance train need much more education in proper nutritional practices. When individuals consume too few calories and make poor food choices, all the hard work in a well-designed program may be lost.[63,102,103] Since the cost of supplements can exceed $400 a month,[79] it is important to know about efficacy of use. Care must also be taken to know the signs and symptoms of toxicity.[103] The information is out there; one who resistance trains needs to seek it and incorporate it into daily living.

References

1. Jackson, C. G. R. and Simonson, S., The relationships between human energy transfer and nutrition, in *Nutrition for the Recreational Athlete*, Jackson, C. G. R. (Ed.), CRC Press, Inc., Boca Raton, 1995, chap 2.
2. Jackson, C. G. R., Nutritional concerns of the female recreational athlete, in *Nutritional Concerns of Women*, Wolinsky, I. and Klimis-Tavantzis, D. (Eds.), CRC Press, Boca Raton, 1996, chap 13.

3. Jackson, C. G. R., Overview of human bioenergetics and nutrition, in *Energy-Yielding Macronutrients and Energy Metabolism in Sports Nutrition*, Driskell, J. A. and Wolinsky, I. (Eds.), CRC Press, Boca Raton, 2000, chap. 2.
4. Groff, J. L. and Gropper, S. W., *Advanced Nutrition and Human Metabolism*, 3rd ed., Wadsworth, Belmont, CA, 1999.
5. Groff, J. L. and Gropper, S. W., Macrominerals, in *Advanced Nutrition and Human Metabolism*, 3rd ed., Wadsworth, Belmont, CA, 1999, chap 11.
6. Groff, J. L. and Gropper, S. W., Microminerals, in *Advanced Nutrition and Human Metabolism*, 3rd ed., Wadsworth, Belmont, CA, 1999, chap 12.
7. Kurtzweil, P., An FDA guide to dietary supplements, *FDA Consumer*, 32(5), 28, 1998.
8. Armstrong, L. and Maresh, C., Vitamin and mineral supplements as nutritional aids to exercise performance and health, *Nutr. Rev.*, 54, S148, 1996.
9. Singh, A., Moses, F. M., and Deuster, P. A., Chronic multivitamin-mineral supplementation does not enhance physical performance, *Med. Sci. Sports Exerc.*, 24(6), 726, 1992.
10. Telford, R., Catchpole, E., Deakin, V., Hahn, A., and Plank, A., The effect of 7 to 8 months of vitamin/mineral supplementation on athletic performance, *Int. J. Sport Nutr.*, 2, 135, 1992.
11. Williams, M. H., *Nutrition for Health, Fitness, and Sport*, WCB/McGraw Hill, Dubuque, IA, 1998.
12. Grunewald, K. K. and Bailey, R. S., Commercially marketed supplements for bodybuilding athletes, *Sports Med.*, 15(2), 90, 1993.
13. Philen, R. M., Ortiz, D. I., Auerbach, S. B., and Falk, H., Survey of advertising for nutritional supplements in health and body building magazines, *JAMA*, 268(8), 1008, 1992.
14. Kreider, R. B., Dietary supplements and the promotion of muscle growth with resistance exercise, *Sports Med.*, 27(2), 97, 1999.
15. Grandjean, A. C., Macronutrient intake of U.S. athletes compared with the general population and recommendations made for athletes, *Am. J. Clin. Nutr.*, 449, 1070, 1989.
16. Kleiner, S. M., Calabrese, L. H., Fiedler, K. M., Naito, H. K., and Skibinski, C. I., Dietary influences on cardiovascular disease risk in anabolic steroid-using and non-using bodybuilders, *J. Am. Coll. Nutr.*, 8, 109, 1989.
17. Andersen, R. E., Barlett, S. J., Morgan G. D., and Brownell, K. D., Weight loss, psychological, and nutritional patterns in competitive male body builders, *Int. J. Eat. Dis.*, 18(1), 49, 1995.
18. Tipton, C. M., Consequences of rapid weight loss, in *Nutrition and Athletic Performance*, Haskell, W., Skala, J., and Whittam, J. (Eds.), Bull Co., Palo Alto, CA, 176, 1982.
19. Welsh, S. and Guthrie, J. F., Changing American diets, in *Micronutrients in Health and in Disease Prevention*, Bendich, A. and Butterworth, C. E. (Eds.), Marcel Dekker, New York, 1991.
20. Food and Nutrition Board Commission on Life Sciences National Research Council, *Recommended Dietary Allowances*, 10th ed., National Academy Press, Washington, D.C., 1989.
21. Haymes, E. M., Vitamin and mineral supplementation of athletes, *Int. J. Sport Nutr.* 1, 146, 1991.

22. Kleiner, S. M., Bazzarre, T. L., and Litchford, M. D., Metabolic profiles, diet and health practices of championship male and female bodybuilders, *J. Am. Diet. Assoc.*, 90, 962, 1990.

23. Kleiner, S. M., Bazzarre, T. L., and Ainsworth, B. E., Nutritional status of nationally ranked elite bodybuilders, *Int. J. Sport Nutr.*, 4, 54, 1994.

24. Bazzarre, T. L., Nutrition and strength, in *Nutrition in Exercise and Sport*, 3rd ed., Wolinsky, I. (Ed.), CRC Press, Boca Raton, 1998, chap 14.

25. Lamar-Hildebrand, N., Saldanha, L., and Endres, J., Dietary and exercise practices of college-aged female body builders, *J. Am. Diet. Assoc.*, 89, 1308, 1989.

26. Sandoval, W. M., Heyward, V. H., and Lyons, T. M., Comparison of body composition, exercise and nutritional profiles of female and male bodybuilders at competition, *J. Sports Med. Phys. Fitness*, 29(1), 63, 1989.

27. Faber, M. and Spinnlerbenade, A. J., Nutrient intake and dietary supplementation on body builders, *S. Afr. Med. J.*, 72, 831, 1987.

28. Burke, L. M., Gollan, R. A., and Read, R. S., Dietary intakes and food use of groups of elite Australian male athletes, *Int. J. Sport Nutr.*, 1, 378, 1991.

29. Sobal, J. and Marquart, L. F., Vitamin/mineral supplement use among athletes: a review of the literature, *Int. J. Sport Nutr.*, 4, 320, 1994.

30. Wolf, E. M. B., Wirth, J. C., and Lohman, T. R., Nutritional practices of coaches in the Big Ten, *Phys. Sportsmed.*, 7(2), 112, 1979.

31. Graves, K. L., Farthing, M. C., Smith, S. A., and Turchi, J. M., Nutrition training, attitudes, knowledge, recommendations, responsibility and resource utilization of high school coaches and trainers, *J. Am. Diet. Assoc.*, 91, 321, 1991.

32. Barry, A. T., Cantwell, T., Doherty, F., Folan, J. C., Ingoldsby, M., Kevany J. P., O'Broin, J. D., O'Connor, H., O'Shea, B., Ryan, B. A., and Vaughan, J., A nutritional study of Irish athletes, *Br. J. Sports Med.*, 15, 99, 1981.

33. Clark, N., *Sports Nutrition Guidebook*, Human Kinetics, Champaign, IL, 1997.

34. Jackson, C. G. R., *Nutrition for the Recreational Athlete*, CRC Press, Inc., Boca Raton, 1995.

35. Kleiner, S. M., *Power Eating*, Human Kinetics, Champaign, IL, 1998.

36. Williams, M., *Nutrition for Fitness and Sport*, William C. Brown, Dubuque, IA, 1998.

37. Wolinsky, I. and Driskell, J. A., *Sports Nutrition, Vitamins and Trace Elements*, CRC Press, Inc., Boca Raton, 1997.

38. Wolinsky, I. (Ed.), *Nutrition in Exercise and Sport*, CRC Press, Boca Raton, 1998.

39. Lukaski, H. C., Micronutrients (magnesium, zinc, and copper): are mineral supplements needed for athletes?, *Int. J. Sport Nutr.*, 5, S74, 1995.

40. Smith, N. J., Food fraud and the athlete, in *Nutrient Utilization During Exercise*, Ross Laboratories, Columbus, OH, 1983, 31.

41. Williams, M. H., Vitamin supplementation and physical performance, in *Nutrient Utilization During Exercise*, Ross Laboratories, Columbus, OH, 1983, 26.

42. Williams, M. H., Nutritional supplements for strength trained athletes, in *Sports Science Exchange*, 6(6), #47, Gatorade Sport Science Institute, Chicago, IL, 1993.

43. Berning, J., Coyle, E. F., Garcia, P. R., O'Connor, H., Orbeta, S., and Terrados, N., Sports foods for athletes: What works?, in *Sports Science Exchange*, 9(2), #32, Gatorade Sport Science Institute, Chicago, IL, 1998.

44. Krumbach, C. J., Ellis, D. R., and Driskell, J. A., A report of vitamin and mineral supplement use among university athletes in a division 1 institution, *Int. J. Sport Nutr.*, 9, 416, 1999.

45. Rogozkin, V. A., Weight lifting and power events, in *Nutrition in Sport*, Maughan, R. J. (Ed.), Blackwell Science, Malden, MA, 2000, chap. 47.

46. Callaway, C. W., McNutt, K. W., Rivlin, R. S., Ross, A. C., Sandstead, H. H., and Simopoulos, A. P., Statement on vitamin and mineral supplements, the Joint Public Information Committee of the American Society for Nutritional Sciences and the American Society for Clinical Nutrition, *FASEB*, 2000.

47. Beltz, S. D. and Doering, P. L., Efficacy of nutritional supplements used by athletes, *Clin. Pharm.*, 12, 900, 1993.

48. Bucci, L., Nutritional ergogenic aids, in *Nutrition in Exercise and Sport*, 2nd ed., Wolinsky, I. and Hickson, J. F., Jr. (Eds.), CRC Press, Boca Raton, 1994.

49. Williams, M. H., Ergogenic aids, in *Sports Nutrition for the 90's: The Health Professional's Handbook*, Berning, J. R. and Steen, S. N. (Eds.), Aspen Publishers, Gaithersburg, MD, 1991.

50. Lui, N. and Roels, O., Vitamin A and carotene, in *Modern Nutrition in Health and Disease*, Goodhart, R. and Shils, M. (Eds.), Lea & Febiger, Philadelphia, 1980.

51. Wald, G., Brouha, L., and Johnson, R., Experimental human Vitamin A deficiency and ability to perform muscular exercise, *Am. J. Physiol.*, 137, 551, 1942.

52. Wolinsky, I. and Driskell, J. A., *Sports Nutrition, Vitamins and Trace Elements*, CRC Press, Inc., Boca Raton, 1997, chap 8.

53. Wolinsky, I. and Driskell, J. A., *Sports Nutrition, Vitamins and Trace Elements*, CRC Press, Inc., Boca Raton, 1997, p. 101.

54. Wolinsky, I. and Driskell, J. A., *Sports Nutrition, Vitamins and Trace Elements*, CRC Press, Inc., Boca Raton, 1997, p. 111.

55. Evans, W. J., Muscle damage: Nutritional considerations, *Int. J. Sport Nutr.*, 1, 214, 1991.

56. Wolinsky, I. and Driskell, J. A., *Sports Nutrition, Vitamins and Trace Elements*, CRC Press, Inc., Boca Raton, 1997, p. 119

57. Wolinsky, I. and Driskell, J. A., *Sports Nutrition, Vitamins and Trace Elements*, CRC Press, Inc., Boca Raton, 1997, p. 111.

58. Cerny, L. and Cerny, K., Can carrots be addictive: an extraordinary form of drug dependence, *Brit. J. Addiction*, 87, 1195, 1992.

59. Hathcock, J. N., Safety of vitamin and mineral supplements, in *Micronutrients in Health and in Disease Prevention*, Bendich, A. and Butterworth, C. E. (Eds.), Marcel Dekker, Inc., New York, 1991.

60. Hathcock, J. N., Hattan, D. G., Jenkins, M. Y., Mcdonald, J. T., Sundaresan, P. R., and Wilkening, V. L., Evaluation of vitamin A toxicity, *Am. J. Clin. Nutr.*, 52, 183, 1990.

61. van Dam, M. A., The recognition and treatment of hypervitaminosis A., *Nurse Pract.*, 14, 28, 1989.

62. Aronson, V., Vitamins and minerals as ergogenic aids, *Phys. Sportsmed.*, 14(3), 209, 1986.

63. Walberg-Rankin, J., A review of nutritional practices and needs of bodybuilders, *J. Str. Cond. Res.*, 9(2), 116, 1995.

64. Linseisen, J., Metges, C. C., and Wolfram, G., Dietary habits and serum lipids of a group of German amateur bodybuilders, *Z. Ernährungswiss*, 32(4), 289, 1993.

65. Kris-Ethertton, P. M., The facts and fallacies of nutritional supplements for athletes, *Sports Science Exchange*, 2(18), Gatorade Sport Science Institute, Chicago, IL, 1989.

66. Fogelholm, M., Micronutrient status in females during a 24-week fitness-type exercise program, *Ann. Nutr. Metab.*, 36, 209, 1992.
67. Fogelholm, M., Vitamins: Metabolic functions, in *Nutrition in Sport*, Maughan, R. J. (Ed.), Blackwell Science, Malden, MA, 2000, chap. 20.
68. Chen, J. D., Some sports nutrition researches in China, in *China's Sports Medicine, Medicine and Sport Science*, Qu, M. Y. and Yu, C. L. (Eds.), Karger, Basel, 28, 94, 1988.
69. Kanter, M. M., Free radicals, exercise and antioxidant supplementation, *Int. J. Sport Nutr.*, 4, 205, 1994.
70. Chen, J., Vitamins: effects of exercise on requirements, in *Nutrition in Sport*, Maughan, R. J. (Ed.), Blackwell Science, Malden, MA, 2000, chap. 21.
71. Williams, M. H., Vitamin supplementation and physical performance, *Nutrient Utilization During Exercise*, Ross Laboratories, Columbus, OH, 26, 19.
72. Gerster, H., Review: the role of vitamin C in athletic performance, *J. Am. Coll. Nutr.*, 8, 636, 1989.
73. Williams, M. H., Nutritional ergogenic aids and athletic performance, *Nutr. Today*, Jan./Feb. 7, 1989.
74. Oakley, G. P., Jr., Adams, M. J., and Dickinson, C. M., More folic acid for everyone, now, *J. Nutr.*, 126, 751S, 1996.
75. Evans, W. J., Muscle damage: nutritional considerations, *Int. J. Sport Nutr.*, 1, 214, 1991.
76. Brooks, G., Gilliam, I., Kanter, M., and Packer, L., Antioxidants and the elite athlete, *Proceedings of the Panel Discussion*, Henkel Corporation, La Grange, IL, 1992.
77. Blumberg, J., Jenkins, R., Clarkson, P., Ji, L. L., and Goldfarb, A., Exercise, nutrition and free radicals: what's the connection? *Gatorade Sports Sci. Exch.*, 5(1), 1, 1994.
78. McBride, J. M. and Kraemer, W. J., Free radicals, exercise and antioxidants, *J. Str. Cond. Res.*, 13(2), 175, 1999.
79. Williams, M. H., Nutritional supplements for strength trained athletes, *Sports Science Exchange*, 6(6), Gatorade Sport Science Institute, Chicago, IL, 1993.
80. Sen, C. K., Sashwati, R., and Packer, L., Exercise-induced oxidative stress and antioxidant nutrients, in *Nutrition in Sport*, Maughan, R. J. (Ed.), Blackwell Science, Malden, MA, 2000, chap. 22.
81. Hathcock, J. N., Safety of vitamin and mineral supplements, in *Micronutrients in Health and in Disease Prevention*, Bendich, A. and Butterworth, C. E. (Eds.), Marcel Dekker, Inc., New York, 1991, 99.
82. Snow-Harter, C. and Marcus, R., Exercise, bone mineral density, and osteoporosis, in *Exercise and Sport Science Reviews*, 19, 351, 1991.
83. Block, J. E., Genant, H. K., and Mack, D., Greater vertebral bone mineral mass in exercising young men, *West. J. Med.*, 145, 39, 1986.
84. Heinrich, C., Going, S. B., Pamenter, R. W., Perry C. D., Boyden, T. W., and Lohman, T. G., Bone mineral content of cyclically menstruating female resistance and endurance trained athletes, *Med. Sci. Sports Exerc.*, 22, 558, 1990.
85. Meema, H. E. and Meema, S., Cortical bone mineral density versus cortical thickness in the diagnosis of osteoporosis: a roentgenological–densitometric study, *J. Am. Geriatric Soc.*, 17, 120, 1969.
86. Frusztajer, N. T., Dhuper, S., Warren, M. P., Brooks-Gunn, J., and Fox, R. P., Nutrition and the incidence of stress fractures in ballet dancers, *Am. J. Clin. Nutr.*, 51, 779, 1990.

87. Dalsky, G., Effect of exercise on bone: Permissive influence of estrogen and calcium, *Med. Sci. Sport Exerc.*, 22, 281, 1990.

88. Osteoporosis Prevention, Diagnosis, and Therapy. *NIH Consensus Statement Online*, 17(2), 1, 2000.

89. Cook, J. D., Dassenko, S. A., and Whittaker, P., Calcium supplementation: effect on iron absorption, *Am. J. Clin. Nutr.*, *53*, 106, 1991.

90. Stearns, M. R., Jackson, C. G. R., Landauer, J. A., Frye, S. D., Hay, W. W., Jr., and Burke, T. J., Small for gestational age: a new insight? *Med. Hypotheses*, 53(3), 186, 1999.

91. McDonald, R. and Keen, C. L., Iron, zinc and magnesium nutrition and athletic performance, *Sports Med.*, 5(3), 171, 1988.

92. Brilla, L. R. and Haley, T. F., Effect of magnesium supplementation on strength training humans, *J. Am. Coll. Nutr.*, 11(3), 326, 1992.

93. Stricker, P. R., Other ergogenic aids, *Clin. Sport Med.*, 17(2), 283, 1998.

94. Lukaski, H. C., Micronutrients (magnesium, zinc, and copper): are mineral supplements needed for athletes? *Int. J. Sport Nutr.*, 5, S74, 1995.

95. Eichner, E. R., King, D., Myhal, M., Prentice, B., and Ziegenfuss, T. N., Muscle builder supplements, *Sports Science Exchange*, 10(3), Gatorade Sport Science Institute, Chicago, IL, 1999.

96. Pearl, J. M., Severe reaction to "natural testosterones": how safe are ergogenic aids? p. 188.

97. Chu, D., Satterwhite, Y., Wathen, D., Reeland, D., and Schmidt, J., Strength and conditioning programs: answers from the experts, *Sports Science Exchange*, 6(5), Gatorade Sport Science Institute, Chicago, IL, 1995.

98. Clarkson, P. M., Nutritional supplements for weight gain, *Sports Science Exchange*, 11(2), Gatorade Sport Science Institute, Chicago, IL, 1998.

99. Berning, J., Coyle, E. F., O'Connor, H., Orbeta, S., and Terrados, N., Sport foods for athletes? What works? *Sports Science Exchange*, 9(2), Gatorade Sport Science Institute, Chicago, IL, 1998.

100. Coleman, E., Vitamin/mineral supplements—use and abuse, *Sports Med. Digest*, 10(6), 5, 1988.

101. Singh, V. N., A current perspective on nutrition and exercise, *J. Nutr.*, 122, 760, 1992.

102. Brownell, K. D., Nelson-Steen, S., and Wilmore, J. H., Weight regulation practices in athletes: analysis of metabolic and health effects, *Med. Sci. Sports Exerc.*, 19, 546, 1987.

103. Reynolds, R. D., Vitamins supplements: current controversies, *J. Am. Coll. Nutr.*, 13(2), 118, 1994.

5

Trace Minerals

Emily M. Haymes and Keith C. DeRuisseau

CONTENTS

5.1 Introduction

Trace minerals are those minerals stored in the human body in quantities of 5 grams or less. Thirteen trace minerals are considered essential for body functions. However, the role of only a few of these in resistance exercises has been examined. This review will examine the role of four trace minerals: iron, zinc, copper, and chromium, in resistance training as well as show the evidence of nutritional and biochemical deficiencies among athletes who engage in resistance training as a part of their conditioning programs. Limited data for two other minerals, boron and vanadium, also will be discussed.

5.2   Iron

Of the essential trace minerals, iron has received the most attention by far within the athlete population. Among the various roles of iron within the body is its critical function in aerobic energy metabolism. Iron is a component of hemoglobin (Hb), myoglobin, and serves as a factor for numerous enzymes. Total body iron in healthy adults is normally in the range of 3 to 5 grams.[1] Iron in the body that is not performing a functional role, approximately 30 to 40% of total body iron, is incorporated into the protein ferritin for storage.[2] Ferritin is located primarily within tissues of the liver, bone marrow, and spleen. A small amount of ferritin can be measured in the serum and is an indicator of total body iron stores; 1 μg/L indicates approximately 8 to 10 mg of storage iron.[3,4] Mean serum ferritin concentration in men is roughly three times higher than that of menstruating women due to much larger iron stores in men.[3]

5.2.1   Nutritional Iron Status

Current recommendations for iron intake by the Food and Nutrition Board were published in 1989.[5] The RDAs for adolescent and adult males are 12 and 10 mg Fe/d, respectively. Adolescent and nonpregnant adult females are recommended to consume 15 mg Fe/d, with the recommendation decreasing to 10 mg Fe/d in the 51+ age category. The extent of absorption of iron depends upon current iron status and composition of the diet.[6] An inverse relationship exists between the iron status of the individual and the amount of iron that is absorbed.[4] Absorption of iron increases as body stores become depleted. Iron in the diet can be in one of two forms, heme and non-heme iron. Food sources of heme and non-heme iron consist primarily of animal and plant products, respectively. Heme iron is a more absorbable form of iron than non-heme iron. Also, unlike non-heme iron, the absorption of heme iron is not affected by composition of the diet.[4] The typical North American and European diet contains approximately 6 mg of iron per 1000 calories and provides approximately 10 to 15% absorption of dietary iron.[7]

   Studies that have examined iron consumption of male strength and power athletes have generally demonstrated adequate intakes. Table 5.1 lists average

TABLE 5.1

Dietary Iron Intake from Food of Male and Female Athletes in Selected Sports

Sport	Age (yr)	Iron Intake (mg/d) Males	Females	Reference
Bodybuilding*	31	20.0		19
Bodybuilding*	28	16.0	24.0	15
Bodybuilding*	29.5	24.0	16.5	20
Bodybuilding*	26.4	18.8	13.6	17
Bodybuilding*	18–30		12.8	27
Bodybuilding			15.0	
Bodybuilding	24.6	22.0		14
Bodybuilding	26	36.5		13
Bodybuilding	27	25.0		9
Bodybuilding		29.0		8
Bodybuilding		20.7	11.3	18
Judo		14.6		
Weightlifting		14.2		
Gymnasts			10.7	
Hockey		15.5	11.5	
Soccer		14.0		
Volleyball			12.3	
Gymnasts		12.0		8
Track & Field		17.0		
Wrestling		15.7		
Football		29.3		
Defensive backs		15.0		
Soccer		15.0		
Crew		24.5	15.0	
Basketball		27.7	15.0	
Swimming			15.0	
Lacrosse		20.0	14.0	
Volleyball			11.3	
Throwing	22.2	22.0	13.3	9
Karate	19		12.7	28
Team handball	20		12.9	
Basketball	20		15.8	
Wrestling & judo	21.6	20.0		25
Weightlifting, wrestling, throwing	23.7	21.3		10
Soccer, hockey, basketball, swimming	21.8	22.3		
Football	12–14	15.0		22
	15–18	20.0		

* = Precompetition

iron intakes for male and female athletes participating in various sports. Male track and field[8] and throwing athletes[9] have demonstrated adequate iron intakes. A combined group of weightlifting, wrestling, and throwing athletes have been shown to consume similar intakes.[10]

Iron intake of male bodybuilders has been reported to be adequate, spanning a wide range from 16 to 42 mg/d with[11,12] and without[8,9,11–13,15–20] nutritional supplementation. It should be noted that not all studies have indicated the particular phase of training in which nutrient intake was assessed. In particular, competitive bodybuilders alter exercise and dietary practices depending on their phase of training.[11,21,22] Although adequate, mean iron intakes of bodybuilders from food sources during precompetition are slightly lower compared to bodybuilders during the noncompetitive phase of training. In one group of bodybuilders, mean iron intake from both food and nutritional supplements did not change significantly from baseline in the 12 weeks prior to competition (30.9 and 33.2 mg Fe/d, respectively) despite a significant decrease in caloric consumption (2811 vs. 2041 kcal/d).[11]

Nutritional analysis of various athletic teams was conducted for a 4-year period at Syracuse University.[8] Mean iron intake for football teams within the study period ranged from 220 to 360% of the RDA, with a slightly lower intake reported for defensive backs. There was no report of any player consuming less than the RDA for iron. A comparable intake was reported in a team of Australian football players.[23] Adolescent football players have also been reported to have adequate iron intakes.[24]

During a period of weight maintenance, iron intake of wrestlers and martial artists (judo) was approximately twice the RDA.[25] During periods of gradual and rapid weight loss, mean iron intake has been shown to decrease to approximately 14 and 9 mg/d, respectively.[25] In close agreement with these findings, during five out of six seasons wrestlers at Syracuse University had adequate iron intakes ranging from a mean of 11 to 21 mg/d.[8] In only one season was there an iron intake below the RDA. Van Erp-Baart and colleagues[18] reported mean iron intakes from two groups of martial artists to be 16.1 and 13.1 mg/d.

Female strength and power athletes do not achieve adequate iron intakes to the extent of their male counterparts. In general, iron consumption is close to the RDAs, either slightly above or below the recommendations. Two studies reported an increased iron intake of 24 mg/d among bodybuilders during precompetition,[12,15] with one study including use of nutritional supplements in the analysis.[12] A lower intake of 15.4 mg/d, however, was reported in a group of six female bodybuilders during precompetition, despite the report of multivitamin or iron supplementation among three of the athletes.[26] Among the various athlete groups in Table 5.1, basketball players,[28] swimmers, and crew [8] have been reported to achieve recommended iron intakes.

5.2.2   Responses to Exercise and Training

Several mechanisms by which resistance exercise may potentially influence measures of iron status and metabolism have been proposed.[29,30] Resistance exercise could lead to the development of iron deficiency if rates of iron absorption or iron loss are affected. A limited number of studies have investigated the effects of exercise on iron absorption, all of which have involved endurance-trained athletes.[31–33] Conflicting results have been reported, most likely due to differences in methodology and subject characteristics. The effect of resistance exercise on iron absorption has not been investigated.

Urinary iron loss resulting from an 8-week resistance-training program has been reported.[34] Thirty-six males were randomly assigned to either chromium (picolinate or chloride) supplement or placebo groups. Subjects who consumed the placebo experienced the greatest urinary iron excretion, which increased up to Week 5 ($p < 0.05$), followed by a decrease to baseline levels at Week 8. Baseline urinary iron excretion was approximately 0.7 μmol/d and increased to approximately 1.1 μmol/d at the end of Week 5, equivalent to 0.04 and 0.06 mg/d. Resistance training therefore was only responsible for an increased urinary iron excretion of 0.02 mg Fe/d. This is a small amount of iron in comparison to the approximate 1 mg total iron loss per day in males.[1]

Increased iron loss through sweat[35,36] and the gastrointestinal (GI) tract[37,38] has been investigated as a contributing factor in iron deficiency in athletes, but has not been investigated in response to resistance training. Additional proposed mechanisms in which resistance training may affect iron metabolism include: mechanical trauma to red blood cells, increased red blood cell osmotic fragility, and changes in renal pressure.[29,30] Measures of red cell synthesis and lysis during resistance training have been examined and are discussed in the next section.

5.2.3 Resistance Training Studies

Resistance training studies that have reported measures of iron status are listed in Table 5.2. There is limited evidence to suggest that resistance training has a negative impact on measures of iron status. One study involved 12 healthy non-strength-trained males and demonstrated impaired iron status during a 12-week resistance-training program.[29] Following 6 weeks of training, reductions in Hb, mean corpuscular hemoglobin (MCH), and mean corpuscular hemoglobin concentration (MCHC) were observed. Accompanying this change was a significant decrease in haptoglobin (Hp) between Weeks 3 and 6, and an increase in reticulocyte count following 6 weeks of training. Decreased Hp and increased reticulocyte count indicate an increased rate of red cell hemolysis and new red cell synthesis, respectively. The training program significantly reduced serum ferritin (sFerr) by 35% but had no effect on measures of iron transport. Decreases in Hb and sFerr were not attributed to hemodilution due to a significant increase in packed cell volume and red cell counts.[29] It was concluded that resistance training placed mechanical stress on the red cells, leading to an increased lysis and erythropoiesis and resulting in a decline in body iron stores.[29] The impact of dietary iron intake on measures of iron status was not assessed.

Another study of young males also demonstrated a significant decrease in sFerr following resistance training.[34] This investigation was designed to assess the effects of supplemental chromium on strength and body composition. Subjects were assigned to one of three groups: chromium picolinate,

TABLE 5.2

Effect of Resistance Training on Indices of Iron Status in Males and Females

Reference (#)	39	40		29	34	30	
	M	M	F	M	M	C	S
Iron(μmol/L)							
pre	11.5	WNR	WNR	17.3	22.8	—	—
post	11.1			15.3	21.2		
TIBC(μmol/L)							
pre	38.2*	38.5*	52.3	—	59.1*	—	—
post	26.5	28.0	55.2	—	62.0		
TS(%)							
pre	30.6*	41.0*	21.0	35.6	39.0*	ND	
post	42.0	49.0	21.0	30.5	34.0		
sFerr(μg/L)							
pre	134.5	133.0	123.0*	74.8*	70.0*	~110	~80
post	112.9	125.0	97.0	49.3	54.0		
Hb(g/dL)							
pre	15.1	WNR	WNR	15.8*	WNR	ND	
post	14.9			15.2			
Hct							
pre	0.44	WNR	WNR	0.479*	WNR	ND	
post	0.44			0.493			
MCV(fl)							
pre	88.6	—	—	NC	—	ND	
post	88.0					ND	
MCH(pg)							
pre	30.3	—	—	29.6*	—	ND	
post	30.0	—	—	27.7	—		
MCHC(g/L)							
pre	342.0	—	—	329.2*	—	ND	
post	341.0	—	—	309.8	—		
TfR(mg/L)							
pre	—	3.6*	5.3	—	—	—	—
post	—	4.9	5.3	—	—		

* = significant differences between pre and post measurements.

Key:

Capacity; TS = Transferrin Saturation; sFerr = Serum Ferritin; Hb = Hemoglobin Concentration; Hct = Hematocrit; MCV = Mean

Corpuscular Volume; MCH = Mean Corpuscular Hemoglobin; MCHC = Mean Corpuscular Hemoglobin Concentration; TfR = Transferrin Receptor

M = Male; F = Female; C = Control; S = Strength; WNR = Within Normal Range; ND = No difference between Control and Strength; NC = No Change between pre and post measurements.

chromium chloride, or placebo supplementation. Following an intensive 8-week program, all groups experienced a significant decline in sFerr and measures of iron transport. Serum iron (SI), however, only tended to decrease as a result of training. While it appeared that measures of iron transport and storage were adversely affected by resistance training, Hb and hematocrit (Hct) were within the normal range and did not change during the 8-week program. No measures of red cell hemolysis or erythropoiesis were obtained, thus not allowing for the assessment of red cell lysis and synthesis.

In contrast to the above-mentioned studies, results from the following investigations did not demonstrate adverse effects of resistance training on iron status, but rather demonstrated an increase in iron transport following training.[39,40] Campbell et al.[39] measured indices of iron status in stored blood samples from moderately overweight, older men who had participated in a 13-week resistance training program. Samples had been obtained at baseline and following 6 and 12 weeks of supplemental chromium picolinate or placebo. Following training there were no significant differences in red cell indices, including Hb and Hct, or indices of iron status between groups. In the placebo group, a significant decrease in TIBC and increase in transferrin saturation following training indicated an increase in iron transport, although there was no change in the serum iron. In contrast to the findings of Schobersberger et al.,[29] no differences in MCH or MCHC were detected. No measures of hemolysis or erythropoiesis were obtained.

Preliminary findings of Murray et al.,[40] also involving older men, reported results similar to those of Campbell et al.[39] Following a 12-week resistance training program, the subjects demonstrated a significant increase in transferrin saturation and a decrease in TIBC. This has been the only investigation to examine the effect of resistance-training on the transferrin receptor concentration (TfR), an index of body iron stores. Despite an elevation in transferrin saturation and adequate storage iron, a significant increase in TfR was observed following the 12-week resistance-training program. An increase in the TfR is an unexpected finding. The TfR normally increases during iron deficiency as the erythroid mass, cells involved with red cell production, attempts to increase iron uptake to support erythropoiesis.[41] No effect was observed in serum iron or red cell count values. Differences in subjects' ages may be a factor explaining some of the observed differences in iron status in the response to resistance training.

Compared to those for males, even fewer studies have examined the effects of resistance exercise on indices of iron metabolism in women.[40,42] Two preliminary studies report conflicting results with respect to the influence of resistance exercise on measures of iron transport and storage. A 12-week resistance training program in older women reported a significant decrease in sFerr with no significant changes in other iron-related parameters.[40] Assessments of red cell lysis, synthesis, or dietary iron intake may have provided insight into the mechanism behind the reduced sFerr; however, this information was not reported.

In contrast to these findings, Matsuo et al.[42] studied women who performed aerobic resistance exercise every day for 12 weeks. The exercise program utilized 2-lb dumbbells and incorporated 11 exercises (10 upper body) for 15 minutes per day. The exercise protocol utilized resulted in little or no weight gain due to muscle hypertrophy.[43] Iron deficient subjects (sFerr < 12 mg/L) demonstrated an increase in iron status at the end of the study period, but hemoglobin, hematocrit (Hct), and red cell count remained unchanged. The non-iron-deficient control group demonstrated significant improvement in all of the blood measures. It was concluded that young women who incorporate 15 minutes of dumbbell exercise per day may actually prevent iron deficiency anemia.[42]

5.2.4   Resistance Exercise and Iron Status

Evidence from a cross-sectional investigation did not demonstrate impaired sFerr values or red cell indices among elite strength-trained male athletes (wrestlers, judo) compared to a group of healthy controls.[30] Hemoglobin concentration was in the normal range for both groups; however, sFerr was a nonsignificant 11% lower in the strength-trained athletes. Measures of hemolysis (Hp, plasma Hb) were not different between groups. A possibility that a greater length of time elapsed between the last exercise session and blood collection may explain the differences between this study[30] and that of Schobersberger et al.[29] In contrast to the study by Schobersberger et al.[29] but in agreement with Campbell et al.,[39] no differences in red cell indices were observed due to strength training. However, a greater activity of erythrocyte glutamo-oxacetate transaminase (GOT) was noted in the strength-trained group compared to the controls, which indicated younger red cells in the strength-trained group.[30] Changes in GOT activity were not detected in the investigation by Schobersberger et al.[29]

Additional studies have assessed indices of iron status in strength-trained athletes.[10,13,15,20,25,28,44] Table 5.3 includes selected indices of iron status of males and females within various sports. Serum ferritin values among male athletes generally demonstrate adequate iron status. Mean sFerr of wrestling (and judo) athletes was reported to be within the range of 36.4 and 67.6 µg/L,[25] slightly lower than the mean sFerr value reported for wrestlers by Karamizrak and colleagues.[44] Serum ferritin values of wrestlers were shown to be unaffected by gradual or rapid weight loss.[10]

Assessment of SI among a group of steroid-using bodybuilders indicated that 79% of the athletes were reported to be within the normal range (mean 15.6 mmol/L), while the remaining 21% of the athletes (n = 3) fell below the range.[13] Hemoglobin and hematocrit of 11 male bodybuilders during precompetition were 21 g/dL and 50%, respectively.[15] Fluid restriction during the precompetition phase of training was believed to have been responsible for the elevated values.[15] Elevated values, however, were not observed in a group of elite bodybuilders during precompetition in a subsequent study.[20]

Serum ferritin values of strength-trained females are lower than values reported for male athletes. A sFerr of 13.6 µg/L denotes iron depletion in a group of female handball players, although SI, Hb, Hct, and transferrin saturation (28.9%) values were within the normal range.[28] In this study, iron intake for the athlete groups, with the exception of basketball players, was below the RDA. The recommended heme iron intake of 1.5 mg Fe/d was not achieved by the martial artists.

TABLE 5.3

Indices of Iron Status in Strength Trained Athletes

Sport	sFerr (µg/L)	SI (mmol/L)	Hb (g/dL)	Hct (%)	Reference
Males					
Football	68.0	18.0	15.0	44.0	44
Wrestling	79.5	18.7	14.5	45.5	
Bodybuilding	81.1	20.8	15.4	45.6	
Swimming	58.4	18.0	15.5	46.3	
Basketball	77.9	18.5	15.3	45.7	
Bodybuilding	100.0	≤	≤	≤	20
Weightlifting, wrestling, throwing	77.0	21.3	15.1	≤	10
Soccer, hockey, swimming, basketball	75.0	22.3	15.0	≤	
Wrestling, judo	36.4–67.6	≤	≤	≤	25
Females					
Karate	26.7	11.6	12.9	39.9	28
Handball	26.7	15.6	13.2	39.9	
Basketball	28.1	13.2	12.8	39.7	
Handball	13.6	18.5	13.0	39.3	44
Swimming	35.7	14.3	13.0	41.0	

Key: sFerr = Serum Ferritin; SI = Serum Iron; Hb = Hemoglobin; Hct = Hematocrit

Two female bodybuilders during precompetition showed elevated levels of both Hb and Hct.[15] Hemoglobin values of the women were 19 and 21 g/dL, with Hct values of 43 and 48%, respectively. As was stated for the men, it was believed that fluid restriction during the precompetition phase of training was responsible for the elevated values.[15] Elite female bodybuilders did not demonstrate elevations in Hb during precompetition, but Hct was slightly elevated (44%).[15] The same group of athletes had a mean sFerr value of 65 mg/L.

5.3   Zinc

Zinc is the second most prevalent trace mineral found in the human body, averaging approximately 2 grams in the adult. It plays an essential role in the functioning of more than 200 enzymes. Included among the zinc-dependent enzymes is lactate dehydrogenase (LDH), needed by skeletal muscles to convert pyruvate to lactate and by several tissues (liver, cardiac muscle, Type I muscle fibers) to convert lactate to pyruvate. Other enzymes that require zinc as part of their structure include carbonic anhydrase, superoxide dismutase, and alkaline phosphatase.

5.3.1   Nutritional Zinc Status

The recommended dietary allowance (RDA) for zinc is 15 mg/day in adult males and 12 mg/day in adult females.[5] Several studies have reported dietary zinc intakes of athletes participating in sports that rely on strength and power (Table 5.4). Most of the male athletes participating in weight lifting, wrestling, the throwing and sprinting events in track and field, and basketball consumed adequate dietary zinc; however, 4 to 15% of these athletes consumed less than the RDA.[9,10] Slightly lower zinc intakes have been reported for male professional volleyball players,[45] collegiate swimmers,[46] and youth ice hockey players.[47] Male bodybuilders were reported to have elevated zinc intakes in one study[13] and marginal intakes in another study.[20] Figure skaters were reported to have the lowest zinc intakes among male athletes.[48]

TABLE 5.4

Dietary Zinc Intake of Male and Female Athletes in Selected Sports

Sport	Age (yr)	Zinc Intake (mg/d)		Reference
		Males	Females	
Ice Hockey	12–13	15 ± 3		47
Gymnastics, figure skating, track and field	11–12		11 ± 3	47
Figure skating	16.5	11 ± 6	7 ± 5	48
Karate			9 ± 2.5	50
Team handball			10 ± 2.2	50
Basketball			11.9 ± 2.1	50
Basketball	18.9	17 ± 6	7.3 ± 3	49
Volleyball	25.9	14.4 ± 4		45
Swimming	19–22	15.6 ± 0.8	10.4 ± 0.8	46
Weightlifting, wrestling, sprinting, throwing	23	17.8 ± 0.7		10
Throwing	22.2	24.5 ± 10	13.1 ± 3.1	9
Bodybuilding	29.5	14.3 ± 5.4	9.1 ± 4.9	20
Bodybuilding		24.7 ± 13		13
Bodybuilding	27.3		8.1 ± 3.8	26

Female athletes are reported to have dietary zinc intakes that fall well below the RDA. Mean zinc intakes of female collegiate swimmers,[46] basketball players,[49] and female bodybuilders[20,26] are below 12 mg/d. Nuviala and colleagues[50] reported that more than 90% of female karate participants, 75% of the team handball players, and more than half the basketball players did not consume 12 mg of zinc per day. More than one third of the young female gymnasts, skaters, and track and field athletes had inadequate zinc intakes,[47] and 75% of elite figure skaters consumed less than two thirds the RDA for zinc.[48] Although female throwers had a mean zinc intake greater than the RDA, 40% of the throwers consumed less than the RDA.[9]

5.3.2 Responses to Exercise and Training

The normal range for plasma zinc is 11.5 to 18.5 μmol/L. Low plasma zinc levels have been reported in some athletes.[51,52] Most strength and power athletes have plasma zinc concentrations that are within the normal range.[10,20,47] However, plasma zinc may not be a particularly good indicator of body zinc stores because it represents only 0.1% of the total body zinc.[53] Most of the zinc in the blood is found inside the cells, such as erythrocytes and leukocytes.

Immediately following high-intensity exercise ($\geq$ 80% VO_2 max) plasma zinc levels are significantly increased.[54-56] During the recovery period following exercise, plasma zinc has been found to fall below pre-exercise levels.[54-56] Increased plasma zinc during exercise is thought to be a result of zinc mobilization as a part of the acute stress response. Part of the increase in plasma zinc, however, may be due to the hemoconcentration that accompanies high-intensity exercise bouts. The decline in plasma zinc following exercise may be due to zinc uptake by the tissues, especially the liver.[54] Excretion of zinc in the urine is elevated during the 24 hours following high-intensity exercise[54] and resistance training.[34] Increased excretion of zinc in the sweat has also been observed during moderate-to-high intensity exercise bouts.[57,58]

Reductions in plasma zinc have been reported in athletes following high-intensity exercise training.[59] Decreased plasma zinc may be due to elevated zinc loss in the sweat and urine during training.[45] However, Lukaski and colleagues[34] observed no significant changes in the plasma zinc of males undergoing 8 weeks of resistance training. Although urinary zinc did not increase significantly during resistance training, there was a trend toward higher zinc losses as training progressed.

5.3.3 Zinc Depletion and Supplementation

Van Loan and colleagues[60] examined the effects of a very low zinc diet on muscular strength and endurance. Eight males were placed on a diet containing $\leq$0.05 mg of zinc per day for 1 month, which resulted in a significant decrease in plasma zinc to 24 μg/dl. No significant changes in peak isokinetic force of the knee and shoulder flexors and extensors were observed following depletion. On the other hand, isokinetic endurance of the shoulder flexors and extensors and knee extensors was significantly reduced by zinc depletion and was still significantly below baseline after 3 weeks of zinc repletion. The authors suggested zinc depletion might inhibit LDH.[60] A reduction in the LDH isoform that converts lactate back to pyruvate could result in lactate accumulation in muscle fibers.

The effects of zinc supplementation on muscular strength and endurance of women was studied using a double-blind crossover design.[61] Subjects consumed supplements containing 135 mg zinc/day or a placebo for 2 weeks between the pretest and posttest followed by a 2-week washout period before the crossover trial. Significant increases in isometric endurance and isokinetic torque of the knee extensors at 180°/second were found following zinc supplementation. There were no significant changes in isometric strength, isokinetic torque of the knee extensors at slower velocities, or isokinetic endurance with zinc supplementation.[61]

Athletes should use caution when consuming zinc supplements. Supplements containing large amounts of zinc (160 mg) have been found to decrease high-density lipoprotein (HDL) cholesterol[62] and even reverse the positive effects of exercise on HDL.[63] Furthermore, supplements containing 50 mg zinc/day have been observed to reduce superoxide formation by polymorphonuclear leukocytes (part of the respiratory burst) and depress T-lymphocyte activity following exercise.[64] Because both responses are important in fighting infections, supplements containing large amounts of zinc may suppress the immune response. It is recommended that athletes not consume supplements containing more than 15 mg of zinc per day.

5.4   Copper

Another trace mineral that could affect exercise performance is copper. It is an essential part of one of several metalloenzymes which include cytochrome oxidase in the electron transport system, superoxide dismutase in the cytoplasm of cells, and lysyl oxidase needed in forming cross-links in collagen fibers.[65] Copper also plays an important role in the absorption and transport of iron. Most of the copper in the plasma is bound to the protein ceruloplasmin, which functions as a ferrioxidase that changes iron from its Fe (II) to Fe (III) state, a necessary step for transferrin to transport iron in the plasma.

5.4.1   Nutritional Intake

Copper has no RDA; instead, an estimated safe and adequate daily dietary intake has been established for copper between 1.5 and 3.0 mg/day.[5] Several studies of female athletes have reported mean copper intakes below 1.5 mg/day including bodybuilders,[20] field athletes,[9] swimmers,[46] and team handball players.[50] Nuviala and colleagues[50] found that 65% or more of the participants in karate and team handball and more than 40% of the basketball players consumed less than adequate amounts of dietary copper. More than 50% of the female athletes participating in gymnastics, figure skating, and track and field also consumed less than 1.5 mg of copper/day.[47]

Most male athletes consume diets containing more than an adequate amount of copper. Male athletes in field events such as discus, hammer, javelin, and shot, and bodybuilders have mean copper intakes of 2.7 mg/d[9] and 2.1 mg/d,[20] respectively. Adolescent ice hockey players[47] and collegiate swimmers[46] have dietary copper intakes averaging 1.6 mg/d.

5.4.2 Biochemical Status and Exercise Responses

The normal range for serum copper is 11 to 22 μmol/L. Adolescent male ice hockey players had mean serum copper levels of 19.6 μmol/L, while adolescent female gymnasts, ice skaters, and track and field athletes had mean serum copper levels of 20.3 μmol/L.[47] Kleiner and colleagues[20] found female bodybuilders had somewhat higher serum copper levels (18.1 μmol/L) than male bodybuilders (14.8 μmol/L). Similar results were reported by Lukaski and colleagues[46] for collegiate female and male swimmers.

Few studies have examined the effects of training on copper status. Lukaski et al.[46] found no significant changes in plasma copper and ceruloplasmin concentrations over a competitive swimming season. However, they observed significant increases in erythrocyte superoxide dismutase activity in both male and female swimmers over the 6-month season. Plasma copper concentration decreased significantly during 8 weeks of resistance training.[34] No significant changes in erythrocyte superoxide dismutase were found during resistance training. Serum copper concentration has been found to both increase[54] and decrease[55] following short, high-intensity exercise bouts. More research is required to explain the disparate results during exercise and training on serum copper levels.

5.5 Chromium

Chromium supplements have attracted much interest among weightlifters over the past decade due to its purported enhancement of muscle mass. Chromium is known to enhance glucose tolerance and appears to reduce the amount of insulin needed for glucose uptake by the cells. Thus, chromium supplements may be particularly beneficial in lowering blood glucose levels in noninsulin-dependent diabetics.[66]

5.5.1 Chromium Intake

The estimated safe and adequate daily dietary intake of chromium is 50 to 200 μg/day.[5] It has been suggested that the low average dietary chromium intake (5 to 150 μg/day) in the U.S. population is due to the intake of highly processed foods. Meats, whole grains, nuts, and cheese are some of the best food sources of chromium.

Very few studies have attempted to measure dietary chromium intake among athletes. Kleiner and colleagues[20] found elite female bodybuilders consumed 21 ± 30 μg chromium/day, less than the ESADDI, while elite male bodybuilders consumed 143 ± 194 μg/day. In a group of middle-aged men who consumed the American Heart Association Phase I diet, which is high in complex carbohydrates, mean chromium intake was 30 ± 4 μg/day.[67] When these men undertook a 16-week resistance-training program, urinary chromium excretion was increased. The results suggest that absorption of dietary chromium is enhanced by both acute and chronic resistance exercise.[67]

5.5.2   Chromium Supplementation and Resistance Training

Chromium picolinate supplements are one of the ergogenic products advertised as beneficial for increasing muscle mass. Numerous studies have examined the effects of chromium picolinate on changes in body composition of resistance-training athletes and nonathletes. Several studies conducted by Gary Evans have reported beneficial effects of chromium picolinate supplements on lean body mass.[66,68] In one study, students enrolled in a weight training class received either chromium picolinate (200 μg Cr) or a placebo for 40 days. Significant increases in lean body mass were found in the students who received the chromium supplement.[66] Another study examined the same supplement given to football players during a 6-week weight training program. Football players who received the chromium supplement had greater increases in lean body mass than those who received the placebo.[66] In a third study, 6 males received 400 μg Cr and 6 females received 200 μg Cr as chromium tripicolinate, while 6 males received 400 μg Cr and 6 females received 200 μg Cr as chromium dinicotinate during a 12-week aerobics class. Lean body mass was significantly increased in the males and females who received chromium picolinate but not in the subjects who received chromium nicotinate.[68] Use of the skinfold technique to measure body fat in the first two studies has been questioned by other investigators.[69] Bioelectrical impedance was used to measure lean body mass in the Evans and Pounchnik study.[68]

Hasten and colleagues[70] attempted to replicate the aforementioned weight training study. Male and female students enrolled in a 12-week weightlifting class were given chromium picolinate (200 μg Cr) or a placebo. Significantly greater increases in lean body mass were observed only in the females who received the chromium supplement. However, no significant differences in muscle strength increases were observed between the chromium supplemented and placebo groups.

Several recent studies have failed to replicate the results of the Evans studies. Clancy and colleagues[71] found no significant effects of 200 μg Cr in chromium picolinate supplements on lean body mass, body fat, or strength of football players following 9 weeks of strength training compared to a placebo. Hallmark and colleagues[72] also failed to find any significant effects of chromium supplementation (200 μg Cr) on lean body mass, body fat, or strength of males participating in weight training for 12 weeks. Both of these studies used the hydrostatic weighing technique to measure changes in lean body mass. Urinary chromium excretion was significantly greater in the supplemented subjects in both studies.

Lukaski and colleagues[34] used dual X-ray absorptiometry (DXA) to examine changes in body composition in male subjects who consumed chromium (200 μg Cr) supplements during resistance training. There were no significant differences in strength gain, fat-free mass, or body fat changes between groups who consumed chromium picolinate, chromium chloride, or a placebo. Serum chromium and urinary chromium levels were elevated in the chromium supplemented groups.

One possible explanation for the lack of significant differences between chromium supplemented and placebo treatments is that 200 μg Cr may not be the optimal amount needed to increase muscle mass. Campbell and colleagues[73] supplemented the diet of older men (ages 56 to 69) with 924 μg Cr/day during a 12-week resistance-training program. Both hydrostatic weighing and total body water (deuterium oxide) methods were used to assess changes in body fat and fat-free mass. No significant differences were found in strength gains or fat and fat-free mass changes between the chromium picolinate and placebo groups. Interestingly, both groups significantly increased fat-free mass calculated from hydrostatic weighing, but decreased fat-free mass calculated from the total body water method following the resistance-training program. The failure of more recent well-controlled studies to replicate the results of the early chromium supplement studies led Anderson[69] to conclude that the effects of chromium "will be small compared with those of exercise and a well-balanced diet."

5.6 Other Trace Minerals

Two other trace minerals have stimulated interest among strength training athletes as potential ergogenic aids to increase muscle mass and muscular strength. Boron supplements have been marketed as a potential substitute for anabolic steroids because boron has been found to increase serum estrogen and testosterone levels in postmenopausal females.[74] Vanadium also has been suggested to have anabolic effects because in large doses it has been found to mimic the action of insulin in diabetes.[75]

5.6.1   Boron

The effects of boron supplements during resistance training were examined by Ferrando and Green.[76] Ten male bodybuilders received a 2.5 mg boron supplement per day and 9 received a placebo during the 7-week training program. Plasma boron was increased in the supplemented group and decreased in the placebo group following training. Total plasma testosterone increased significantly in both groups during training, but no differences were found between the boron supplement and placebo groups. Significant increases in lean body mass determined by the hydrostatic weighing technique, and muscular strength (1 RM) in the bench press and squat were found in both groups following training, but the increases were not significantly different between the two groups. The authors suggested that boron supplements are not effective in increasing strength and lean body mass in male bodybuilders.[76]

5.6.2   Vanadium

Vanadium is an ultratrace mineral that has received attention from athletes as being a potential ergogenic aid. Evidence demonstrating the ability of pharmacological doses of vanadium to mimic the action of insulin in diabetes[75] has fostered beliefs among athletes that supplementation of vanadium may induce anabolic effects. Vanadium intake from the diet is within the range of 5 to 20 mg/d, with shellfish, mushrooms, parsley, dill seed, and black pepper as good sources.[77]

To examine claims that vanadyl sulfate supplementation exerts anabolic effects in athletes, Fawcett et al.[78] utilized dual energy X-ray absorptiometry (DEXA) along with 1 and 10 repetition maximum testing to evaluate body composition and strength performance in resistance-trained athletes. Subjects who consumed 0.5 mg/kg/d of vanadyl sulfate did not demonstrate improvements in body composition or strength compared to a placebo group over a 12-week period. However, slight differences in anthropometric measures and strength were noted between groups at Week 4, which suggested an initial but modest treatment effect.[78] Body weight and skinfold thickness measures increased in the vanadyl sulfate group, with no differences observed in those consuming a placebo. The authors suggest that vanadyl sulfate supplementation may have enhanced short-term fat deposition.[78] A treatment by time interaction for the leg extension 1-repetition maximum showed an improvement in the vanadyl sulfate group compared to the placebo, which suggested a short-term ergogenic effect.[78] Additional effects of vanadyl supplementation included elevated fasting glucose and insulin levels, and reports of tiredness. Further studies are clearly needed to shed light on the potential short-term (1-month) effects of vanadyl sulfate on body composition and strength performance.

5.7 Summary

Iron intakes of male strength-trained athletes are above the RDA of 10 mg/d and appear to maintain adequate iron status among these athletes. Female strength-trained athletes, on the other hand, do not appear to achieve recommended iron intakes and need to be aware of the adverse implications of iron deficiency anemia on performance. The impact of resistance training on iron status is far from clear, due to the general lack of research on the topic. The potential for long-term resistance training to adversely affect red cell indices and iron transport deserves further study.

Most male athletes appear to consume adequate zinc in their diets, however, many female athletes consume less zinc than the RDA of 12 mg/d. The only study that has examined the effects of resistance training on plasma zinc found no changes over an 8-week period. Consumption of a diet containing less than 0.05 mg Zn/d for 1 month had no effect on muscular strength, but significantly reduced isokinetic endurance of the knee and shoulder extensors.

Some female athletes have copper intakes below the recommended range of 1.5 to 3.0 mg/d, while most male athletes have intakes within the recommended range. The effects of resistance training on copper status have been examined in only one study. Although plasma copper decreased, erythrocyte superoxide dismutase did not change after 8 weeks of training.

Numerous studies have examined the effects of chromium supplementation during resistance training. Three studies reported significantly greater increases in lean body mass following 12 weeks of chromium picolinate supplements, while four studies reported no significant differences between chromium supplemented and placebo groups. Furthermore, no significant difference in strength gains between chromium supplemented and placebo groups following resistance training were found in five studies.

References

1. Clarkson, P. M. and Haymes, E. M., Exercise and mineral status of athletes: calcium, magnesium, phosphorus, and iron, *Med. Sci. Sports Exerc.*, 27, 831, 1995.
2. Clement, D. B. and Sawchuk, L. L., Iron status and sports performance, *Sports Med.*, 1, 65, 1984.
3. Cook, J. D., Clinical evaluation of iron deficiency, *Semin. Hematol.*, 19, 6, 1982.
4. Finch, C. A. and Huebers, H., Medical progress: perspectives in iron metabolism, *N. Engl. J. Med.*, 306, 1520, 1982.

5. Food and Nutritional Board, *National Academy of Sciences, Recommended Dietary Allowances*, 10th ed., National Academy Press, Washington, D.C., 1989.

6. Groff, J. L, Groper, S. S., and Hunt, S. M., Microminerals, in *Advanced Nutrition and Human Metabolism*, 2nd ed., West Publishing Company, St. Paul, 1995.

7. Finch, C. A. and Cook, J. D., Iron deficiency, *Am. J. Clin. Nutr.*, 39, 471, 1984.

8. Short, S. H. and Short, W. R., Four-year study of university athletes' dietary intake, *J. Am. Diet. Assoc.*, 82, 632, 1983.

9. Faber, M. and Benade, A. J., Mineral and vitamin intake in field athletes (discus-, hammer-, javelin- throwers and shotputters), *Int. J. Sports Med.*, 12, 324, 1991.

10. Fogelholm, G. M., Himberg, J. J., Alopaeus, K., Gref, C. G., Laakso, J. T., Lehto, J. J., and Mussalo-Rauhamaa, H., Dietary and biochemical indices of nutritional status in male athletes and controls, *J. Am. Coll. Nutr.*, 11, 181, 1992.

11. Bamman, M. M., Hunter, G. R., Newton, L. E., Roney, R. K., and Khaled, M. A., Changes in body composition, diet, and strength of bodybuilders during the 12 weeks prior to competition, *J. Sports Med. Phys. Fitness*, 33, 383, 1993.

12. Bazzarre, T. L., Kleiner, S. M., and Litchford, M. D., Nutrient intake, body fat, and lipid profiles of competitive male and female bodybuilders, *J. Am. Coll. Nutr.*, 9, 136, 1990.

13. Keith, R. E., Stone, M. H., Carson, R. E., Lefavi, R. G., and Fleck, S. J., Nutritional status and lipid profiles of trained steroid-using bodybuilders, *Int. J. Sport Nutr.*, 6, 247, 1996.

14. Linseisen, J., Metges, C. C., and Wolfram, G., Dietary habits and serum lipids of a group of German amateur bodybuilders, *Z. Ernahrungswiss.*, 32, 289, 1993.

15. Kleiner, S. M., Bazzarre, T. L., and Litchford, M. D., Metabolic profiles, diet, and health practices of championship male and female bodybuilders, *J. Am. Diet. Assoc.*, 90, 962, 1990.

16. Faber, M. and Benade, A. J., Nutrient intake and dietary supplementation in body-builders, *S. Afr. Med. J.*, 72, 831, 1987.

17. Sandoval, W. M., Heyward, V. H., and Lyons, T. M., Comparison of body composition, exercise and nutritional profiles of female and male body builders at competition, *J. Sports Med. Phys. Fitness*, 29, 63, 1989.

18. van Erp-Baart, A. M., Saris, W. M., Binkhorst, R. A., Vos, J. A., and Elvers, J. W., Nationwide survey on nutritional habits in elite athletes. Part II. Mineral and vitamin intake, *Int. J. Sports Med.*, 10 Suppl 1, S11, 1989.

19. Manore, M. M., Thompson, J., and Russo, M., Diet and exercise strategies of a world-class bodybuilder, *Int. J. Sport Nutr.*, 3, 76, 1993.

20. Kleiner, S. M., Bazzarre, T. L., and Ainsworth, B. E., Nutritional status of nationally ranked elite bodybuilders, *Int. J. Sport Nutr.*, 4, 54, 1994.

21. Andersen, R. E., Barlett, S. J., Morgan, G. D., and Brownell, K. D., Weight loss, psychological, and nutritional patterns in competitive male body builders, *Int. J. Eat. Disord.*, 18, 49, 1995.

22. Hickson, J. F. and Johnson, T. E., Nutrition and the precontest preparations of a male bodybuilder, *J. Am. Diet. Assoc.*, 90, 264, 1990.

23. Burke, L. M. and Read, R. S. D., A study of dietary patterns of elite Australian football players, *Can. J. Spt. Sci.*, 13, 15, 1988.

24. Hickson, J. F., Duke, M. A., Risser, W. L., Johnson, C. W., Palmer, R., and Stockton, J. E., Nutritional intake from food sources of high school football athletes, *J. Am. Diet. Assoc.*, 87, 1656, 1987.

25. Fogelholm, G. M., Koskinen, R., Laakso, J., Rankinen, T., and Ruokonen, I., Gradual and rapid weight loss: effects on nutrition and performance in male athletes, *Med. Sci. Sports Exerc.*, 25, 371, 1993.
26. Walberg-Rankin, J., Edmonds, C. E., and Gwazdauskas, F. C., Diet and weight changes of female bodybuilders before and after competition, *Int. J. Sport Nutr.*, 3, 87, 1993.
27. Lamar-Hildebrand, N., Saldanha, L., and Endres, J., Dietary and exercise practices of college-aged female bodybuilders, *J. Am. Diet. Assoc.*, 89, 1308, 1989.
28. Nuviala, R. J., Castillo, M. C., Lapieza, M. G., and Escanero, J. F., Iron nutritional status in female karatekas, handball and basketball players, and runners, *Physiol. Behav.*, 59, 449, 1996.
29. Schobersberger, W., Tschann, M., Hasibeder, W., Steidl, M., Herold, M., Nachbauer, W., and Koller, A., Consequences of 6 weeks of strength training on red cell O2 transport and iron status, *Eur. J. Appl. Physiol.*, 60, 163, 1990.
30. Spodaryk, K., Haematological and iron-related parameters of male endurance and strength trained athletes, *Eur. J. Appl. Physiol.*, 67, 66, 1993.
31. Ehn, L., Carlmark, B., and Hoglund, S., Iron status in athletes involved in intense physical activity, *Med. Sci. Sports Exerc.*, 12, 61, 1980.
32. Clement, D., Taunton, J., McKenzie, D., Lyster, D., Wiley, J., and Sawchuk, L., Iron absorption in iron deficient, endurance trained females, *Med. Sci. Sports Exerc.*, 16, 164, 1984.
33. Dallongeville, J., Ledoux, M., and Brisson, G., Iron deficiency among active men, *J. Am. Coll. Nutr.*, 8, 195, 1989.
34. Lukaski, H. C., Bolonchuk, W. W., Siders, W. A., and Milne, D. B., Chromium supplementation and resistance training: effects on body composition, strength, and trace element status of men, *Am. J. Clin. Nutr.*, 63, 954, 1996.
35. Lamanca, J. J., Haymes, E. M., Daly, J. A., Moffatt, R. J., and Waller, M. F., Sweat iron loss of male and female runners during exercise, *Int. J. Sports Med.*, 9, 52, 1987.
36. Paulev, P., Jordal, R., and Pedersen, N. S., Dermal excretion of iron in intensely training athletes, *Clin. Chim. Acta*, 127, 19, 1983.
37. McMahon, L. F., Ryan, M. J., Larson, D., and Fisher, R. L., Occult gastrointestinal blood loss in marathon running, *Ann. Intern. Med.*, 100, 846, 1984.
38. Stewart, J. G., Ahlquist, D. A., McGill, D. B., Ilstrup, D. M., Schwartz, S., and Owen, R., Gastrointestinal blood loss and anemia in runners, *Ann. Int. Med.*, 100, 843, 1984.
39. Campbell, W. W., Beard, J. L., Joseph, L. J., Davey, S. L., and Evans, W. J., Chromium picolinate supplementation and resistive training by older men: effects on iron-status and hematologic indexes, *Am. J. Clin. Nutr.*, 66, 944, 1997.
40. Murray, L. E., Beard, J. L., Joseph, L. J., and Davey, S. L., Evans, W. J., and Campbell, W. W., Resistance training affects iron status in older men and women, *FASEB J.*, 12, A847, 1998.
41. Baynes, R. D., Skikne, B. S., and Cook, J. D., Circulating transferrin receptors and assessment of iron status, *J. Nutr. Biochem.*, 5, 322, 1994.
42. Matsuo, T. and Suzuki, M., Dumbbell exercise improved iron deficient stores in young women without iron supplementation, *FASEB J.*, 12, A847, 1998.
43. Matsuo, T. and Suzuki, M., Effects of low-calorie diet therapy with and without dumbbell exercise on body fat reduction in obese young women, *J. Clin. Biochem. Nutr.*, 25, 49, 1998.

44. Karamizrak, S. O., Islegen, C., Varol, S. R., Taskiran, Y., Yaman, C., Mutaf, I., and Akgun, N., Evaluation of iron metabolism indices and their relation with physical work capacity in athletes, *Br. J. Sports Med.*, 30, 15, 1996.

45. Cordova, A. and Navas, F. J., Effect of training on zinc metabolism: changes in serum and sweat zinc concentrations in sportsmen, *Nutr. & Metab.*, 42, 274, 1998.

46. Lukaski, H. C., Hoverson, B. S., Gallagher, S. K., and Bolonchuk, W. W., Physical training and copper, iron and zinc status of swimmers, *Am. J. Clin. Nutr.*, 51, 1092, 1990.

47. Rankinen, T., Fogelholm, M., Jujala, U., Rauramaa, R., and Uusitupa, M., Dietary intake and nutritional status of athletic and nonathletic children in early puberty, *Int. J. Sport Nutr.*, 5, 136, 1995.

48. Ziegler, P. J., Nelson, J. A., and Jonnalagadda, S. S., Nutritional and physiological status of U.S. National Figure Skaters, *Int. J. Sport Nutr.*, 9, 345, 1999.

49. Nowak, R. K., Knudsen, K. S., and Schulz, L. O., Body composition and nutrient intakes of college men and women basketball players, *J. Am. Diet. Assoc.*, 88, 575, 1988.

50. Nuviala, R. J., Lapieza, M. G., and Bernal, E., Magnesium, zinc, and copper status in women involved in different sports, *Int. J. Sport Nutr.*, 9, 295, 1999.

51. Haralambie, G., Serum zinc in athletes in training, *Int. J. Sports Med.*, 2, 135, 1981.

52. Singh, A., Deuster, P. A., and Moser, P. B., Zinc and copper status of women by physical activity and menstrual status, *J. Sports Med. Phys. Fitness*, 30, 29, 1990.

53. Cousins, R. J., Zinc, in *Nutrition Reviews' Present Knowledge in Nutrition,* 7th ed., ILSI Press, Washington, D.C., 1996, 293.

54. Anderson, R. A., Bryden, N. A., and Polansky, M. M., Acute exercise effects on urinary losses and serum concentrations of copper and zinc of moderately trained and untrained men consuming a controlled diet, *Analyst*, 120, 867, 1995.

55. Bordin, D., Sartorelli, L., Bonanni, G., Mastrogiacomo, I., and Scalco, E., High intensity physical exercise induced effects on plasma levels of copper and zinc, *Biol. Trace Elem. Res.*, 36, 129, 1993.

56. Van Rij, A. M., Hall, M. T., Dohm, G. L., Bray, J., and Pories, W. J., Changes in zinc metabolism following exercise in human subjects, *Biol. Trace Elem. Res.*, 10, 99, 1986.

57. Aruoma, O. I., Reilly, T., MacLaren, D., and Halliwell, B., Iron, copper, and zinc concentrations in human sweat and plasma: the effects of exercise, *Clin. Chim. Acta*, 177, 81, 1988.

58. Tipton, K., Green, N. R., Haymes, E. M., and Waller, M., Zinc loss from athletes exercising at high or neutral temperatures, *Int. J. Sport Nutr.*, 3, 261, 1993.

59. Couzy, F., Lafargue, P., and Guezennec, C. Y., Zinc metabolism in the athlete: influences of training, nutrition and other factors, *Int. J. Sports Med.*, 11, 263, 1990.

60. Van Loan, M. D., Sutherland, B., Lowe, N. M., Turnlund, J. R., and King, J. C., The effects of zinc depletion on peak force and total work of knee and shoulder extensor and flexor muscles, *Int. J. Sport Nutr.*, 9, 125, 1999.

61. Krotkiewski, M., Gudmundsson, M., Backstrom, P., and Mandroukas, K., Zinc and muscle strength and endurance, *Acta Physiol. Scand.*, 116, 390, 1982.

62. Hooper, P. L., Visconti, L., Garry, P. J., and Gohnson, G. E., Zinc lowers high-density lipoprotein cholesterol levels, *JAMA*, 244, 1960, 1980.
63. Goodwin, J. S., Hunt, W. C., Hooper, P., and Garry, P. J., Relationship between zinc intake, physical activity, and blood levels of high-density lipoprotein cholesterol in a healthy elderly population, *Metabolism*, 34, 519, 1985.
64. Singh, A., Failla, M. L., and Deuster, P. A., Exercise-induced changes in immune function: effects of zinc supplementation, *J. Appl. Physiol.*, 76, 2298, 1994.
65. O'Dell, B. L., Copper, in *Nutrition Reviews' Present Knowledge in Nutrition*, 5th ed., The Nutrition Foundation, Washington, D.C., 1984, 506.
66. Rubin, M. A., Miller, J. P., Ryan, A. S., Treuth, M. S., Patterson, K. Y., Pratley, R. E., Hurley, B. F., Veilion, C., Moser-Veilion, P. B., and Anderson, R. A., Acute and chronic resistive exercise increase urinary chromium excretion in men as measured with an enriched chromium stable isotope, *J. Nutr.*, 128, 73, 1998.
67. Evans, G. W., The effect of chromium picolinate on insulin controlled parameters in humans, *Int. J. Biosocial Med. Res.*, 11, 163, 1989.
68. Evans, G. W. and Pounchnik, D. J., Composition and biological activity of chromium-pyridine carboxylate complexes, *J. Inorgan. Biochem.*, 49, 177, 1993.
69. Anderson, R. A., Effects of chromium on body composition and weight loss, *Nutr. Rev.*, 56, 266, 1998.
70. Hasten, D. L., Rome, E. P., Franks, B. D., and Hegsted, M., Effects of chromium picolinate on beginning weight training students, *Int. J. Sport Nutr.*, 2, 177, 1992.
71. Clancy, S. P., Clarkson, P. M., DeCheke, M. E., Nosaka, K., Freedson, P. S., Cunningham, J. J., and Valentine, B., Effects of chromium picolinate supplementation on body composition, strength, and urinary chromium loss in football players, *Int. J. Sport Nutr.*, 4, 142, 1994.
72. Hallmark, M. A., Reynolds, T. H., DeSouza, C. A., Dotson, C. O., Anderson, R. A., and Rogers, M. A., Effects of chromium and resistive training on muscle strength and body composition, *Med. Sci. Sports Exer.*, 28, 139, 1996.
73. Campbell, W. W., Joseph, L. J. O., Davey, S. L., Cyr-Campbell, D., Anderson, R. A., and Evans, W. J., Effects of resistance training and chromium picolinate on body composition and skeletal muscle in older men, *J. Appl. Physiol.*, 86, 29, 1999.
74. Nielsen, F., Hunt, C., Mullen, L., and Hunt, J., Effect of dietary boron on mineral, estrogen, and testosterone metabolism in postmenopausal women, *FASEB J.*, 1, 394, 1987.
75. Verma, S., Cam, M. C., and McNeill, J. H., Nutritional factors that can favorably influence the glucose/insulin system: vanadium, *J. Am. Coll. Nutr.*, 17, 11, 1998.
76. Ferrando, A. A. and Green, N. R., The effect of boron supplementation on lean body mass, plasma testosterone levels and strength in male bodybuilders, *Int. J. Sport Nutr.*, 3, 149, 1993.
77. Nielsen, F., Nutritional requirements for boron, silicon, vanadium, nickel, and arsenic: current knowledge and speculations, *FASEB J.*, 5, 2661, 1991.
78. Fawcett, J. P., Farquahar, S. J., Walker, R. J., Thou, T., Lowe, G., and Goulding, A., The effect of oral vanadyl sulfate on body composition and performance in weight-training athletes, *Int. J. Sport Nutr.*, 6, 382, 1996.

6

Dietary Supplements and Strength-Trained Athletes

Tausha Robertson

CONTENTS

6.1   Introduction

Resistance training is a component of conditioning and training for almost any sport. It is critical for athletes participating in sports that require increased lean body mass (LBM). Increased LBM is important for enhancing strength and power production, improving stability, and enhancing aesthetic appearance through muscle hypertrophy. In the past and continuing to the present, substances such as human growth hormone (hGH) and anabolic/androgenic steroids were used in the hope of circumventing genetic limitations in hormonal status and in the ability to build muscle. These substances have been associated with a number of health risks and are banned by most athletic governing agencies.[1] As a result, many competitive and recreational athletes have turned to dietary supplements marketed to enhance strength training and performance. For example, Brill and Keane documented supplement use patterns in 309 male and female bodybuilders.[2] Protein powders and amino acids were utilized when building bulk was desired, while fat-burners were utilized during the "cutting" phase prior to competition. Over half of the subjects spent $25 to 100 per month on supplements, while 4.9% reported spending over $150 per month. Supplement use can be very costly for athletes.

A 1992 survey of nutritional supplements in health and bodybuilding magazines reported that there were 89 separate brands, 311 products, and 235 unique ingredients, most of which were promoted as aids to muscle growth.[3] Over the years the number of products, as well as the number of ingredients, has increased, creating a multibillion dollar supplement industry. Because these products are classified as dietary supplements and therefore are considered foods, not drugs, regulation is limited. Some of these products contain potentially harmful drugs or substances that may contribute to positive drug tests in competitive athletes.[4] The purpose of this chapter is to provide current research information on several supplements commonly used by strength-trained athletes. These products can be divided into three major categories: anabolic agents (supplements marketed to increase anabolic hormone levels or decrease catabolic processes so that there is an increase in muscle mass and bulk), energy delivery enhancers (agents which allow more work to be accomplished), and thermogenic agents (supplements marketed to decrease body fat).

6.2   Anabolic Agents

6.2.1   Amino Acid Supplements

The majority of products targeted for strength-trained athletes contain amino acids, the building blocks of protein, and claim to promote weight gain and/or muscular growth.[5] Studies have been conducted on amino acids such as arginine, citrulline, histidine, leucine, lysine, methionine, ornithine, phenylalanine, and valine. These amino acids are involved in numerous metabolic processes of interest to strength-trained athletes. It has been shown that these particular amino acids are involved in protein synthesis, release of human growth hormone (hGH) or somatotropin, creatine synthesis, removal of ammonia, and the release of insulin.[4] It is the effect on the release of hGH which is of primary concern. The majority of studies, however, have used infusions of amino acids and have not used oral supplementation, the method strength-trained athletes choose. It is known that amino acids are destroyed in stomach acids, thereby making questionable their availability for protein synthesis and muscle growth.

6.2.1.1 Arginine

Oral dosages at 5 to 250 g/kg body weight of arginine, arginine aspartate, or arginine glutamate have been shown to elicit the following metabolic responses in humans: increased somatotropin and insulin release or response, increased creatine stores, and decreased exercise-induced blood-ammonia.[4,6–9] Of the studies noted, it is important to point out that only Fluckey et al. included resistance training for the subjects.[7] Hawkins et al. reported no benefit of oral arginine supplementation on measures of muscle function or body composition.[10] Arginine use has not been shown to enhance muscle development.

6.2.1.2 Glutamine

Much of the research on glutamine has focused on the relationship between glutamine and stress hormones related to catabolism. The catabolic states studied included burns, trauma, surgery, or infections. Under stress the increase in glucocorticoid synthesis activates muscle catabolism and intracellular amino acid oxidation.[11,12] Physiological stress is marked by declines in protein synthesis and increases in glutamine efflux from skeletal muscle related to muscle atrophy. Glutamine supplementation has been utilized successfully to counteract the cortisol-induced muscle atrophy. Intense exercise can elicit a glucocorticoid stress response similar to physiological stress. As a result, researchers have investigated glutamine use in overtraining and exercise recovery related to glycogen repletion. Oral glutamine supplementation of 2g increased somatotropin release and increased muscle glycogen replenishment.[13] An infusion of glutamine increased glycogen replenishment after intense exercise.[14] It is important to note that many of the studies reporting positive benefits of glutamine supplements utilized parenteral or enteral feeding methods.[15,16] To date, little research has been conducted on oral ingestion of glutamine, which would be the most likely method used by strength-trained athletes.

6.2.1.3   Ornithine

Ingestion of 170mg/kg body weight of ornithine increased somatotropin release in male bodybuilders. However, the high dosage of ornithine caused osmotic diarrhea in the subjects. No effects on somatotropin levels were noted at the lower doses of 70mg/kg or 100mg/kg.[17] It is not clear that the increased growth hormone secretion had any muscle mass potentiating effect.

6.2.1.4   Ornithine Alpha Ketoglutarate

Ornithine alpha ketoglutarate (OKG) is composed of two ornithine molecules bound to one α–ketoglutarate molecule. Oral doses of 10 to 20g/day has aided the treatment of burns, sepsis, postsurgical healing, malnutrition, liver disease, renal disease, and immunosuppression.[18,19] In addition, oral doses of OKG have been associated with increased protein synthesis, glutamine production, and insulin levels.[18,19] The metabolic pathways associated with observed increases are unclear. A number of metabolic responses affected by OKG use are desired outcomes for strength training. Unfortunately, there is no published research that reports positive responses in strength-trained athletes.

6.2.2   Combinations of Amino Acids — Evaluation of Synergistic Effects

Researchers have attempted to evaluate whether or not there would be synergistic effects of amino acid combinations. Fogelholm et al. noted no significant increases in human growth hormone (hGH) or insulin secretion following supplementation with a combination of arginine and lysine in competitive weightlifters.[20] In another study by Lambert et al., serum growth hormone concentrations in male bodybuilders were not increased by supplementation of 2.5g of an arginine/lysine mix or 1.85g of an ornithine/tyrosine mix as compared to a placebo.[21] Suminski et al. reported that supplementation with 1500 mg arginine and 1500 mg lysine immediately before resistance exercise did not alter exercise-induced changes in hGH levels in male weightlifters. However, under basal conditions ingestion of the same amino acid mixture increased the acute secretion of hGH.[22] Whether or not acute secretion of hGH has any physiological effect on potentiation of muscle mass remains to be seen. It has been shown that mixtures of amino acids do not enhance the development of muscle mass.

6.2.3   Gamma Hydroxybutyric Acid (GHB)

As of February 2000, GHB was classified as a federally controlled, Schedule 1 substance. The U.S. Drug Enforcement Administration officially cites more than 45 deaths and 5500 emergency room visits associated with GHB. Persons who possess, manufacture, or distribute GHB could face prison terms of up to 20 years.[23] GHB is most commonly used as a party drug. However, strength-trained athletes have used GHB for its purported ability to raise growth hormone levels as reported in a 1977 study by Takahara et al.[24] It is important to note that no research regarding anabolic effects of GHB in strength-trained athletes has been published.

Although GHB is illegal, some states allow the sale of products containing gamma butyrolactone (GBL) or 1,4-butanediol (BD). Both of these substances are converted by the body to GHB, producing the same potential for harm. GBL is a chemical intermediate used as a solvent and is part of the manufacture process for pesticides and herbicides.[25] Unfortunately, GBH, GBL, and BD are available for purchase over the internet, and some web sites provide instructions for home preparation.[26] There is no known performance-enhancing use for these substances.

6.3   Anabolic Agents — Herbs and Plant-Based Substances

6.3.1   Gamma Oryzanol

Gamma oryzanol, a plant sterol, has been marketed to strength-trained athletes as an alternative to anabolic steroids. Fry et al.[27] reported no changes in strength or hormone levels (testosterone, cortisol, estradiol, growth hormone, insulin) in resistance-trained athletes supplemented with 500 mg/day gamma oryzanol as compared to a placebo group. A review of gamma oryzanol and metabolism by Wheeler and Garleb reported that such plant sterols are poorly absorbed. This review also suggested that gamma oryzanol may increase catabolic or muscle breakdown activity.[28] There is no research to support anabolic effects in humans.

6.3.2   *Tribulus terrestris*

Tribulus terrestris is an herb which has been utilized in herbal medicine as a remedy for impotence and for increasing libido. The supplement is marketed as an anabolic agent that will increase testosterone levels and promote protein synthesis. Bucci reported that the only study showing increased testosterone levels was conducted on rams.[4] No published studies have investigated the effects of *Tribulus terrestris* on testosterone levels in humans.

6.3.3   Yohimbine

Yohimbine, a substance extracted from the bark of the yohimbe tree, increases sympathetic nerve activity in humans and animals.[29,30] This substance has been used to treat obesity and impotence.[31] It has been marketed to strength-trained athletes as a means of increasing testosterone levels. To date, no published research has reported a link between yohimbine and increased testosterone levels or increased muscle mass in humans.

6.3.4   Beta-Hydroxy-Beta-Methylbutyrate (HMB)

Beta-hydroxy-beta-methylbutyrate (HMB) is a metabolite of leucine catabolism. It is utilized and produced by body tissues. Because it is found in food products such as catfish and in some citrus fruits, it meets the criteria of a dietary or food supplement. Research has not shown that HMB is a necessary nutrient for humans. Studies indicate that HMB may counteract the effects of stress and increase the growth of animals.[32–35]

HMB is of interest to strength-trained athletes because there is evidence that it affects protein synthesis and lean body mass.[36] For example, Nissen et al.[37] studied the effects of dietary supplementation of HMB on strength-trained athletes. One group of 41 untrained subjects who had not participated in resistance training for at least 3 months was randomly separated into three groups receiving different levels of HMB supplementation (0 g, 1.5 g, or 3 g) and two levels of protein supplementation (117g/day or 175g/day). Each of the three groups weightlifted for 1.5 hours, 3 days per week for 3 weeks. The groups receiving HMB showed significant decreases in the expected exercise-induced rise in muscle proteolysis as measured by 3-methylhistidine during the first 2 weeks of exercise. The amount of weight lifted by subjects receiving HMB supplementation increased during each week of the study as compared to the unsupplemented subjects. In addition, plasma creatine phosphokinase was decreased with HMB supplementation. The second part of the Nissen et al. study examined the effects of HMB supplementation on untrained subjects participating in high-volume resistance training. The 28 subjects who were fed 0 or 3g of HMB weightlifted 2 to 3 hours, 6 days/week, for 7 weeks. Fat-free mass was significantly increased in the subjects receiving 3g of HMB as compared to the unsupplemented subjects. The authors concluded that supplementation with 1.5 g to 3.0 g of HMB could prevent exercise-induced proteolysis and result in larger gains in muscle function in weight-trained subjects.[37]

Kreider et al.[38] investigated the effects of HMB on experienced resistance-trained subjects. This study examined the effects of HMB supplementation during weight training which averaged 6.9 hours/week for 28 days on markers of protein catabolism, body composition, and strength. The 40 subjects were matched and randomly assigned to one of three groups. These groups supplemented their diets, while weight training, with a carbohydrate/protein powder containing 0, 3, or 6 g of HMB for 28 days. Fasting venous blood and urine, dual energy X-ray absorptiometer-determined body composition, isotonic bench press and leg press (one repetition maximum) were measured before and after the 28-day supplementation period. The results showed that serum and urinary HMB concentrations were raised by supplementation. However, no statistically significant differences were observed in the markers of whole-body anabolic/catabolic status, muscle and liver enzyme efflux, percentage body fat, or 1 RM strength. Thus it was concluded that 28 days of HMB supplementation did not reduce catabolism or affect training-induced changes in body composition and strength in experienced resistance-trained males.[38]

HMB has also been marketed to strength-trained athletes for its ability to increase the oxidation of fatty acids during exercise. The data for these claims are based on *in vitro* studies of muscle cell preparations such as one published by Cheng et al.[39] The study extrapolated the results found in cells to the whole body and suggested that HMB may provide an oxidative advantage during exercise that could account for some of the decrease in muscle fat observed with HMB intake in humans. To date, no studies have been done in intact humans to validate this claim.

Other researchers have investigated possible synergistic effects of the combined intake of creatine monohydrate and HMB. Almada et al.[40] investigated the effects of HMB supplementation with or without creatine on strength and sprint capacity in college football players. The results indicated a positive change in strength and/or aerobic capacity.

6.4 Anabolic Agents — Minerals

6.4.1 Vanadium

Vanadium salts have been successfully used to induce insulin-mimetic metabolic changes in animal models and diabetic humans.[41,42] It is marketed to strength-trained athletes for potential insulin-like anabolic effects. However, Fawcett et al.[43] reported no changes in body composition or performance in weight-trained athletes supplemented with .05 mg/kg/day of oral vanadyl sulfate for 12 weeks. In addition, Tsiani et al.[44] reported that although vanadate supplementation produced positive changes in glucose metabolism, it inhibited amino acid uptake. The possibility of toxicity from vanadium supplementation is unknown.[44]

6.4.2 Boron

Nielson et al.[45] published a study on the effects of dietary boron on mineral, estrogen, and testosterone levels in postmenopausal women. After the women were fed a diet deficient in boron, their hormone levels declined. They were then supplemented with 3 mg/day sodium borate. The investigators reported that testosterone levels increased after supplementation. It is important to note that the testosterone along with estrogen returned to pre-diet levels.[45] Supplement companies have marketed boron based on an inaccurate interpretation of these results suggesting that boron supplementation could raise serum testosterone levels. Supplementing bodybuilders with 2.5 mg/day of boron produced no changes in serum testosterone, lean body mass, or strength as compared to a placebo group.[46]

6.5   Energy Delivery Enhancers — Inosine

Inosine is a nucleotide involved in the formation of purines such as adenine. Adenine can play a role in replenishing or preventing the decline of ATP levels during intense exercise, or improving oxygen utilization in erythrocytes.[47,48] As a result of these findings, supplement companies have marketed inosine as a method of increasing ATP formation in muscle, which could benefit strength-trained athletes by permitting more rapid energy delivery. MacNaughton et al.[49] found no increase in anaerobic or aerobic performance in cyclists supplemented with inosine. No peer-reviewed studies have reported any ergogenic benefits of inosine supplementation in humans.[47]

6.6   Thermogenic Agents

6.6.1   Ephedrine

Ephedrine is a potent sympathomimetic agent that simulates epinephrine effects. It is sold in the herbal form as Ma Huang, Chinese Ephedra, or other ephedra species that contain a mixture of closely related alkaloids such as ephedrine, pseudoephedrine, norephedrine, or pseudonorephedrine.[50] Ephedrine alkaloids have been associated with increased mental function rather than enhancement in performance or physiological parameters affecting exercise.[51] Studies investigating ephedrine combined with caffeine, with or without aspirin, have reported increased weight loss in subjects.[52] Users theorize that such cocktails promote lipolysis while decreasing muscle breakdown. The limited research on the subject has not produced conclusive evidence that the theory is correct.

Consuming high doses (>25 mg/day) of ephedrine alkaloids has been linked to a number of adverse side effects including nervousness, light-headedness, heart palpitations, tachycardia, increased blood pressure, interference with MAO inhibitor drugs, hyperthermia, and death.[50] A number of these adverse affects can be produced by combining ephedrine alkaloids with other stimulants. Many sports-governing bodies ban the use of substances in this family of drugs.[4] Athletes should be aware that consuming legal herbal supplements or over-the-counter medicines that contain ephedrine alkaloids can result in positive drug tests.[52] The number of deaths attributed to ephedrine consumption has reached alarming proportions and points to the fact that the risks do not outweigh the perceived benefits of the consumption of this substance for the enhancement of performance. There is a current move in the U.S. to have ephedrine products available only by prescription as they are in other countries.

6.6.2 Caffeine

Researchers have published numerous studies related to the ergogenic effects of caffeine. Some studies have concluded that caffeine can benefit weight loss, endurance performance, strength, sprints, repetitive anaerobic work, reaction time, and perception of fatigue. Bucci's summary of 10 review articles on caffeine and exercise performance found 39 studies that show ergogenic effects of caffeine and 35 studies finding no ergogenic effects.[4] Caffeine is primarily used by strength-trained athletes as a thermogenic agent in conjunction with ephedrine and/or aspirin rather than for its other potential ergogenic effects. Very little research exists examining caffeine use in strength-trained athletes, making effective dose guidelines difficult to provide.

Sports-governing bodies allow caffeine levels of up to 15 mcg/ml urine. Such levels can be obtained using doses of 9 to 10 mg/kg. An athlete must take care not to exceed this dose prior to competition because disqualification may occur. Large doses of caffeine (>10 mg/kg) can produce adverse side effects such as gastric upset, anxiety, insomnia, and increased heart rate and blood pressure.[53,54]

6.7 Summary

Many of the positive metabolic responses to amino acids were observed in nontrained subjects. When studied in the targeted population, strength-trained athletes, arginine has failed to produce conclusive anabolic benefits. The dosage of ornithine needed to produce increases in somatotropin levels caused osmotic diarrhea, thus making it an impractical ergogenic aid. Preliminary research suggests that glutamine supplementation may increase somatotropin levels, aid glycogen repletion, and decrease protein catabolism. More research on strength-trained athletes utilizing oral supplements is needed to produce conclusive results and dosing schedules. Arginine and lysine together produce increases in hGH at rest but not with resistance training. There are no published studies indicating anabolic properties of gamma oryzanol, tribulus, and yohimbine.

Some HMB studies in strength-trained athletes have produced positive results, while others have produced no change. More research is needed to provide conclusive results. Purported anabolic effects of GHB have not been substantiated by published research. Classification as a Schedule 1 controlled substance indicates the danger of this substance. The mineral supplements vanadium and boron fail to provide anabolic affects in strength-trained subjects.

Thermogenic combinations of ephedrine, caffeine, and/or aspirin produced weight loss in obese subjects. These results have not been duplicated in trained subjects. This combination is impractical to most athletes because it contains an NCAA- and IOC-banned substance, ephedrine, and caffeine, which is banned in high concentrations.

References

1. Williams, M. H., *Nutrition for Fitness and Sport*, 4th ed., Brown and Benchmark, Dubuque, IA, 1995, 12.
2. Brill, J. B. and Keane, M. W., Supplementation patterns of competitive male and female bodybuilders, *Int. J. Sport Nutr.*, 4, 398, 1994.
3. Philen, R. M., Ortiz, D. I., Auerbach, S. B., and Falk, H., Survey of advertising for nutritional supplements in health and bodybuilding magazines, *JAMA*, 268, 1008, 1992.
4. Bucci, L. R., Dietary supplements as ergogenic aids, in *Nutrition in Exercise and Sports*, 3rd ed., Wolinsky, I. (Ed.), CRC Press, Boca Raton, FL, 1998, chap. 6.
5. Bazzarre, T. L., Nutrition and strength, in *Nutrition in Exercise and Sports*, 3rd ed., Wolinsky, I. (Ed.), CRC Press, Boca Raton, FL, 1998, chap. 14.
6. Besset, L., Increase in sleep related growth hormone and prolactin secretion after chronic arginine aspartate administration, *Acta Endocrinol.*, 99, 18, 1982.
7. Fluckey, J. D., Gordon, S. E., Kraemer, W. J., and Farrell, P. A., Arginine stimulated insulin secretion from pancreatic islets is increased following resistance exercise, *Med. Sci. Sports Exer.*, 26 (5 Suppl.), S22, 1994.
8. Denis, C., Dormois, D., Linossier, M. T., Eychenne, J. L., Hauseux, P., and Lacour, J. R., Effect of arginine aspartate on the exercise-induced hyperammonemia in humans: a two periods cross-over trial, *Arch. Int. Physiol. Biochim. Biophys.*, 99, 123, 1991.
9. Eto, B., Peres, G., and Le Moel, G., Effects of and ingested arginine salt on ammonemia during and after long lasting cycling, *Arch. Int. Physiol. Biochim. Biophys.*, 102, 161, 1994.
10. Hawkins, C., Walberg-Rankin, J., and Sebolt, D., Oral arginine does not effect body composition or muscle function in male weightlifters, *Med. Sci. Sports Exer.*, 23, S15 abstract, 1991.
11. Di Pasquale, M. G., *Amino Acids and Proteins for the Athlete: The Anabolic Edge*, CRC Press, Boca Raton, FL, 1997, 134.

12. Wing, S. S. and Goldberg, A. L., Glucorticoids activate the ATP-ubiquitine-dependent proteolytic system in skeletal muscle during fasting, *Am. J. Physiol.*, 264, E668, 1993.

13. Welbourne, T. C., Increased plasma bicarbonate and growth hormone after an oral glutamine load, *Am. J. Clin. Nutr.*, 61, 1058, 1995.

14. Varnier, M., Leese, G. P., Thompson, J., and Rennie, M. J., Stimulatory effect of glutamine on glycogen accumulation in human skeletal muscle, *Am. J. Physiol.*, 269, E309, 1995.

15. Wernerman, J., Hammarkvist, F., Ali, M. R., and Vinnars, E., Glutamine and ornithine-alpha-ketoglutarate but not branched-chain amino acids reduce the loss of muscled glutamine after surgical trauma, *Metabolism*, 38, 63, 1989.

16. Blomqvist, B. I., Hammarqvist, F., von der Decken, A., and Wernerman, J., Glutamine and alpha-ketoglutarate prevent the decrease in muscle free glutamine concentration and influence protein synthesis after total hip replacement, *Metab. Clin. Exp.*, 44, 1215, 1995.

17. Bucci, L. R., Hickson, J. F., Pivarnik, J. M., Wolinsky, I., McMahon, J. C., and Turner, S. D., Ornithine ingestion and growth hormone release in bodybuilders, *Nutr. Res.*, 10, 239, 1990.

18. Cynober, L., Ornithine α-ketoglutarate in nutritional support, *Nutrition*, 7, 1, 1991.

19. Silk, D. B. A. and Payne-James, J. J., Novel substrates and nutritional support: possible role of ornithine α-ketoglutarate, *Proc. Nutr. Soc.*, 49, 381, 1990.

20. Fogelholm, M., Naveri, H., Kiilavuori, K., and Harkonen, M., Lose-dose amino acid supplementation: no effects on serum human growth hormone and insulin in male weightlifters, *Int. J. Sport Nutr.*, 3, 290, 1993.

21. Lambert, M. I., Hefer, J. A., Millar, R. P., and Macfarlane, P. W., Failure of commercial oral amino acid supplements to increase serum growth hormone concentrations in male body-builders, *Int. J. Sport Nutr.*, 3, 298, 1993.

22. Suminski, R. R., Robertson, R. J., Goss, F. L., Arslanian, S., Kang, J., DaSilva, S., Utter, A. C., and Metz, K. F., Acute effect of amino acid ingestion and resistance exercise of plasma growth hormone concentration in young men, *Int. J. Sport Nutr.*, 7, 48, 1997.

23. Nordenburg, T., The death of the party: all the rave, GHB's hazards go unheeded, *FDA Consumer Magazine*, March-April, 2000.

24. Takahara, J., Yunoki, S., Yakushiji, W., Yamauchi, J., Yamane, Y., and Ofuji, T., Stimulatory effects of gamma-hydroxybutyric acid of growth hormone and prolactin release in humans, *J. Clin. Endocrinol. Metab.*, 44, 1014, 1977.

25. BASF Technical Data Sheet, Feb, 1997.

26. FDA warns about products containing gamma butyrolactone or GBL and asks companies to issue a recall, *FDA Talk Paper*, Jan., 1999.

27. Fry, A. C., Bonner, E., Lewis, D. L., Johnson, R. L., Stone, M. H., and Kraemer, W. J., The effects of gamma-oryzanol supplementation during resistance exercise training, *Int. J. Sport Nutr.*, 7, 318, 1997.

28. Wheeler, K. B. and Garleb, K. A., Gamma oryzanol-plant sterol supplementation: metabolic, endocrine, and physiological effects, *Int. J. Sport Nutr.*, 1, 170, 1991.

29. Mazza, E., Ghigo, E., and Bellone, J., Effects of alpha and beta adrenergic antagonists and antagonists on growth hormone secretion in man, *SO Endocrinol. Exp.*, 24, 211, 1990.

30. Grossman, E., Rea, R. F., Hoffman, A., and Goldstein, D. S., Yohimbine increases sympathetic nerve activity and norepinephrine spill over in normal volunteers, *Am. J. Physiol.*, 260, R142, 1991.

31. Williams, M. H., Nutritional supplements for strength trained athletes, *Sports Science Exchange*, 6, 6, 1993.

32. Nissen S., Fuller, J. C., Sell, J., Ferket, P. R., and Rives, D. V., The effect of beta-hydroxy-beta-methylbutyrate on growth, mortality, and carcass qualities of broiler chickens, *Poult. Sci.*, 73, 137, 1994.

33. Gatnau, R., Zimmerman, D. R., Nissen, S. L., Wannemuehler, M., and Ewan, R. C., Effects of dietary leucine and leucine catabolites of growth and immune responses in weanling pigs, *J. Anim. Sci.*, 73, 159, 1995.

34. Nissen, S., Faidley, T. D., Zimmerman, D. R., Izard, R., and Fisher, C.T., Colostral milk fat percentage and pig performance are enhanced by feed the leucine metabolited beta-hydroxy-beta-methylbutyrate to sows, *J. Anim. Sci.*, 71, 2331, 1994.

35. Van Koevering, M. T., Dolezal, H. G., Gill, D. R., Owens, F. N., Strasia, C. A., Buchanan, D. S., Lake, R., and Nissen, S., Effects of beta-hydroxy-beta-methylbutyrate on performance and carcass quality of feedlot steers, *J. Anim. Sci.*, 72, 1927, 1994.

36. Di Pasquale, M. G., *Amino Acids and Proteins for the Athlete: The Anabolic Edge*, CRC Press, Boca Raton, FL, 1997, 112.

37. Nissen, S., Sharp, R., Ray, M. et. al., Effects of leucine metabolite beta-hydroxy-beta-methylbutyrate on muscle metabolism during resistance-exercise training, *J. Appl. Physiol.*, 81, 2095, 1996.

38. Kreider, R. B., Ferreira, M., Wilson, M., and Almada, A. L., Effects of calcium beta-hydroxy-beta-methylbutyrate supplementation during resistance-training on markers of catabolism, body composition, and strength, *Int. J. Sport Nutr.*, 20, 503, 1999.

39. Cheng, W., Phillips, B., and Abumrad, N., Beta-hydroxy-beta-methylbutyrate increases fatty acid oxidation by muscle cells, *FASEB J.*, 11, A381, 1997.

40. Almada, A. L., Krieder, R. B., Ferreira, M., Wilson, M., Grindstaff, P. et al., Effects of calcium beta-hydroxy-beta-methylbutyrate supplementation with or without creatine during training on strength and sprint capacity, *FASEB J.*, 11, A374, 1997.

41. Heyliger, C. E., Tahiliani, A. G., and McNeil, J. H., Effect of vanadate on elevated blood glucose and depressed cardiac performance in diabetic rats, *Science*, 227, 1474, 1985.

42. Ramanadham, S., Mongold, J. J., Brownsey, R. W., Cros, G. H., and McNeil, J. H., Oral vanadyl sulfate in the treatment of diabetes mellitus in rat, *Am. J. Physiol.*, 257, H904, 1989.

43. Fawcett, J. P., Farquhar, S. J., Robert, J. W., Thou, T., Lowe, G., and Goulding, A., The effect of oral vanadyl sulfate on body composition and performance in weight-training athletes, *Int. J. Sport Nutr.*, 6, 382, 1996.

44. Tsiani, E., Abdullah, N., and Fantus, I. G., Insulin-mimetic agents vanadate and pervanadate stimulate glucose but inhibit amino acid uptake, *Am. J. Physiol.*, 272, C156, 1997.

45. Nielsen, F., Hunt, C., Mullen, L., and Hunt, J., Effect of dietary boron on mineral, estrogen, testosterone metabolism in postmenopausal women, *FASEB J.*, 1, 394, 1987.

46. Ferrando, A. A. and Green, N. R., The effect of boron supplementation on lean body mass, plasma testosterone, levels and strength in male bodybuilders, *Int. J. Sport Nutr.*, 3, 140, 1993.

47. DiPasquale, M. G., Inosine, *Drugs Sports*, 3, 6, 1995.

48. Bucci, L. R., Micronutrient supplementation and ergogenesis-metabolic intermediates, in *Nutrients as Ergogenic Aids for Sports and Exercise*, Bucci, L. R. (Ed.), CRC Press, Boca Raton, FL, 1993, 41.

49. McNaughton, L., Dalton, B., and Tarr, J., Inosine supplementation has no effect on aerobic or anaerobic cycling performance, *Int. J. Sport Nutr.*, 9, 333, 1999.

50. Kalix, P., Pharmacology of psychoactive alkaloids from Ephedra and Catha, *J. Ethnopharmacol.*, 32, 201, 1991.

51. Daly, P., Krieger, D., Dulloo, A., Young, J., and Landsberg, L., Ephedrine, caffeine, and aspirin: safety and efficacy for treatment of human obesity, *Int. J. Obesity*, 17, S73, 1993.

52. Ros, J. J., Pelders, M. G., and De Smet, P. A., A case of positive doping associated with a botanical food supplement, *Pharm. World Sci.*, 21, 44, 1999.

53. Bucci, L. R., Nutritional ergogenic aids, in *Nutrition in Exercise and Sports*, Wolinsky, I. and Hickson, J. F. (Eds.), CRC Press, Boca Raton, FL, 1994, 295.

54. Bucci, L. R., Dietary substances not required in human metabolism, in *Nutrients as Ergogenic Aids for Sports and Exercise*, Bucci, Luke R. (Ed.), CRC Press, Boca Raton, FL, 1993, 83.

7

Overview of Anabolic/Androgenic Hormones and Strength

M. Brian Wallace

CONTENTS

0-8493-8198-3/01/$0.00+$.50
© 2001 by CRC Press LLC

7.1   Anabolic/Androgenic Hormones and Strength

7.1.1   Introduction

The pursuit to be bigger, stronger, more powerful seems intrinsic to the male mentality and is indelibly woven into the fabric of modern sport. Since the introduction in the early 1950s of anabolic–androgenic steroids (AAS), the use of anabolic hormones and other ergogenic aids has become increasingly popular among athletes as a means of increasing strength, improving body composition, and enhancing performance. Today, their use by athletes has reached almost epidemic proportions. A recent exposé regarding government-directed systematic AAS abuse chronicled three decades of secret hormonal doping of East German athletes.[1] The report provided considerable detail regarding drug dosages, side effects, performance enhancement, and the extent of abuse, and left little doubt of both their efficacy and use by both male and female athletes in virtually all sports. Further, the advent of "nutritional supplements," such as the prohormones, dehydroepiandrosterone (DHEA), and androstenedione, and of recombinant DNA technology is increasing the availability of additional hormones to either replace AAS or supplement their use, including growth hormone (GH) and insulin-like growth factor-1 (IGF-1).

There has also been increasing interest in the use of these anabolic interventions to promote increased muscle mass and strength in aging men and women. Aging is associated with numerous physiological and metabolic changes that include a progressive decrease in strength, skeletal muscle mass, and bone mineral density.[2] Age-associated sarcopenia, an involuntary loss of skeletal muscle mass and strength, typically begins by the third decade of life in both men and women, progressing slowly at first and then more rapidly after the ages of 41 and 60.[2,3] Sarcopenia is associated with changes in several trophic factors which include a parallel decrease in male sex hormones (andropause) and decreased function of the somatotrophic axis (somatopause). In fact, many of the catabolic sequelae seen in normal aging have been attributed to a decrease in these hormone levels.[2,4] Testosterone, GH, IGF-1, androstenedione, and DHEA are among the super hormone candidates or supplements eagerly being pursued as means to prevent or reverse aging-related loss of strength and lean body mass. Maintaining and promoting strength in athletes as well as in the aging population are topics of major interest to science, the public, and the media. In this chapter, the use of these anabolic interventions for maintaining and promoting strength in athletes, healthy adults, and hormone-deficient individuals will be presented and examined.

7.2 Testosterone — The Principal Androgen

7.2.1 General Concepts

Testosterone is the principal biologically active androgen circulating in the blood of both men and women, although women produce only about one twentieth of the amount produced by men. Anabolic–androgenic steroids (AAS) are synthetic analogues of testosterone and were developed in an attempt to dissociate the androgenic, masculinizing, from the anabolic, growth-promoting, effects. As yet it has been impossible to completely disso-ciate the two major actions into pure compounds which are either solely ana-bolic or androgenic. In the early 1950s, scientists found that by slightly changing the steroidal configuration of testosterone by the addition of a methyl group on the 17th carbon, they were able to produce a compound with a tremendously increased half-life that enhanced the anabolic effect of syn-thetic testosterone.[5] Testosterone is not only the parent molecule of AAS, it is also becoming increasingly popular as a hormone replacement strategy itself. A basic knowledge of testosterone biochemistry is critical to understanding the many ramifications AAS and hormone replacement strategies possess.

7.2.2 Synthesis and Regulation

All androgens are steroid compounds, and all steroids are related to a char-acteristic molecular structure composed of 17 carbon atoms, arranged in four rings (A–D). The steroid nucleus, cyclopentanoperhydrophenanthrene, is a basic four-ring carbon skeleton which may be modified in practically an unlimited number of ways by removal, replacement, or addition of a few atoms at a time (Figure 7.1).

Naturally occurring steroids differ in the number of carbon atoms attached to the number-17 carbon atom in the skeleton, and in the way in which hydro-gen, oxygen, and hydroxyl groups attach to the carbon atoms. Both in the male testes and in adrenal glands, the immediate precursor of steroid synthe-sis is cholesterol, and the rate-limiting step is cholesterol side-chain cleavage.

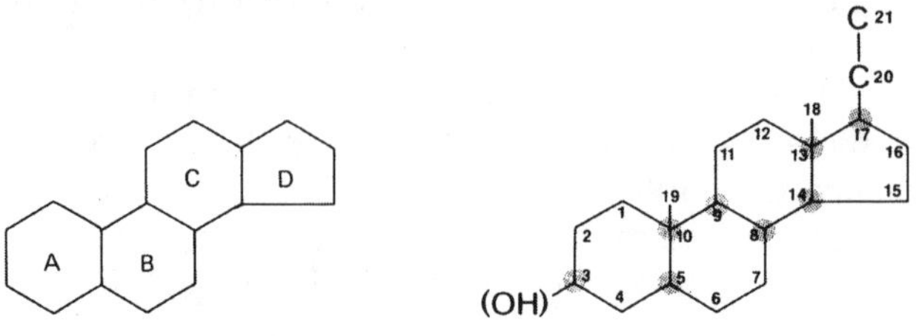

Cyclopentanoper-
hydrophenanthrene
nucleus

(OH)

Numbering of the carbon
atoms. Asymmetric car-
bons are shaded.

FIGURE 7.1
Structural features of steroid molecules. (From Murray, R. et al., *Harper's Review of Biochemistry*, 25th ed., McGraw-Hill, New York, 2000. With permission.)

Cholesterol is converted to pregnenolone in the gonads and in the adrenal gland. Pregnenolone, in turn, can be converted to testosterone via two pathways: the progesterone pathway, which is the preferred direction, or via the DHEA pathway (Figure 7.2). About 95% of plasma testosterone in men is produced by the Leydig cells of the testes and released into the circulation in a pulsatile manner. The remainder of plasma testosterone comes from conversion of adrenal androgens, largely androstenedione and DHEA. In addition to testosterone, the testes also secrete several androgens including dihydrotestosterone (DHT) and androstenedione.[6,7]

Testosterone synthesis and release is controlled by the hypothalamic–pituitary–gonadal axis (HPG). This process begins in the hypothalamus which, when stimulated by low testosterone levels, synthesizes and releases in a pulse-like fashion, gonadotropin-releasing hormone (GnRH). GnRH acts directly on the anterior pituitary to synthesize and secrete the gonadotropins, follicle-stimulating hormone (FSH), and luteinizing hormone (LH), the primary hormonal mediators of testicular function. LH stimulates the Leydig cells in the testes to synthesize testosterone, while FSH acts on the Sertoli cells to stimulate spermatogenesis.[6–8]

7.2.3 Metabolism and Transport

Under control of LH, testosterone is secreted at the rate of ~4 to 9 mg/day (13.9 to 31.2 nmol/day) in normal adult men. The testosterone produced by the testes and the adrenal cortex act to control blood concentrations (free plus bound: male ~525 ng/ml [~20 nmol/L], female ~30 ng/ml: [~1.0 nmol/L]) by feedback inhibition of both LH and GnRH. After secretion by the testes, 97 to 99% of testosterone circulates in blood bound to two proteins, sex hormone-binding globulin (SHBG), for which it has a high affinity, and albumin, for which it has a weaker affinity. Only a small fraction (1 to 2%) is in the free or biologically active form. The testosterone/SHBG ratio is often used as an index of bioavailable testosterone.[6,7]

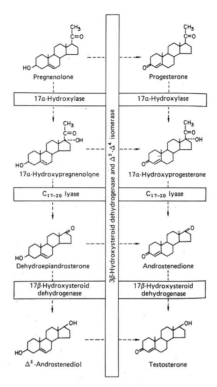

FIGURE 7.2
Pathways of testosterone biosynthesis. The pathway on the left side of the figure is called the Δ^5 or dehydroeplandrosterone pathway; the pathway on the right side is called the Δ^4 or progesterone pathway. (From Murray, R. et al., *Harper's Review of Biochemistry*, 25th ed., McGraw-Hill, New York, 2000. With permission.)

Once secreted into the circulation, testosterone exerts a negative feedback on the hypothalamus and anterior pituitary suppressing GnRH and LH release, thereby controlling the production of testosterone. This explains why the exogenous administration of AAS can cause testicular atrophy. Exogenous AAS elevates plasma steroid levels, which inhibits the hypothalamic–pituitary–testicular axis and, as a consequence, the endogenous synthesis of testosterone is suppressed, leaving the testes somewhat dormant. Depending on tissue needs and enzyme activity, circulating testosterone can be converted to estradiol via aromatization, largely in adipose tissue and the brain, converted to DHT in androgen-dependent tissues such as prostate, seminal vesicles, and external genitalia or converted to androstanediol, another potent androgen.[5–7]

7.2.4 Mechanism of Androgen Action

At the target cells (e.g., muscle, bone, kidney, and brain), free testosterone (androgens) enters the cells through the plasma membrane within a few minutes after secretion and binds with a cytoplasmic steroid receptor protein. The biologic functions of androgens are mediated through this androgen receptor (AR) protein at the cell (Figure 7.3). This protein can bind both testosterone (androgens) and DHT, although it has a much higher affinity for the latter in those cells with the highest 5 α-reductase activity such as prostate, seminal vesicles, and external genitalia. Once the steroid enters the cell and binds to the AR there is a conformational change exposing the DNA binding domain on the AR that can then interact with specific sequences of DNA which are termed androgen-responsive elements (AREs). Binding of the AREs regulates transcription of mRNA inducing the DNA–RNA transcription process and protein synthesis.[9]

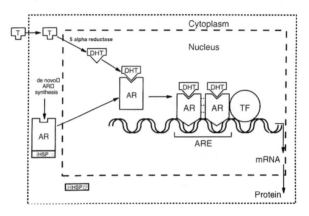

FIGURE 7.3
Mechanism of androgen action. Testosterone (T) enters the cell and is converted by 5α-reductase to 5α-dihydrotestosterone (DHT). DHT binds to the androgen receptor (AR) leading to a conformational change in the protein and the dissociation of several accessory proteins, including heatshock proteins (HSP). Binding of the AR to the androgen response element (ARE), along with other transcription factors (TF), regulates the transcription of mRNAs. (From Lindzey, J, Kumar, M. V., Grossmann, M., Young, C., Tindall, D.J., Molecular mechanisms of androgen action, in Litwack, G. (Ed.), *Vitamins and Hormones*, Academic Press, Orlando, FL, 1995, 49:383-432. With permission.)

Of particular importance in adaptations to strength training, the protein synthesis just described mediates many of the functions of testosterone, both androgenic or masculinizing and anabolic or growth promoting. The androgenic functions promote such male secondary sex characteristics as the stimulation of the growth of facial and body hair, the enhancement of male sexual behavior and aggressiveness, and the maintenance of spermatogenesis and tissues of the reproductive tract. The anabolic functions are associated with tissue growth including skeletal muscle and, thus, influence the expression and development of strength.[5-7]

7.2.5   Testosterone Replacement Therapy (TRT)

There is an age-associated decrease in serum total and free testosterone levels in healthy men. At the onset of puberty, testosterone production increases rapidly under the stimulus of anterior pituitary gonadotropic hormones, peaks in the second decade, and ultimately decreases beyond the age of 40 to 50 to become 20 to 50% of the peak value by the age of 80.[2–4] This decline is a result of changes at multiple levels of the hypothalamic–pituitary–testicular axis in that the testicular response to gonadotropins is diminished, the pituitary gonadotrope responsiveness to androgen suppression is attenuated, and the pulsatility of the hypothalamic GnRH pulse generation is altered.[2,4] Disease, malnutrition, and medications can also affect serum testosterone levels. Although there is no consensus on the serum testosterone levels that can be used to define androgen deficiency, in aging males, total testosterone levels below 200 ng/dl or bioavailable testosterone levels below 60 ng/dl warrant replacement, especially if associated with symptoms suggestive of androgen deficiency.[2] If classified based on bioavailable testosterone, it is believed the prevalence of deficiency would be as high as 50% in aging males.[2]

TRT has been shown to increase fat-free mass (FFM), bone density, and maximal voluntary strength in young, androgen-deficient men as well as aging males with low testosterone. A composite of currently published trials suggests that male TRT may have a significant benefit in terms of improved bone mineral density, increased muscle mass and strength, and in some, improved libido and mood.[2,4] However, scientific information regarding hormone replacement therapy in the aging population is only in its nascent stages. Whether physiological testosterone replacement can induce clinically meaningful changes in muscle function or strength, reduce falls and fractures, or improve quality of life in the aging population remains to be determined.

In the short term, considered up to 3 years, the adverse effects of TRT seem predictable and manageable; but, the long-term safety, particularly with respect to the risk of cardiovascular disease and prostate cancer, remains to be established. Thus, the risk/benefit ratio for TRT remains equivocal. Research regarding the dose–response relationship between serum testosterone levels and muscle strength is needed to optimize the clinical efficacy and safety of testosterone regimens for use in aging males. Ultimately, the effect of TRT will depend on individual genetics, training (type, intensity, frequency, duration, and volume), nutrition quantity and composition, plus starting hormone levels. The potential benefits and risks of testosterone therapy in aging men are listed in Table 7.1.

7.3 Anabolic–Androgenic Steroids

7.3.1 General Concepts

Anabolic–androgenic steroids (AAS) are synthetic analogues of testosterone which were developed in an attempt to minimize the androgenic effects

TABLE 7.1

Potential Benefits and Risks of Testosterone Therapy in
Aging Men

Benefits	Risks
↑ Bone mineral density	Fluid retention
↑ Lean body mass	Induce sleep apnea
↑ Strength and stamina	Develop gynecomastia
↑ Physical function	Produce polycythemia
Improve well-being	↑ Risk of prostate problems
↓ Cardiovascular risk	↑ Cardiovascular risk

while maintaining the anabolic effects of the drugs. The extent to which the androgenic–anabolic ratio may be altered has been referred to as the therapeutic or anabolic index (TI). In the past, androgens have been referred to as having a high anabolic index if they produce less of an effect on reproductive tissues (seminal vesicles) than on the levator ani muscle of the rat; these observations are compared with the relative effects of various testosterone compounds.[10] The anabolic effect is associated with the extent to which a particular steroid compound causes nitrogen retention, known to be a reasonably good index of the protein metabolism capacity of the steroid. The term anabolic steroid, in fact, originated to describe the nitrogen-retaining action of AAS as a marker of the muscle- or protein-building effect. The SPAI (Steroid–Protein Activity Index) has been used to describe the effect of a steroid on nitrogen retention and therefore protein synthesis. However, there is little information comparing the variable anabolic vs. androgenic effects of different AAS in humans.

7.3.2 Types of Anabolic–Androgenic Steroids

AAS can be categorized into those that are administered parentally by injection and those taken orally. Most of the orally active steroids are produced by adding an alkyl group at C-17 of the D-ring in the basic testosterone nucleus. Alkylation at the C17 position reduces hepatic metabolism and enhances the longevity of the steroid.[5,10,11] The injectable preparations are suspended in an oil base and are given in prolonged release forms, called "depot" injections, which are administered intramuscularly typically by deep gluteal injections. They have become popular because they are administered less frequently than the oral preparations and are associated with less toxicity to liver function inasmuch as they are not typically alkylated at the C17 position. As a rule, they are also believed to be more potent than oral steroids because of their route of delivery. Parenterally active anabolic steroids include testosterone esters and two esters of 19-nortestosterone–nandrolone decanoate (deca-durabolin) and nandrolone phenpropionate (durabolin). Esters of testosterone attached to the 17 carbon are long-acting preparations and include testosterone propionate, testosterone enanthate, and testosterone cypionate.[5,10,11] Principle oral and injectable AAS are listed in Table 7.2 with both trade and generic names.

TABLE 7.2

Trade and Generic Names for Commonly Used
Anabolic–Androgenic Steroids (AAS)*

Oral AAS

Anadrol (Oxymetholone)
Anavar (Oxandrolone)
Dianabol (Methandrostenolone)
Metandren (methyltestosterone)
Primobolin (Methenolone)
Winstrol (Stanozolol)

Injectable AAS

Deca-durabolin (Nandrolone decanoate)
Delatestryl (Testosterone enanathate)
Depo-testosterone (Testosterone cypionate)
Parabolan (Trenbolone acetate)

---

* Trade names are listed first with generic names in parentheses.

7.3.3 Effects of Anabolic–Androgenic Steroids on Strength and Muscle Mass

Despite their reputation, AAS have had some important clinical applications. For example, they have been used in treatment of osteoporosis, recovery from illness or injury, treatment of muscular dystrophy, balance therapy for hypogonadal individuals, treatment of chronic anemias, treatment of muscle wasting-diseases such as AIDS and, more recently, as a male contraceptive.[4,5,11] Ironically, it was their potential use as a male contraceptive which led to their initial synthesis as drugs; we have come full circle and are exploring again the reasons they were researched in the first place. Although they have been in use for over five decades, there is considerable confusion regarding the efficacy of their use as ergogenic aids. This is largely a result of critical weaknesses in the research designs used to study their effects including: a lack of proper controls and study design; the use of variable types of drugs, dosage, method of administration, and treatment duration; lack of nutritional control for such items as additional supplements consumed, calorie or energy intake, and protein intake; variable training experience of the subjects; different training intensity/volume used; measurement techniques such as nonspecific strength testing; genetic variability of receptors, hormones, and enzymes; and the inability to have research projects approved by human subjects committees who focus on the risks of steroid use. This makes it virtually impossible to precisely quantify the effects of AAS on body composition and strength.

Despite these problems, there is little doubt among strength-training athletes that AAS can have a dramatic impact on body composition and strength levels. These effects have been most recently confirmed by a study that controlled not only dietary factors but also the type of exercise and the weightlifting experience of the subjects.[12] Male subjects were randomly assigned to one of four groups: (1) placebo with no strength training, (2) testosterone ester with no strength training, (3) placebo with strength training, and (4) testosterone ester with strength training. The two testosterone groups received a supraphysiological dose (600 mg) every week for 10 weeks. The men who received testosterone but did no strength training gained significantly more muscle size and strength than the placebo group who did no strength training. The subjects receiving both testosterone and strength training experienced increased muscle size and strength that was far greater than effects in the other three groups. AAS seem to have their greatest effect in athletes who participate in a strength-training program and who continue this training during the steroid treatment. This suggests that anabolic steroids will consistently result in significant strength increases if they are given to athletes intensively trained in weightlifting immediately before the start of the steroid regimen and who continue this intensive weight training during the steroid regimen.[5]

Three primary mechanisms have been proposed to explain the ability of AAS to effect changes in muscle mass and strength. Coupled with their anabolic effects, AAS have both anticatabolic and psychological effects. The anabolic effects of AAS are mediated via enhanced protein synthesis in target tissues such as skeletal muscle if protein intake is adequate. The anticatabolic effects, which may be the most important, are mediated in two ways: reversal of the catabolic effects of glucocorticosteroids that are released during periods of stress, and conversion of a negative nitrogen balance by improved use of ingested protein, thereby increasing nitrogen retention. Intense weightlifting can force an athlete into a catabolic state, first by stressing the body causing the release of glucocorticosteroids, and second by substantially increasing nitrogen utilization. As a result intensively trained athletes are often in a chronic catabolic state. AAS, given to athletes in a negative nitrogen balance, would enhance the use of the ingested protein and result in a positive nitrogen balance, if there is adequate protein intake. Conversely, an athlete not intensively trained in weightlifting prior to anabolic steroid treatment would not be expected to be in a catabolic state or in a negative nitrogen balance and the net effect would be diminished.

The psychological effects of AAS have been well documented and may be manifest through increased motivation, reduced fatigue, increased aggressiveness, and/or the placebo effect. Athletes who use AAS often experience a state of euphoria and reduced fatigue which enhances motivation, self confidence, and amount of training. There are numerous anecdotal and case reports regarding the effects of AAS on increased aggressiveness.[13] Appropriately channeled increased aggression is a part of most sports and therefore would improve performance. High levels of aggression and the hormone release associated with this type of response may also increase the capacity to tolerate the pain and discomfort associated with training. Studies which have demonstrated that AAS can affect both the central nervous system and neuromuscular junction suggest there could be a biochemical foundation for aggressive behavior. Finally, the placebo effect cannot be eliminated. Simply taking something an athlete thinks will help often provides the psychological motivation for the athlete to show increased strength beyond what would have been expected in the absence of an AAS. It seems likely that the effects are, at least in part, mediated through each of the aforementioned mechanisms.[5,11,13,14]

7.3.4 Adverse Effects and Risks of Anabolic–Androgenic Steroids

Are the potential gains worth the possible risks associated with the use of AAS? These drugs are illegal, and athletes risk being banned from their sports if they use them. More important are the medical risks associated with steroid use, especially with the excessive doses often used by athletes. AAS use has been associated with a considerable number of adverse side effects. Of major concern are the effects on the liver, cardiovascular system, reproductive system, and psychological status.

7.3.4.1 *Reproductive System Effects*

Although AAS can dramatically improve sexual function and reproductive capability in hypogonadal individuals, these drugs can elicit the opposite reactions in normal healthy males. In healthy young men, prolonged high dosages, which are often 10 to 200 times therapeutic recommendations, can lead to long-term impairment of the hypothalamic–pituitary–testicular axis, testosterone endocrine function leading to testicular atrophy, decrease in spermatogenesis, reduced testosterone levels, and possibly gynecomastia[5,11,13,14] (Appendices I and J). Though many steroid users report increased libido initially, a diminished sex drive is associated with prolonged use. Most men who self-administer high doses of steroids become infertile during the period of use and for some time afterwards, perhaps 6 months or more. There is a risk of sterility with prolonged use at high dosage levels, but no case has ever been reliably documented.

7.3.4.2 *Cardiovascular System Risk*

The steroid-induced effects on the cardiovascular system may prove to be the most profound. AAS have a dramatic effect on risk factors associated with the development of cardiovascular disease (CVD) including: hyperinsulinemia, altered glucose tolerance, elevated blood pressure, decreased HDL, and elevated LDL. Changes in serum lipid profiles of users indicate that steroids may be some of the most potent atherogenic drugs known. Coupled with other reported adverse effects that include fluid retention, blood platelet aggregation (clotting abnormalities), and functional alterations in myocardial cell cultures, the potential for devastating effects on the cardiovascular system is clear[3,5,11,13,14] (Appendix J).

7.3.4.3 Human Liver Risk

AAS use of specifically the 17α-alkylated oral steroids has been associated with blockage of bile flow causing jaundice and an increased risk of liver tumors. Prolonged use could lead to cell death and cirrhosis, which will impair normal liver function. The most serious liver complications associated with AAS use are peliosis hepatitis, blood filled cysts in the liver, and liver tumors. Peliosis hepatitis is a potentially life-threatening condition in which blood-filled cysts develop in the liver and has been reported in individuals treated with AAS for various medical conditions. Before the development of steroids, this condition was seen almost exclusively in patients with pulmonary tuberculosis. These cysts may rupture and cause painful abdominal bleeding and possible death. However, despite these risks and the widespread abuse of AAS, the critical side effects on the liver have been primarily documented only in those patients who have been previously ill and have received 17-α-alkylated steroids over prolonged periods.[14] Notably, one bodybuilder died of liver cancer after having abused a variety of AAS for at least 4 years[3,5,11,13,14] (Appendix J).

7.3.4.4 Psychological Status Effects

In both sexes, psychological effects of AAS include increases or decreases in libido, mood swings, and aggressive behavior, sometimes uncontrollable called "roid rage," which is related to high testosterone levels. AAS may cause an indirect increase in neurotransmitters in the central nervous system thus producing stimulation effects which in turn could possibly cause changed sex drive and increased excitability, irritability, and insomnia.[3,5,11] In some people the psychological changes can emerge as reckless behavior and loss of judgment. Psychosis may occur in some susceptible individuals possibly at doses that also activate corticosteroid-specific responses, since corticosteroid use has been known to produce psychosis. Ultimately the effects of AAS will be determined by individual genetics, previous and current training programs, nutrition, age, sex, and type, dose, and duration of steroid use. The reader is referred to the American College of Sports Medicine position statement on the use and abuse of anabolic–androgenic steroids (Appendix I), which the author of this chapter and professionals in the field endorse.

7.4 Growth Hormone

7.4.1 General Concepts

Growth hormone (GH) currently competes with anabolic–androgenic steroids as the next "magic pill" in performance-enhancing drugs for athletes and anti-aging strategies for aging baby-boomers. Discovery of recombinant human growth hormone (rhGH) in the possession of Chinese swimmers heading for the 1998 World Swimming Championships and similar discoveries at the Tour de France cycling event in 1998 and the 1996 Olympic Summer Games in Atlanta, which are sometimes referred to as the "growth hormone games," strongly suggest the abuse of rhGH at the elite level.[13,15] This problem extends into the broader community and includes high school students and aging adults who continue to search for the next "fountain of youth."

GH, also known as somatotropin, is a polypeptide hormone secreted from the anterior pituitary under a complex regulatory mechanism involving stimulation by hypothalamic growth hormone releasing hormone (GHRH) and inhibition by hypothalamic somatostatin. The intermittent, pulse-like secretion of GH is intricately regulated by neural, metabolic, and hormonal feedback mechanisms.[16] Major stimuli leading to GH release include sleep, fasting, stress, exercise, hypoglycemia, and certain amino acids. It may be inhibited by hyperglycemia, circulating IGF-1, obesity, and body fat distribution.[17] Abdominal obesity and increased visceral fat have been associated with hyperinsulinemia, lower serum IGF-1 concentrations, and decreased spontaneous 24-hr GH release.[18]

Once in the circulation, GH exerts many of its anabolic effects by stimulating the liver to produce and release small polypeptides called insulin-like growth factors, IGF-1 and IGF-2. A small amount of IGF-1 circulates freely, but most (~99%) circulates bound to a series of binding proteins, IGFBP 1-6. The regulation of the biological effects of GH and IGF-1 by binding proteins is currently an area of intensive investigation which may help explain the variable metabolic effects reported during GH administration.[19,20]

GH is fundamentally involved in the growth process of skeletal muscle and many other tissues as it promotes cell division and cellular proliferation throughout the body. It is implicated as affecting somatic growth during childhood and is also known to have widespread physiologic activity in adults, such as the maintenance of muscle mass and strength, body composition, and energy metabolism.[19] On the surface, GH appeals to the strength athlete because at physiologic levels it stimulates amino acid uptake and protein synthesis by muscle while it enhances fatty acid oxidation, thus conserving glycogen stores,[21] and it also enhances bone and cartilage growth.[19] Not only is GH important for normal development, but it also appears to play a vital role in adaptation to the stress of strength training and may improve recovery following musculoskeletal injuries.[11,19]

7.4.2   Exercise and GH

Acute exercise is generally associated with an increase of both GH pulse frequency and amplitude. Exercise stimulates the production of endogenous opiates which facilitate GH release by an inhibition of liver production of somatostatin, a hormone that blunts the release of GH.[19] When the GH response to exercise is evaluated, attention must be given to program design variables. It appears that GH is differentially sensitive to variable strength-training protocols. With increasing exercise intensity there is a dramatic rise in GH production and total secretion, theoretically optimizing the anabolic environment, which would include increased protein synthesis leading to subsequent muscle hypertrophy, skeletal growth, and cell proliferation. It is thought that the stimulus for increased GH release is elevated hydrogen ion levels.[22] The most dramatic, acute, increases in GH have been observed in high-volume, short-rest programs (10 repetitions × 3 sets × 1-minute rest periods) as opposed to low-volume, longer-rest programs typically used by Olympic and power lifters.[11] Therefore, differential GH responses will occur depending on load, rest periods, and volume of exercise which, in turn, may impact anabolic responses. The long-term chronic adaptations of serum GH to strength training have not been extensively studied, but reports of normal resting GH concentrations in elite lifters suggest there is little change with training.[23] Strength training, however, may increase the sensitivity to stimuli, such as the amino acid arginine, which promotes the release of GH.

7.4.3   GH Use

The recent availability of recombinant human GH (rhGH) has provided investigators the opportunity to examine the prospect that GH treatment might enhance lean body mass (LBM) or muscle protein accretion during anabolic conditions such as growth and exercise or suppress protein wasting associated with catabolic conditions such as age-related sarcopenia. In young, hypopituitary adults, GH replacement therapy improves muscle volume, isometric strength, and exercise capacity.[24] Athletes use GH to increase muscle mass, train harder, longer, and more frequently, and to recover faster after training.[15] Anecdotal reports suggest that strength athletes and body-builders self-administer large doses of rhGH despite strict security and distribution regulations and experience dramatic increments in muscle mass and strength. However, attributing these effects specifically to rhGH would be virtually impossible because these athletes typically administer a number of "anabolic" agents simultaneously in a somewhat indiscriminate manner. It has been estimated that athletes who self-administer rhGH undertake three 6- to 8-week cycles of rhGH treatment each year and use 1 to 2 IU or more every other day during a particular cycle. The cost per year on the black market is about $3000.[15]

7.4.4   GH Effects in Normal, Healthy Adults

Few studies have actually examined whether rhGH administration enhances the anabolic effects of strength training by stimulation of further muscle hypertrophy and/or strength in physically active individuals with normal GH secretory function. Several studies have reported similar increases in muscle protein synthesis, muscle cross-sectional area, and muscle strength in placebo and rhGH-treated exercising young adults alike, which suggests it is unlikely that the nitrogen retention associated with daily rhGH treatment results in an increase in contractile protein, improved muscle function, strength, and athletic performance.[19] GH recipients who participated in a 12 week resistance-training program demonstrated a greater increase in fat-free mass (FFM), total body water, and whole-body protein synthesis than a placebo group. However, there were no significant differences between groups in fractional rate of protein synthesis in skeletal muscle, torso, or limb circumference, or strength measures.[25] The greater increase in whole-body protein synthesis in the rhGH group was attributed to a possible increase in nitrogen retention in lean tissue (e.g., connective tissue, fluid, and noncontractile protein) other than skeletal muscle. An extensive review concluded that daily rhGH treatment modestly increases nitrogen retention in most normal adults, probably by permissive mechanisms, but only for a short period of time (~1 month). During prolonged rhGH administration, resistance to the anabolic actions of GH seems to occur.[19]

The observed lack of a greater anabolic effect of prolonged GH treatment combined with strength training is in agreement with earlier animal studies[19] as is the observation that the initial nitrogen-sparing effect of GH dissipates with prolonged treatment. This in part may be related to the fact that GH works best synergistically with other hormones. Thus, rhGH is considerably more effective when combined with hormones needed to maximize the anabolic effect, such as insulin and thyroid hormone,[14] both of which usually decrease when rhGH is taken. Only under these circumstances can the liver produce and release an optimal amount of insulin-like growth factors. For example, too little insulin, such as occurs during dieting, may reduce the anabolic effects of rhGH, whereas frequent feedings during the day would create an anabolic environment for potentiating the effect of GH. Anecdotal evidence from athletes who have used rhGH concur that its effects on promoting muscle growth and strength are disappointing. However, when rhGH and AAS are administered together, there appears to be a synergistic effect in increased anabolism and strength. Combining low doses of AAS with rhGH is more effective than either substance alone.[15] The effect of excess GH on body composition and strength may best be exemplified in untreated acromegaly where body weight, FFM, and extracellular water content are increased while fat mass is reduced. Interestingly, although acromegalics have larger than normal muscles, they do not have stronger than normal muscles.

7.4.5   GH Replacement Therapy: Aging and
Growth Hormone Deficiency (GHD)

The activity of the GH/IGF-1 axis declines significantly with advancing age; both GH secretion and serum IGF-1 decrease, which is termed the somatopause. Many of the catabolic sequelae seen in normal aging, which include reduced LBM and strength, decreased protein synthesis, increased adiposity, and decreased bone mass, have been attributed to decreased function of the GH/IGF-1 axis.[2] In order to provide hormone replacement therapy for the somatopause, aging subjects and patients have been treated with rhGH, IGF-1, or both hormones together. Whereas numerous beneficial effects on body composition, strength, and quality of life have been reported in some studies, other studies have reported only marginal functional improvement.[19]

GH administration, with dosage based on IGF-1 levels, to healthy older men (61 to 81 years) increased LBM (+8.8%), decreased body fat (–14.4%), and increased bone density in the lumbar spine (+1.6%), but improvements in muscle mass and strength were not assessed.[26] Growth hormone deficiency (GHD) in adults and somatopause often share many of the same characteristics, such as increased fat mass, reduced lean mass, osteopenia, impaired fibrinolysis, altered cardiac structure and function, unfavorable glucose and lipid metabolism, reduced exercise capacity, and reduced quality of life.[2,19] Since the introduction of rhGH, several clinical trials have examined the characteristics of GHD. Adults with GHD appear to have muscle weakness caused by decreased muscle mass that can be improved with rhGH therapy.[27] Several observations suggest that rhGH administration may have an important role in body composition and bone density in aging adults and GHD patients. Using physiologic doses adjusted according to IGF-1 levels in patients with GHD, long-term GH therapy improved body composition (increased LBM and decreased fat mass), bone mineral density, psychological well-being, and increased (or reduced the age-related decline of) muscle strength.[27-29] Specific guidelines regarding the use of serum IGF-1 to individualize GH replacement therapy have not been established.

7.4.6   Adverse Effects and Risks of GH Use

As with steroids, there are *potential* medical risks associated with the use of GH. The extent of any side effect would be directly related to the amount of rhGH used and the starting GH levels of the individual. For example, low doses administered to individuals over the age of 60 with low starting levels do not appear to cause any side effects,[28] while high doses administered to athletes may cause more dramatic side effects.[14] Acromegaly can result from taking GH after bones have fused, which results in bone thickening that causes broadening of the hands, feet, and face; in skin thickening and soft tissue growth; and in enlarged internal organs. Cardiomyopathy, glucose intolerance, diabetes, hypertension, and an increased incidence of additional side effects such as arthralgias, myalgias, edema, and carpal tunnel syndrome can also result from GH use in already mature adults.[14,19,20] Some athletes report headaches, nausea, vomiting, and visual disturbances during the first weeks of administration, which disappear in most cases with continued use. It remains to be seen whether rhGH use impairs the ability of the body to produce GH naturally.

7.4.7 Conclusions Regarding GH Use

Despite the availability of rhGH and subsequent research, no unifying thesis regarding the effects of GH treatment on muscle mass and strength has evolved. In general, the anabolic or anticatabolic effects of GH treatment observed to date have been inconsistent, which is related to the variable doses, regimens, populations, and conditions under which it has been administered. Further, understanding of the interactions among all the components of the somatotropic axis is incomplete. Optimizing the anabolic effects of rhGH treatment will require a better understanding of the interactions among GH, IGF-1 production, IGFBP, the dose regimen, and other hormones and regulatory factors.

7.5 The Insulin-Like Growth Factor System

7.5.1 General Concepts

There has been a growing interest in the insulin-like growth factor system (IGF) as a result of its numerous known functions and widespread distribution throughout the body. Of interest to strength training, the primary indirect or IGF-1 mediated action of GH on body protein metabolism is believed to be the stimulation of protein synthesis that results in skeletal and somatic growth. This effect is mediated by both circulating and locally produced IGF-1.[20,30] In addition to GH, insulin levels and nutritional status, such as acute changes in nitrogen balance and protein intake, influence IGF transport, production, and regulatory control. Circulating IGF-1, in turn, exerts an inhibitory feedback on GH synthesis and release.

The IGF system consists of IGF-1 and 2, multiple binding proteins (1 to 6), and three well-described receptor systems.[20,31] It has been traditionally recognized that IGF-1 (somatomedin C) is a component of the GH control axis with much of the research emphasis placed on its insulin-like anabolic and metabolic effects. IGFs are secreted by the liver following GH stimulated synthesis. In the circulation, they attach to binding proteins (IGFBPs), which regulate their action and bioavailability. Release from the binding protein is signaled by the availability of the receptor site on the cell. Circulating levels of IGF-1 are thought to reflect GH-mediated production by the liver. However, it also appears that IGF-1 may be released from nonhepatic tissue independent of GH. Cells, including muscle and fat cells, may produce and keep IGFs without their being released into the circulation. IGF-1 expression in skeletal muscle increases during hypertrophy in response to increased loading without concomitant increased plasma IGF-1 levels.[11,20,31]

7.5.2   Anabolic Effects of IGF-1

It is generally agreed that IGF-1 exerts an anabolic action similar to that produced by insulin[17-19] as it stimulates protein synthesis, suppresses protein degradation and increases amino acid uptake. The well-established ability of IGF-1 to mediate anabolism represents one attribute of this growth factor that could clearly contribute to the hypertrophy process in skeletal muscle. A number of studies demonstrate that GH treatment results in significant increased circulating IGF-1, resulting in increased LBM without improvement in muscle-related measures such as strength and muscle mass.[19] Even when GH doubled IGF-1 concentration, the measured strength gains elicited by the resistance-training program in young and older subjects were not increased. The majority of human and animal studies suggest that *circulating* IGF-1 levels are of minimal importance in the adaptation of specific muscles to changes in loading.[19] On the other hand, there is evidence pointing to a cause and effect relationship between hypertrophy and increased GH *independent* IGF-1 expression in skeletal muscle — contributing to the hypertrophy process via the mobilization of satellite cells during remodeling[20]. The exact relationship between tissue specific IGF-1 expression and circulating IGF-1 remains to be elucidated.

7.5.3   Recombinant Human IGF-1 Replacement Therapy

IGF-1 has just recently become available in sufficient amounts for systemic supplementation. Clinically, recombinant human IGF-1 (rhIGF-1) has considerable promise for the management of many different conditions including diabetes, wound healing, osteoporosis, and amyotrophic lateral sclerosis. In contrast to GH treatment, IGF-1 decreases plasma glucose in normal and in diabetic patients.[33] When both GH and IGF-1 were used simultaneously, a marked enhancement of anabolism was demonstrated as well as a dramatic decrease in fat mass, suggesting the potential for combination therapy.[34] However, the incidence of side effects was also greater with combined therapy. Clearly, strength athletes considering combination administration must be aware of these increased risks. Clinical use is in doubt since trials have been suspended due to concerns regarding side effects. Though the safety of repeated injections of rhIGF-1 has been demonstrated in both young and elderly, there may be a connection between circulating IGF-1 levels and cancer. This has stimulated interest in the role of the IGF-1 system in tumorigenesis and the possibility of manipulating this system for therapeutic reasons.[19,20,33]

The regulation of the biological effects of GH and IGF-1 by binding proteins is currently an area of intensive investigation which may eventually help explain the variable metabolic effects reported during GH administration.[35]

7.6 Prohormones: DHEA and Androstenedione

Considerable media attention has been given to the prohormones dehydroepiandrosterone (DHEA) and androstenedione. Both are steroid hormones produced primarily by the adrenal glands and gonads of both sexes. The hormones act as intermediates in the endogenous production of both testosterone and estrogens.[36] In the adrenal cortex, DHEA is converted to androstenedione, which in turn can either be dehyrogenated in the liver to testosterone or aromatized to estrone.[37] It is, in fact, the prohormone role in testosterone synthesis which has stimulated much of the recent interest in their potential as anabolic or ergogenic aids. Like testosterone, the production of these hormones peaks in the mid-20s and then declines steadily with age after the third decade of life.[38] It has been speculated, therefore, that supplementation with these "precursor" hormones may help keep androstenedione and/or testosterone levels elevated, thereby optimizing the anabolic state. Ironically, DHEA and androstenedione are currently available without a prescription as "dietary supplements" (Dietary Supplement Health and Education Act, 1994) and are marketed primarily to athletes and bodybuilders as an alternative to AAS use. Despite the legal availability of these substances, the International Olympic Committee, National Collegiate Athletic Association, and the National Football League have banned their use.

Supplementation with androgenic hormones may pose a potential risk for promoting the growth of hormone-sensitive tumors, most notably prostatic hypertrophy, as well as promoting hepatotoxicity and increasing the risk of cardiovascular disease.[4,39,40] Recently, we compared the effects of short-term (12-weeks) DHEA vs. androstenedione supplementation on body composition, strength levels, and hormonal profiles in middle-aged males experienced in weight training.[41] The results demonstrated that supplementation with 100mg/day for 3 months did not significantly increase lean body mass or strength levels, relative to changes observed in the placebo group. These results are consistent with a recent study finding no differences in strength and LBM gains (androstenedione vs. placebo) and with previous studies which reported no increase in LBM or decrease in percent fat.[42] However, the aforementioned results contradict others which reported an increase in both LBM and strength with DHEA supplementation.[43,44] These discrepancies may be related to a number of factors that include the basal physiologic milieu such as the initial hormonal and metabolic profile; body composition, which considers lean body mass vs. fat mass; nutritional status and factors of quantity, composition, and timing; training index of frequency × intensity × volume;

dosing criteria of timing, quantity, and route of administration; and age. Low levels may be critical to inducing a statistically significant response with replacement dose supplementation.

Though there is evidence that androstenedione can raise serum testosterone into normal range from low basal levels,[37,45] short- and long-term supplementation with androstenedione did not increase testosterone levels on a day-to-day basis in more recent studies. However, both testosterone and estrogen levels have recently been shown to increase on a short-term basis (< 8hrs) when androstenedione was administered in larger doses (300 mg/day); testosterone and estrogen levels returned to normal values by the next day.[46] This may be related to the short half-life of testosterone in the circulation, known to be 60 to 80 minutes, as well as the short half-life of androstenedione and its rapid conversion in peripheral tissues. Muscle, along with adipose tissue, is a major source of serum estrogens derived from androstenedione.[47] In fact, serum estradiol levels actually increased, and serum estrone levels were reportedly higher in subjects who received androstenedione.[48] Therefore, increasing androstenedione levels with high doses in men may not provide the anabolic environment desired. Overproduction of androstenedione may cause feminizing effects such as gynecomastia.

In contrast to high-dose administration, supplemental androstenedione in low doses does not exhibit excess elevation of estrogen levels,[37] particularly in hypogonadism. It also appears that a small additional amount of estrogen produced by supplemental androstenedione may trigger formation of more androgen receptors where they are wanted most — skeletal muscles.[49] It is likely that the body rapidly adapts to excess androstenedione and may downregulate its endogenous production and subsequent conversion to testosterone or estrogens as needed. Finally, because androstenedione and DHEA have been shown to decrease with long-term strength training,[45] supplementation may have been "sacrificed" to maintain testosterone levels and prevent overtraining. Replacement therapy may help reduce overtraining syndrome and prevent a deficiency induced by intense training and the delayed strength plateaus normally observed.

Ultimately, the potential benefit of supplementation with prohormones may only be manifest in specific population subsets such as those characterized by low basal hormone levels and/or high-intensity training who use much longer supplementation periods and larger doses. Researchers have, in fact, recently demonstrated the ability of DHEA used as a supplement to undergo biotransformation into potent androgens and estrogens in subjects with panhypopituitarism, a syndrome characterized by the absence of adrenal and gonadal steroid secretion.[50]

Although the precise functions of DHEA, thus the implications of an elevated DHEA level with supplementation, remain unclear,[39] it has been postulated that it may play a role as a discriminator of life expectancy and aging.[50] It has also been reported that DHEA-S level is independently and inversely predictive of death from any cause and from cardiovascular disease.[51,52] Thus, it is tempting to speculate that supplementation with DHEA may help confer some protection against chronic disease and/or premature death. The potential benefits and risks of DHEA and/or androstenedione supplementation may be manifest only with long-term supplementation, higher dosage, and/or in special subset populations with very low initial basal levels or those individuals involved in high-intensity training. Future studies should further delineate the population and dosing criteria.

7.7 Summary

The quest to be bigger and stronger likely goes back to the beginning of mankind. The advent of pharmacologic and dietary anabolic agents used as ergogenic aids have both facilitated and complicated this issue. While there may be a legitimate use for many of these anabolic agents in hormone-deficient and aging individuals, the use and abuse by young, healthy athletes is clearly contraindicated. It is clear that the anabolic ramifications, especially with respect to muscle hypertrophy and strength, in athletes as well as normal and aging adults, requires further study. The interpretation of available research is confounded by the complex interactions among exercise, nutrition, and genetics. Research in the future will need to control for each separate factor to further delineate the specific role of anabolic interventions used for enhancing strength. Evidence to support the use of anabolic hormones and their precursors as supplemental strategies in age-related sarcopenia, and their long-term safety is still in its infancy. Scientific knowledge is far behind public and media interest in this issue. We expect this will be an exciting and intensive area of investigation in the future.

References

1. Frank, W. W. and Berendonk, B., Hormonal doping and androgenization of athletes: a secret program of the German Democratic Republic government, *Clin. Chem.*, 43, 1262, 1997.
2. Bross, R., Javanbakht, M., and Bhasin, S., Anabolic interventions for aging-associated sarcopenia, *J. Clin. Endo. Metab.*, 84, 3420, 1999.
3. McArdle, W. D., Physical activity, health, and aging, in *Exercise Physiology: Energy, Nutrition and Human Performance*, 4th ed., McArdle, W. D., Katch, F. I., and Katch, V. L. (Eds.), Williams and Wilkins, Baltimore, MD, 1996, chap. 30.
4. Tenover, J. L., Testosterone replacement therapy in older adult men, *Int. J. Androl.*, 22, 300, 1999.
5. Haupt, H. A. and Rovere, G. D., Anabolic steroids: A review of the literature, *Am. J. Spt. Med*, 12(6), 469, 1984.

6. Granner, D. K., Hormones of the gonads, in *Harper's Review of Biochemistry*, 20th ed., Lange Medical Publications, Los Altos, CA, 1985, chap. 41.
7. Loebel, C. C. and Kraemer, W. J., A brief review: testosterone and resistance exercise in men, *J. Strength Cond. Res.*, 12(1), 57, 1998.
8. Griswold, M. D., Gonadotropins, steroids and their sites of synthesis, in *Handbook of Andrology*, 2nd ed., American Society of Andrology, San Francisco, CA, 1995.
9. Tindall, D. J., Hormone receptors, signal transduction, in *Handbook of Andrology*, 2nd ed., American Society of Andrology, San Francisco, CA, 1995, chap. 4.
10. Kochakian, C. D., Anabolic–androgenic steroids, in *Handbook of Experimental Pharmacology*, Kochakian, C. D. (Ed.), Berlin, Springer-Verlag, 43, 1976.
11. Friedl, K. E., Performance-enhancing substances: effects, risks, and appropriate alternatives, in *Essentials of Strength Training and Conditioning*, Baechle, T. R. (Ed.), Human Kinetics, Champaign, IL, 1994.
12. Bhasin, S., Storer, T. W., and Berman, N., The effect of supraphysiological doses of testosterone on muscle size and strength in normal men, *N. Engl. J. Med.*, 335, 1, 1996.
13. Yesalis, C. E. and Cowart, V. S., *The Steroids Game*, Human Kinetics, Champaign, IL, 1998.
14. Grunding, P. and Bachman, M., *World Anabolic Review, 1996*. Sport Verlag Ingenohl, D-Heilbronn, M. Bodingbauer, D-Selm, German American Technologies, Inc., San Leandro, CA, 1999.
15. Schnirring, L., Growth hormone doping: the search for a test, *Phys. and Sports Med.*, 28(4), 16, 2000.
16. Thorner, M., Vance, M., Horvath, E., and Kovacs, K., The anterior pituitary, in *Williams Textbook of Endocrinology*, Wilson J. Foster, (Ed.), Philadelphia, Saunders, 1991, 221.
17. Hartman, M. L., Veldhuis, J. D., and Thorner, M. O., Normal control of growth hormone secretions, *Horm. Res.*, 40, 37, 1993.
18. Kanaley, J. A., Weatherup-Dentes, M., Jaynes, E. B., and Hartman, M. L., Obesity attenuates the growth hormone response to exercise, *J. Clin. Endo. Metab.*, 84, 3156, 1999.
19. Yarasheski, K. E., Growth hormone effects on metabolism, body composition, muscle mass, and strength, in *Exercise and Sport Sciences Reviews*, Grayson, T. H. (Ed.), Williams and Wilkins, Philadelphia, 22, 285, 1994.
20. Adams, G. R., Role of insulin-like growth factor-1 in the regulation of skeletal muscle adaptation to increased loading, in *Exercise and Sport Sciences Reviews*, Holloszy, J. O. (Ed.), Williams and Wilkins, Philadelphia, 26, 31, 1998.
21. MacIntyre, J. G., Growth hormone and athletes, *Sports Med.*, 4, 129, 1987.
22. Gordon, S. E., Kraemer, W. J., Vos, N. H., Lynch, J. M., and Kneuttgen, H. G., Effect of acid-base on serum human growth hormone concentration to acute high intensity cycle exercise, *J. Appl. Physiol.*, 76(2), 821, 1994.
23. Hakkinen, K., Pakarinen, A., Alen, M., Kauhanen, H., and Komi, P. V., Daily hormonal and neuromuscular responses to intensive strength training in one week, *Int. J. Sports Med.*, 9, 422, 1988.
24. Jorgensen, J. O. L., Pedersen, S. A., Thuesen, L., Jorgensen, J., and Ingemann-Hansen, T., Beneficial effects of growth hormone treatment in GH-deficient adults, *Lancet*, 1, 1221, 1989.

25. Yarasheski, K. E., Campbell, J. A., Smith, K., Rennie, M. J., Holloszy, J. O., and Bier, D. M., Effect of growth hormone and resistance exercise on muscle growth in young men, *Am. J. Physiol.*, 262, E261, 1992.

26. Rudman, D., Feller, A. G., Nagraj, H. S., Gergans, G. A., Lalitha, P. Y., Goldberg, A. F., Schlenker, R. A., Cohn, L., Rudman, I. W., and Mattson, D. E., Effects of human growth hormone in men over 60 years old, *N. Engl. J. Med.*, 323, 1, 1990.

27. Janssen, Y. J. H., Doornbos, J., and Roelfsema, F., Changes in muscle volume, strength, and bioenergetics during recombinant human growth hormone therapy in adults with GH deficiency, *J. Clin. Endo. Metab.*, 84, 279, 1999.

28. Toogood, A. A. and Shalet, S. M., Growth hormone replacement therapy in the elderly with the hypothalamic-pituitary disease: a dose-finding study, *J. Clin. Endo. Metab.*, 84, 131, 1999.

29. Johansson, A. G., Engstrom, B. E., Ljunghall, S., Karlsson, F. A., and Burman, P., Gender differences in the effects of long term growth hormone treatment on bone in adults with GH deficiency, *J. Clin Endo. Metab.*, 84, 2002, 1999.

30. Czech, M. P., Signal transmission by the insulin-like growth factors, *Cell*, 59, 235, 1989.

31. Clemmons, D. R., IGF binding proteins and their functions, *Mol. Reprod. Dev.*, 35, 368, 1993.

32. Florini, J. R., Ewton, D. Z., and Coolican, S. A., Growth hormone and insulin like growth factor system in myogenesis, *Endo. Rev.*, 17, 481, 1996.

33. Roith, L. R., Insulin-like growth factor, *Horm. Metab. Res.*, 31, 41, 1999.

34. Kupfer, S. R., Underwood, L. E., Baxter, R. C., and Clemmons, D. R., Enhancement of the anabolic effect of growth hormone and insulin-like growth factor-1 by use of both agents simultaneously, *J. Clin. Invest.*, 91, 391, 1993.

35. Ferry, R. J., Cerri, R. W., and Cohen, P., Insulin-like growth factor binding proteins: new proteins, new functions, *Horm. Res.*, 51, 53, 1999.

36. Shackleton, C., Roitman, E., Phillips, A., and Chang, T., Androstenediol and 5-androstenediol profiling for detecting exogenously administered dihydrotestosterone, epitestosterone, and dehydroepiandrosterone: Potential use in gas chromatography isotope ratio mass spectrometry, *Steroids*, 62, 665, 1997.

37. Mahesh, V. B. and Greenblatt, R. B., The *in vivo* conversion of dehydroepiandrosterone and androstenedione to testosterone in the human, *Acta Endocrinol.*, 41, 400, 1962.

38. Orenteich, N., Brind, J. L., Rizer, R. L., and Vogelman, J. H., Age changes and sex differences in serum DHEA-S concentrations throughout adulthood, *J. Clin. Endocrinol. Metab.*, 59, 551, 1984.

39. Gann, P. H., Hennekens, C. H., Longcope, C., Verhoek-Oftedahl, W., Grodstein, W., and Stampfer, M. J., A prospective study of plasma hormone levels, nonhormonal factors, and development of benign prostatic hyperplasia, *Prostate*, 26, 40, 1995.

40. Jones, J. A., Nguyen, A., and Straub, M., Use of DHEA in a patient with advanced prostate cancer: a case report and review, *Urology*, 50(5), 784, 1997.

41. Wallace, M. B., Lim, J., Cutler, A., and Bucci, L., Effects of dehydroepiandrosterone vs. androstenedione supplementation in men, *Med. Sci. Sport Exerc.*, 31(12), 1788, 1999.

42. Welle, S., Jozefowicz, R., and Statt, M., Failure of dehydroepiandrosterone to influence energy and protein metabolism in humans, *J. Clin. Endocrinol.*, 71(5), 1259, 1990.

43. Morales, A. J., Nolan, J. J., and Nelson, J. C., Effects of replacement dose dehydroepiandrosterone in men and women of advancing age, *J. Clin. Endocrinol. Metab.*, 78(6), 1360, 1994.
44. Yen, S. S., Morales, A. J., and Khorram, O., Replacement of DHEA in aging men and women: potential remedial effects, *Ann. N. Y. Acad. Sci.*, 774, 128, 1995.
45. Alen, M., Pakarinen, A., Hakkinen, K., and Komi, P. V., Responses of serum androgenic–anabolic and catabolic hormones to prolonged strength training, *Int. J. Sports Med.*, 9, 220, 1988.
46. Leder, B. Z., Loncope, C. L., Catline, D. H., Ahrens, B., Schomfeld, D. A., and Finkelstein, J. S., Oral androstenedione administration and serum testosterone concentrations in young men, *JAMA*, 283, 779, 2000.
47. Mastrogiacomo, I., Bonanni, G., Menegazzo, E., Santarossa, C., Pagani, E., Gennarelli, M., and Angeli, C., Clinical and hormonal aspects of male hypogonadism in myotonic dystrophy, *Ital. J. Neurol. Sci.*, 17, 59, 1996.
48. King, D. S., Sharp, R. L., Vukovich, M. C., Brown, G. A., Reifenrath, T. A., Uh, N. I., and Parsons, K. A., Effect of oral androstenedione on serum testosterone and adaptations to resistance training in young men: a randomized controlled trial, *JAMA*, 281, 2020, 1999.
49. Chaikovskii, V. S., Evtinova, I. V., and Basharina, O. B., Steroid levels and androgen receptors in skeletal muscles during adaptation to physical effort, *Vopr. Med. Khim.*, 31, 81, 1985.
50. Young, J., Couzinet, B., Nahoul, K., Brailly, S., Chanson, P., Baulier, E., and Schaison, G., Panhypopituitarism as a model to study the metabolism of dehydroepiandrosterone (DHEA) in humans, *J. Clin. Endocrinol. Metab.*, 82 (8), 2578, 1997.
51. Barrett-Connor, E., Khaw, K. T., and Yen, S. S., A prospective study of dehydroepiandrosterone sulfate, mortality, and cardiovascular disease, *N. Eng. J. Med.*, 315(24), 1519, 1986.
52. Barrett-Connor, E. and Goodman-Gruen, D., The epidemiology of DHEAS and cardiovascular disease, *Ann. N. Y. Acad. Sci.*, 774, 259, 1995.

8

Creatine Supplementation and the Strength Athlete

Jeff S. Volek

CONTENTS

8.1 Introduction

Many athletes have experimented with nutritional supplements in an effort to gain an edge on their competition. Scientists have not kept pace with the increasing number of nutritional supplements used by and marketed to athletes. While the effects of many dietary supplements remain uninvestigated, there continues to be widespread interest in creatine research. This chapter will explore the relatively significant body of literature on creatine supplementation accumulated over the last 7 years. Creatine metabolism and function will be overviewed prior to a discussion of the pertinent literature describing the effects of creatine supplementation on body composition, muscular strength, and physiological mechanisms. Emphasis will be placed on short-term creatine supplementation studies examining resistance-exercise performance and long-term weight-training studies examining body composition and muscular strength. The reader is referred to several other review papers on the effects of creatine supplementation on other types of high-intensity performance.[1-3] A brief discussion of possible side effects will conclude the chapter.

8.2. Creatine Background

8.2.1 Sources

Creatine is a natural component of the diet found primarily in animal products. Meat contains approximately 2 to 5 grams of creatine per kilogram. Average intake in omnivores is about 1 gram creatine per day. Creatine supplements are also manufactured in the laboratory, the most common form being creatine monohydrate. Creatine monohydrate is a tasteless and odorless white powder that is moderately soluble in water.

Although creatine can be obtained in the diet from meat products and supplements, our bodies also synthesize creatine. Creatine biosynthesis occurs primarily in the liver, pancreas, and kidney,[4] although nearly all the creatine is stored in skeletal muscle. Creatine biosynthesis is adequate to maintain normal muscle creatine levels without consumption of dietary sources. Thus, creatine is not considered a dietary essential nutrient. In the first step of the biosynthesis of creatine, a guanidino group from arginine is transferred to glycine forming guanidinoacetate. This first step is catalyzed by the enzyme transamidinase. A methyl group (CH_3) is then added to guanidinoacetate by the primary methyl-donor in the body, S-adenosylmethione, to form creatine. This second step is catalyzed by the enzyme methyltransferase.

8.2.2 Metabolism

Creatine from the diet is absorbed unchanged from the intestinal lumen directly into the bloodstream. Creatine synthesized in the liver is also released into the blood circulation. Creatine is transported in the blood to its primary storage site, skeletal muscle, where about 95% of the total creatine in the body is located. A specific sodium-dependent creatine transporter protein on the sarcolemma concentrates creatine in skeletal muscle,[5,6] thereby keeping blood creatine concentrations relatively low (<100 μmol/L). Once inside the sarcoplasm, the majority of creatine is phosphorylated to phosphocreatine, which requires hydrolysis of one molecule of ATP. The reaction is catalyzed by creatine kinase. Phosphocreatine accounts for about two thirds and free creatine one third of the total creatine concentration in resting skeletal muscle. The normal concentration of total creatine in skeletal muscle is 120 mmol/kg dry mass but ranges from about 100 to 140 mmol/kg depending on meat intake, muscle fiber type, training, age, and other unknown factors. Loss of muscle creatine occurs via an irreversible nonenzymatic conversion into creatinine at a relatively constant rate and amounts to about 2 grams per day in a 70-kg person. Thus, muscle creatine concentrations remain relatively stable and are not significantly influenced by intense exercise or other stressors. Creatinine is filtered in the kidney by simple diffusion, but not reabsorbed, and is eventually excreted in the urine.

8.2.3 Function

The final fuel for all muscular work is adenosine triphosphate (ATP), which is hydrolyzed during intense exercise resulting in ADP, inorganic phosphate, and energy for muscle contraction (Rx #1). The primary function of phosphocreatine is as a temporal energy buffer during periods of rapid ATP turnover, such as occurs during resistance exercise. Phosphocreatine participates in the reversible creatine kinase reaction that acts to replenish ATP during intense exercise and in the resynthesis of phosphocreatine during recovery (Rx #2).

$$\text{Rx \#1: ATP} \xrightarrow{\text{(ATPase)}} \text{ADP} + P_i + \text{Energy for muscle contraction}$$

$$\text{Rx \#2: PCr} + \text{ADP} + H^+ \xrightarrow{\text{(creatine kinase)}} \text{Cr} + \text{ATP}$$

Thus, the concentration of phosphocreatine decreases and free creatine increases with resistance exercise, but there is no change in total creatine. The creatine kinase reaction ensures a rapid method of replenishing ATP during intense exercise; however, phosphocreatine stores are relatively small and become depleted quickly during intense exercise (between 10 and 20 seconds). The advantage of using phosphocreatine as an energy source is that it is a very high-power energy system because it produces a large amount of ATP per unit time. Depletion of phosphocreatine coincides with a reduction in force/power output.[7] During recovery from intense exercise or sets of resistance exercise, phosphocreatine resynthesis is rapid, with a half-life of about 30 seconds; about 95% of phosphocreatine is resynthesized after only 3 to 4 minutes.[8] Although the storage capacity of creatine and phosphocreatine in skeletal muscle is small, recent evidence has clearly demonstrated that it can be increased through oral ingestion of the supplement creatine monohydrate.

8.3   Short-Term (<One Week) Supplementation

An important question to be answered regarding creatine supplementation was whether muscle total creatine concentrations could be increased. After evidence was obtained that muscle creatine stores could be increased rapidly, several studies then examined the potential for increased muscle creatine to augment different exercise protocols. These initial studies provide evidence that short-term (less than 1 week) creatine supplementation can help some types of high-intensity, short-duration activities.

8.3.1   Muscle Creatine

Almost a decade ago, a study was published documenting an effective strategy for increasing muscle creatine stores by ingesting large amounts of creatine monohydrate.[9] These researchers reasoned that if blood levels of creatine could be elevated above a certain threshold then perhaps a portion of the creatine might "spill over" into muscle. A 5-gram dose of creatine was determined to significantly elevate blood creatine concentrations peaking about 1 hour after ingestion and returning to baseline levels after 2 to 3 hours. In order to keep creatine elevated throughout the day, a 5-gram dosing regimen every 2 hours for 8 hours was adopted. This creatine dosing protocol, which was maintained for at least 2 days, resulted in significant increases in the total creatine content of the quadriceps femoris muscle. Subsequent studies have confirmed that this creatine dosing strategy is effective in increasing muscle creatine stores.[10–15] Increases in muscle total creatine range from 10 to 37%. The majority of creatine uptake occurs within the first 2 days, and muscle becomes saturated with creatine in less than 7 days at 20 to 25 g/day. The maximal amount of creatine appears to reside near 155 to 160 mmol/L dry muscle, which is attained within 5 to 6 days using this loading regimen.

Not all individuals respond to creatine supplementation by increasing muscle creatine stores, especially individuals with high initial levels.[9,13] Ingestion of a large amount of glucose with creatine during a 5-day loading regimen has been shown to reduce the variability in uptake between individuals and enhance intramuscular creatine accumulation.[12] The enhancement of muscle creatine accumulation in muscle when combined with the simple carbohydrate glucose is thought to be a result of carbohydrate-mediated insulin release. Insulin has been shown to stimulate sodium-dependent muscle creatine transport. Importantly, the amount of glucose consumed in this study was 370 g (almost 1500 kcal) for a daily 20-gram dose of creatine, which might not be advisable for athletes or palatable for some individuals. Subsequent research in humans using the euglycemic clamp technique, a technique that keeps glucose concentrations stable while different amounts of insulin are infused, has indeed shown that insulin can enhance creatine accumulation in muscle but only if insulin levels are present at extremely high or supraphysiological concentrations.[16]

In the initial study demonstrating that creatine supplementation was effective at increasing muscle creatine stores, the impact of exercise on muscle creatine accumulation was also addressed. Creatine supplementation combined with 1 hour of one-legged cycling resulted in a 25% increase in total muscle creatine in the nonexercised leg and a 37% increase in the exercised leg.[9] The authors concluded that regular intense exercise in conjunction with creatine supplementation augments creatine accumulation in the exercised muscles. A single bout of exercise was recently shown to augment subsequent creatine accumulation in the exercised muscle.[17] In this study, carbohydrate ingestion with the creatine also augmented glycogen concentrations in the exercised muscle, indicating a synergistic effect of creatine and carbohydrate on glycogen synthesis.

Since the majority of creatine in the human body is stored within skeletal muscle, arguments have been made that creatine should be consumed relative to body weight or lean body mass (LBM). A common recommendation is 0.3 grams creatine per kilogram body weight.[14] This dose was derived from studies that measured muscle creatine stores in subjects weighing approximately 80 kg and supplemented with a dose of 20 grams per day (20 g creatine/day divided by 80 kg = 0.3 g creatine/kg). While valid in theory, studies have not been performed to confirm whether 0.3 g creatine/kg is effective in individuals with a body weight significantly less than or greater than 80 kg.

8.3.2 Body Composition

The vast majority of short-term creatine loading studies show a significant increase or a small nonsignificant increase in body weight up to about 1.5 to 2.0 kg. This is most likely due to increased retention of body water. Since creatine accumulates in muscle, the opinion of most researchers is that water is accumulating inside the cell, and there is some evidence to support this contention.[18,19]

A recent study reported that creatine supplementation (20 g/day for 5 days) significantly increased body weight (1.6 kg) and LBM (1.4 kg) using dual-energy X-ray absorptiometry (DEXA) in men.[20] Our laboratory recently reported that creatine supplementation (25 g/day for 7 days) significantly increased body weight (1.7 kg) and LBM (1.5 kg) as measured by hydrostatic weighing in men.[15] Thus, at least some of the increase in body weight with acute supplementation could be LBM in addition to water. Because there are limitations in the methods available to detect small changes in LBM and water compartments, any conclusions must be viewed with caution.

8.3.3   Strength Performance

A large number of studies have examined the effects of creatine supplementation on different types of exercise including cycling, running, sprinting, jumping, swimming, and rowing protocols. This section will focus only on studies that examined the acute effects of creatine on muscular strength during resistance exercise protocols. The vast majority of research to date has utilized young men as subjects. However, a sufficient number of projects have utilized women as subjects and indicate that women can also benefit from creatine supplementation. Strength is obviously important to performance of many sports and daily life activities. Increased maximal strength is the reason many individuals use creatine. The effect of typical creatine loading regimens has been examined using isometric,[21–23] isokinetic,[22,24–27] and isotonic[15,28] muscle actions.

Greenhaff et al.[26] had subjects perform an isokinetic protocol consisting of 5 sets of 30 unilateral knee extensions at a constant angular velocity of 180°/second with 1 minute of recovery between each bout. Creatine-supplemented subjects were able to significantly reduce the decline in muscle peak torque production during bouts 2, 3, and 4. Using a similar isokinetic protocol of 5 sets and 30 repetitions, Gilliam et al.[24] reported no beneficial effect of creatine supplementation. Work from our laboratory indicates that muscular performance is enhanced during high-intensity resistance exercise.[28] The testing protocol consisted of 5 sets of bench press using a 10-repetition maximum load and 5 sets of 10 repetitions of squat jumps using 30% of the 1-repetition maximum with 2 minutes recovery between all sets. Creatine-supplemented subjects performed significantly more repetitions during all 5 sets of bench press (Figure 8.1) and achieved significantly higher peak power outputs during all 5 sets of squat jumps (Figure 8.2) after one week of supplementation.

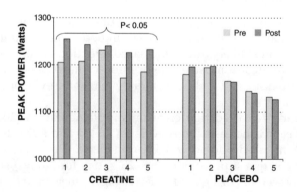

FIGURE 8.1

Total number of bench press repetitions performed during 5 sets using a 10 repetition maximum load before (Pre) and after (Post) 7 days of creatine (25 g/day) or placebo supplementation. (Data from Volek, J. S., Kraemer, W. J., Bush, J. A., Boetes, M., Incledon, T., Clark, K. I., and Lynch, J. M., Creatine supplementation enhances muscular performance during high intensity resistance exercise, *J. Am. Diet. Assoc.*, 97, 765, 1997.)

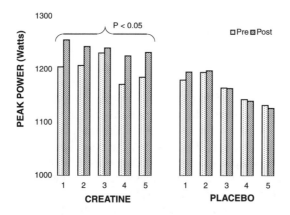

FIGURE 8.2

Peak power output during 5 sets of squat jumps using 30% of the 1 repetition maximum before (Pre) and after (Post) 7 days of creatine (25 g/day) or placebo supplementation. (Data from Volek, J. S., Kraemer, W. J., Bush, J. A., Boetes, M., Incledon, T., Clark, K. I., and Lynch, J. M., Creatine supplementation enhances muscular performance during high intensity resistance exercise, *J. Am. Diet. Assoc.*, 97, 765, 1997.)

There are limited data on the effect of short-term creatine supplementation on 1-repetition maximum strength. We recently reported that 1 week of creatine supplementation slightly increased maximal squat (4.1%) and maximal bench press (5.4%) strength in moderately trained men.[15]

8.3.4   Mechanisms

The ability of creatine supplementation to enhance short-term maximal exercise is hypothesized to be due to an increased availability of muscle creatine that can buffer the rapid accumulation of ADP resulting from ATP hydrolysis, especially in fast type II muscle fibers.[11] The increased availability of muscle creatine allows higher force/power outputs because of a better match between ATP supply and ATP demand as indicated by reduced adenine nucleotide degradation following brief maximal exercise.[29–31] An increase in the rate of phosphocreatine resynthesis during recovery may also benefit high-intensity intermittent exercise protocols by allowing higher phosphocreatine levels at the onset of exercise.[13] However, a recent study provided evidence that phosphocreatine resynthesis was not enhanced after creatine supplementation.[32] Another theory to explain improved performance after creatine supplementation is a decrease in relaxation time, the time needed for a muscle to relax after a contraction.[23] The small increases in 1 RM strength are difficult to explain after short-term creatine supplementation but may be due to functional or biomechanical advantages associated with increased body weight or LBM.

8.4   Long-term (>One Week) Supplementation

8.4.1   Muscle Creatine

Numerous studies indicate that acute creatine loading elevates muscle creatine concentrations. However there is less data on appropriate doses of creatine to maintain elevated creatine stores. While the majority of studies have utilized a "loading" dose of 20 grams creatine per day for 5 to 7 days to rapidly increase muscle creatine stores, consuming lower doses for a longer period of time may also be effective. Ingestion of 3 grams creatine per day for 28 days resulted in a similar increase in muscle creatine concentrations (approximately 20%) compared to a group of subjects supplemented with 20 grams per day for 7 days.[14] Thus, muscle creatine stores can be increased rapidly by consuming 20 grams per day for 6 days or slowly by consuming 3 grams per day for 4 weeks. Consuming less than 3 grams per day may not result in increased muscle creatine uptake. Ingestion of 2 grams of creatine per day for 6 weeks failed to alter muscle phosphocreatine concentrations at rest, during exercise, and recovery from exercise in athletic women.[33]

The majority of studies that have measured muscle creatine stores in response to creatine supplementation have been short-term (less than 1 week) so there is some uncertainty as to the appropriate creatine dose necessary to retain elevated muscle creatine stores after a loading phase. In an average healthy person, approximately 2 grams of creatine are broken down and excreted in the urine per day. In one of the first studies to address maintenance doses, the effects of replacing the normal breakdown of creatine (2 grams) were examined. After a 6-day creatine loading regimen of 20 grams per day, a group of sedentary subjects maintained elevated creatine stores for 1 month while consuming only 2 grams per day.[14] A similar group, who stopped consuming creatine after the loading protocol, slowly reached muscle creatine levels that were not significantly different from baseline values in 4 weeks.[14] This study demonstrates that elevated muscle creatine stores decline at a relatively slow rate after discontinuing creatine supplementation and can be offset by consuming just 2 grams per day. In another study, a daily 5-gram creatine dose following an initial loading dose was sufficient to maintain elevated muscle phosphocreatine stores in untrained women who participated in a 10-week resistance-training program.[34] A 5-gram maintenance dose following an initial loading dose resulted in a small decline in muscle creatine in moderately trained men during 12 weeks of intense resistance training.[15] No studies have been performed to corroborate this finding in athletes training intensely.

As was the case for loading doses of creatine, a maintenance dose has also been recommended relative to body weight. Since 2 grams per day were adequate to maintain elevated muscle creatine stores in individuals weighing approximately 80 kg, a maintenance dose of 0.03 g creatine per kg body weight might be appropriate (2 g creatine/day divided by 80 kg = 0.03 g creatine/kg/day). Once again, this maintenance dose has not been validated in athletes of different body sizes performing different training programs. An ideal maintenance dose may prove elusive based on individual differences in diet composition and meat intake, muscle fiber type distribution, gender, age, and initial total muscle creatine concentrations. Furthermore, creatine requirements may be altered depending on the specific training regimen, exercise configurations, and training adaptation of interest, such as increased muscular strength, speed, or lean body mass. At present however, a maintenance dose of 2 to 5 grams per day seems appropriate.

8.4.2   Body Composition and Strength Performance

Increased lean body mass (LBM) and muscular strength are primary goals of many individuals using creatine and performing weight training. More recently, several studies have examined the effect of creatine supplementation on changes in body composition and muscular strength in response to different weight-training programs. Since the majority of these studies determined body composition and muscular strength, both these responses will be discussed together. Table 8.1 summarizes the effects of long-term creatine supplementation and resistance-training studies on LBM and muscular strength.

The majority of creatine supplementation and training studies have used recreational weight-trained men between 18 and 30 years, although one study reported positive effects on LBM and muscular strength in untrained women.[34] Long-term studies involved resistance training only or resistance training in combination with sprint/agility workouts for 14 to 84 days. Supplementation generally consisted of a loading dose of creatine (15 to 25 g/days) for 5 to 7 days followed by a maintenance dose (2 to 10 g/day) or the same loading dose for the remainder of the training. One study examined creatine with other supplements[35] and is not included. Body composition has been assessed using skin folds, hydrostatic weighing, and dual-energy X-ray absorptiometry (DEXA). Strength testing has typically used 1 RM testing of large muscle group (bench press and squat) and smaller muscle group (preacher curl and leg extensions) exercises. In addition, isokinetic testing and number of repetitions performed using a standard weight (e.g., 70% or 85% of 1 RM) have been evaluated.

In terms of body composition, several studies have shown increases in LBM up to 5.3 kg. Creatine supplementation resulted in larger numerical increases in LBM compared to placebo in every study, with the exception of a study in elderly men and women 67 to 80 years.[36] Our laboratory recently reported that creatine supplementation during 12 weeks of periodized heavy resistance training resulted in significantly greater increases in LBM, which corresponded with significantly greater muscle fiber hypertrophy compared to placebo.[15] None of the long-term creatine supplementation studies have reported any significant effect of creatine on fat mass.

TABLE 8.1 Effects of Long-Term Creatine Supplementation and Resistance Training on Lean Body Mass (LBM) and Strength

Reference	Days	Loading	Maintenance	Method	LBM Change Cr	LBM Change PI	Strength Testing	Change (%) Cr	Change (%) PI
Becque et al. (54)	42	5 d @ 20 g/d	37 d @ 2 g/d	HW	1.6	−0.1	1 RM preacher curl	30	17
Berman et al. (36)	52	5 d @ 20 g/d	47 d @ 3 g/d	SF	0.0	0.4	1 RM chest press	17	12
							12 RM chest press	19	12
							1 RM leg press	17	10
							12 RM leg press	16	20
							1 RM leg extension	19	17
							12 RM leg extension	16	18
Earnest et al. (55)	28	20 g/d		HW	1.6	−0.5	1 RM bench press	6	−2
							Reps @ 70% 1 RM	35	0
Francaux & Poortmans (18)	42	5 d @ 21 g/d	37 d @ 3 g/d	N/A	N/A	N/A	1 RM isokinetic squat	7	6
Kelly et al. (56)	25	5 d @ 20 g/d	20 d @ 5 g/d	SF	2.5	?NS	3 RM bench press	8	2
							Reps @ 85% 1 RM	40	7
Kirksey et al. (57)	42	0.3 g/kg BM/d	0.3 g/kg BM/d	HW	2.6	1.0	Vertical jump	7	2
Kreider et al. (48)	28	15.75 g/d	15.75 g/d	DEXA	2.4	1.3	Bench press volume @ 4-8 RM	Sig	NS
							Squat volume @ 4-8 RM	NS	NS
							Power clean volume @ 4-8 RM	NS	NS
							Total volume	Sig	NS
Noonan et al. (58)	56	5 d @ 20 g/d	51 d @ 0.1 g/kg LBM	HW	3.2	1.5	1 RM bench press	6	1
Noonan et al. (58)	56	5 d @ 20 g/d	51 d @ 0.3 g/kg LBM	HW	2.2	1.5	1 RM bench press	6	1
Pearson et al. (59)	70	5 g/d	5 g/d	SF	0.3	−1.3	1 RM bench press	3	−1
							1 RM squat	11	5
							1 RM power clean	6	−2
Peeters et al. (46)	42	3 d @ 20 g/d	38 d @ 10 g/d	SF	2.7	0.2	1 RM bench press	10	1
							1 RM leg press	12	9
							Curl reps @ 8-10 RM	106	97
Peeters et al. (46)	42	3 d @ 20 g/d	38 d @ 10 g/d	SF	2.2	0.2	1 RM bench press	8	1

Study		Loading	Maintenance				Measure		
Rawson et al. (39)	30	10 d @ 20 g/d	20 d @ 10 g/d	HW	0.6	0.1	1RM leg press	11	9
							Curl reps @ 8–10 RM	120	97
							1 RM isometric preacher curl	32	2
Stone et al. (60)	35	0.22 g/kg BM/d	0.22 g/kg BM/d	HW	5.3	2.0	1 RM bench press		
							1 RM squat		
Stone et al. (60)	35	0.09 g/kg BM/d	0.09 g/kg BM/d	HW	2.9		1 RM bench press		
							1 RM squat		
Vandenberghe et al. (34)	74	4 d @ 20 g/d	70 d @ 5 g/d	HW	2.6	1.6	1 RM bench press	45	38
							1 RM squat	46	25
							1 RM leg press	43	25
							1 RM leg curl	63	39
							1 RM leg extension	85	57
							1 RM shoulder press	31	24
Volek et al. (15)	84	7 d @ 25 g/d	77 d@ 5 g/d	HW	4.3	2.1	1 RM bench press	24	16
							1 RM squat	32	24

# Creatine phosphate
LBM = lean body mass
HW = hydrostatic weighting
SF = skin folds
DEXA = dual-energy X-ray absorptiometry

A few long-term creatine studies have used swim training instead of weight training.[33,37,38] These studies indicate no significant increase in LBM. Thus, weight training should be an integral part of the training program during long-term supplementation if gains in LBM are desired. The majority of evidence does indicate weight training in conjunction with long-term creatine supplementation results in greater gains in LBM. Although increases in LBM are greater with supplementation, the differences are often not excessively larger than gains in the placebo group.

Eight studies have examined the effects of creatine supplementation on 1 RM bench press strength and indicate significant increases ranging from 3 to 45%. Eight studies assessed 1 RM squat or leg press strength and indicate significant increases ranging from 7 to 46%. Preacher curl and leg extension/leg curl 1 RM strength has also been shown to improve with creatine supplementation (30 to 85%). Larger increases have been reported after creatine supplementation in total repetitions performed using a standard weight and range from 16 to 120%. In all studies, the increases in strength were numerically greater in creatine compared to placebo subjects with the exception of a study in elderly men and women 67 to 80 years.[36] Creatine supplementation failed to enhance performance and body composition in elderly men 60 to 82 years[39] and elderly men and women 67 to 80 years[36] during resistance training for 30 and 52 days, respectively, indicating supplementation may be ineffective in elderly subjects.

8.4.3 Mechanisms

The mechanisms linking long-term creatine supplementation to improvements in body composition and strength are more diverse. One theory is that creatine supplementation enhances the intensity of individual resistance exercise workouts,[28] which over time augments muscle strength and body composition responses to resistance training.[15] There is some indication creatine is involved in protein metabolism in differentiating skeletal muscle cells;[40] however, no studies have measured protein synthesis or degradation after creatine supplementation in humans. It has also been suggested that muscle creatine accumulation causes water to move into cells in order to maintain a constant osmolality between the intracellular and extracellular fluid compartments. This accumulation of water in cells or "cellular swelling" is believed to be an anabolic stimulus and promote protein synthesis and a positive nitrogen balance.[41] Once again, no studies have determined if an increase in intracellular water due to creatine supplementation has an influence on skeletal muscle protein synthesis. Hormonal mechanisms are also not a likely mechanism by which creatine enhances performance or muscle mass.[42] Total testosterone, free testosterone, cortisol, sex hormone binding globulin, growth hormone, and insulin-like growth factor-I concentrations were not altered after 12 weeks of creatine supplementation and resistance training (unpublished observations). The exact mechanism(s) responsible for the greater increases in muscular strength and LBM in subjects supplementing with creatine and performing resistance exercise is unclear and requires further research.

8.5 Side Effects

The widespread use of creatine by athletes has led to concerns about potential side effects. Despite a large number of creatine supplementation studies, there is no evidence that supplementation has any serious adverse health effects.

Short-term creatine supplementation has no effect on heart rate at rest or during exercise,[43,44] even when performed in a high heat/humidity environment.[45] There does not appear to be any effect of long-term creatine supplementation on either diastolic or systolic blood pressure.[20,46] Ejection fraction assessed via echocardiography was not affected after creatine supplementation in patients suffering from chronic heart failure.[25] Plasma volume changes during exercise in the heat are not altered with creatine supplementation.[45] Thus, creatine supplementation does not appear to affect the cardiovascular system.

There is some indication creatine supplementation may improve blood lipids. One study demonstrated that creatine supplementation had a positive effect on the blood lipid profiles of physically active middle-aged subjects with total cholesterol concentrations exceeding 200 mg/dL.[47] This study showed that 8 weeks of creatine supplementation reduced plasma total cholesterol (–5%), VLDL-cholesterol (–22%), and triglycerides (–22%). Another study demonstrated that 4 weeks of creatine supplementation in conjunction with an exercise program consisting of resistance exercises and agility/sprint conditioning increased HDL-cholesterol (13%) and reduced VLDL-cholesterol (–13%) in collegiate football players.[48] These findings are in contrast to work in our laboratory where we have not observed any impact of creatine loading (1 week) or long-term supplementation during 12 weeks of heavy resistance training on blood lipids and lipoproteins in healthy moderately trained men.[49]

Short-term oral creatine supplementation (20 g/day for 5 days) does not adversely affect several measures of renal function including glomerular filtration rate and protein and albumin excretion rates in healthy men.[50] Serum and urinary creatine are increased when large amounts of creatine are ingested,[34,50,51] but creatinine is only slightly elevated, within normal ranges, with ingestion of 20 grams per day[20,50,51] or when a 5-gram maintenance dose is consumed for 10 to 12 weeks.[15,34] There is little reason to believe creatine supplementation in healthy adults over a long period of time poses any threat to normal kidney function. In fact, a recent report indicated that compared to controls, athletes consuming creatine (2 to 30 g per day) for

10 months to 5 years demonstrated no differences in plasma concentrations or urine excretion rates for creatinine, urea, and albumin.[52] Further, glomerular filtration rates, tubular reabsorption, and glomerular permeability were normal, indicating no adverse affects of long-term creatine use on renal function.[52] Thus, there is little evidence supplementation will result in renal problems in healthy individuals.

When large doses of creatine are consumed in the diet, synthesis in the body is reduced[4] but returns to normal when creatine is removed from the diet.[14,53] Chronic use of creatine may also result in downregulation of the expression of creatine transporter isoforms in skeletal muscle.[5] This also appears to be reversible when creatine supplementation is discontinued. Thus, there is little evidence indicating that discontinuing creatine will negatively affect the normal production of creatine in the body.

In summary, acute creatine supplementation has been shown to be medically safe in healthy persons. There is insufficient data concerning the potential effects of creatine supplementation over long periods of time to conclude supplementation will have negative health effects. More research is needed in both animal and human studies to thoroughly evaluate any potential deleterious side effects. At this point in time, however, there is no reason to believe creatine supplementation in healthy adults poses any threat to normal physiological functioning.

8.6   Summary

Resistance training is a fundamental component of training programs for a variety of athletes. Much of the research examining creatine supplementation has focused on acute and chronic resistance exercise performance and body composition responses. Muscle creatine concentrations can be increased rapidly in the majority of individuals, and this usually enhances the ability to perform multiple repetitions at a given weight or prevent the normal decline in power; there is less of a benefit on maximal strength. Long-term creatine supplementation and resistance-training studies indicate greater increases in LBM, maximal strength of large and small muscle groups, and fatigue resistance during multiple repetition tests with a standard weight. Creatine supplementation appears to be a safe and legal method to augment muscle mass and muscle strength adaptations to weight training.

References

1. Balsom, P. D., Söderlund, K., and Ekblom, B., Creatine in humans with special reference to creatine supplementation, *Sports Med.*, 18, 268, 1994.
2. Volek, J. S. and Kraemer, W. J., Creatine supplementation: Its effect on human muscular performance and body composition, *J. Str. Cond. Res.*, 10, 200, 1996.
3. Williams, M. H. and Branch, J. D., Creatine supplementation and exercise performance: an update, *J. Am. Coll. Nutr.*, 17, 216, 1998.
4. Walker, J. B., Creatine: biosynthesis, regulation, and function, *Adv. Enzym.*, 50, 177, 1979.
5. Guerrero-Ontiveros, M. L. and Wallimann, T., Creatine supplementation in health and disease. Effects of chronic creatine ingestion *in vivo*: down-regulation of the expression of creatine transporter isoforms in skeletal muscle, *Mol. Cell. Biochem.*, 184, 427, 1998.
6. Loike, J. D., Zalutsky, D. L., Kaback, E., Miranda, A. F., and Silverstein, S. C., Extracellular creatine regulates creatine transport in rat and human muscle cells, *Proc. Nat. Acad. Sci. USA*, 85, 807, 1988.
7. Hultman, E., Bergström, J., and McLennan Anderson, N., Breakdown and resynthesis of adenosine triphosphate in connection with muscular work in man, *Scand. J. Clin. Lab. Invest.*, 19, 56, 1967.
8. Harris, R. C., Edwards, R. H. T., Hultman, E., Nordesjo, L.-O., Nylind, B., and Sahlin, K., The time course of phosphorylcreatine resynthesis during recovery of the quadriceps muscle in man, *Pflugers Arch.*, 367, 137, 1976.
9. Harris, R. C., Söderlund, K., and Hultman, E., Elevation of creatine in resting and exercised muscle of normal subjects by creatine supplementation, *Clin. Sci.*, 83, 367, 1992.
10. Balsom, P. D., Söderlund, K., Sjodin, B., and Ekblom, B., Skeletal muscle metabolism during short duration high-intensity exercise: influence of creatine supplementation, *Acta Physiol. Scand.*, 154, 303, 1995.
11. Casey, A., Constantin-Teodosiu, D., Howell, S., Hultman, E., and Greenhaff, P. L., Creatine ingestion favorably affects performance and muscle metabolism during maximal exercise in humans, *Am. J. Physiol.*, 271, E31, 1996.
12. Green, A. L., Hultman, E., MacDonald, I. A., Sewell, D. A., and Greenhaff, P. L., Carbohydrate ingestion augments skeletal muscle creatine accumulation during creatine supplementation in humans, *Am. J. Physiol.*, 271, E821, 1996.
13. Greenhaff, P. L., Bodin, K., Söderlund, K., and Hultman, E., Effect of oral creatine supplementation on skeletal muscle phosphocreatine resynthesis, *Am. J. Physiol.*, 266, E725, 1994.
14. Hultman, E., Söderlund, K., Timmons, J. A., Cederblad, G., and Greenhaff, P. L., Muscle creatine loading in men, *J. Appl. Physiol.*, 81, 232, 1996.
15. Volek, J. S., Duncan, N. D., Mazzetti, S. A., Putukian, M., Staron, R., Putukian, M., Gómez, A. L., Pearson, D. R., Fink, W. J., and Kraemer, W. J., Performance and muscle fiber adaptations to creatine supplementation and heavy resistance training, *Med. Sci. Sports Exerc.*, 31, 1147, 1999.
16. Steenge, G. R., Lambourne, J., Casey, A., MacDonald, A., and Greenhaff, P. L., Stimulatory effect of insulin on creatine accumulation in human skeletal muscle, *Am. J. Physiol.*, 275, E974, 1998.

17. Robinson, T. M., Sewell, D. A., Hultman, E., and Greenhaff, P. L., Role of submaximal exercise in promoting creatine and glycogen accumulation in human skeletal muscle, *J. Appl. Physiol.*, 87, 598, 1999.
18. Francaux, M. and Poortmans, J. R., Effects of training and creatine supplement on muscle strength and body mass, *Eur. J. Appl. Physiol.*, 80, 165, 1999.
19. Ziegenfuss, T., Lowery, L. M., and Lemon, P. W. R., Acute fluid volume changes in men during three days of creatine supplementation, *J. Exerc. Physiol. Online*, 1, 1998.
20. Mihic, S., MacDonald, J. R., McKenzie, S., and Tarnopolsky, M. A., Acute creatine loading increases fat-free mass, but does not affect blood pressure, plasma creatine, or CK activity in men and women, *Med. Sci. Sports Exerc.*, 32, 291, 2000.
21. Urbanski, R. L., Loy, S. F., Vincent, W. J., and Yaspeelkis, B. B., Creatine supplementation differentially effects maximal isometric strength and time to fatigue in large and small muscle groups, *Int. J. Sport Nutr.*, 9, 136, 1999.
22. Vandenberghe, K., Gillis, N., Van Leemputte, M., Van Hecke, P., Vanstapel, F., and Hespel, P., Caffeine counteracts the ergogenic action of muscle creatine loading, *J. Appl. Physiol.*, 80, 452, 1996.
23. Van Leemputte, M., Vandenberghe, K., and Hespel, P., Shortening of muscle relaxation time after creatine loading, *J. Appl. Physiol.*, 86, 840, 1999.
24. Gilliam, J. D., Hohzorn, C., Martin, D., and Trimble, M. H., Effect of oral creatine supplementation on isokinetic torque production, *Med. Sci. Sports Exerc.*, 32, 993, 2000.
25. Gordon, A., Hultman, E., Kaijser, L., Kristjannsson, S., Rolf, C. J., Nyquist, O., and Sylven, C., Creatine supplementation in chronic heart failure increases skeletal muscle creatine phosphate and muscle performance, *Cardio. Res.*, 30, 413, 1995.
26. Greenhaff, P. L., Casey, A., Short, A. H., Harris, R., Söderlund, K., and Hultman, E., Influence of oral creatine supplementation on muscle torque during repeated bouts of maximal voluntary exercise in man, *Clin. Sci.*, 84, 565, 1993.
27. Vandebuerie, F., Vanden Eynde, B., Vandenberghe, K., and Hespel, P., Effect of creatine loading on endurance capacity and sprint power in cyclists, *Int. J. Sports Med.*, 19, 490, 1998.
28. Volek, J. S., Kraemer, W. J., Bush, J. A., Boetes, M., Incledon, T., Clark, K. I., and Lynch, J. M., Creatine supplementation enhances muscular performance during high intensity resistance exercise, *J. Am. Diet. Assoc.*, 97, 765, 1997.
29. Balsom, P. D., Ekblom, B., Söderlund, K., Sjodin, B., and Hultman, E., Creatine supplementation and dynamic high-intensity intermittent exercise, *Scan. J. Med. Sci. Sports*, 3, 143, 1993.
30. Birch, R., Nobel, D., and Greenhaff, P. L., The influence of dietary creatine supplementation on performance during repeated bouts of maximal isokinetic cycling in man, *Eur. J. Appl. Physiol.*, 69, 268, 1994.
31. Mujika, I., Chatard, J-C., Lacoste, L., Barale, F., and Geyssant, A., Creatine supplementation does not improve sprint performance in competitive swimmers, *Med. Sci. Sports Exerc.*, 28, 1435, 1996.
32. Vandenberghe, K., Van Hecke, P., Van Leemputte, M., Vanstapel, F., and Hespel, P., Phosphocreatine resynthesis is not affected by creatine loading, *Med. Sci. Sports Exerc.*, 31, 236, 1999.

33. Thompson, C. H., Kemp, G. J., Sanderson, A. L., Dixon, R. M., Styles, P., Taylor, D. J., and Radda, G. K., Effect of creatine on aerobic and anaerobic metabolism and skeletal muscle in swimmers, *Br. J. Sports Med.*, 30, 222, 1996.

34. Vandenberghe, K., Goris, M., Van Hecke, P., Van Leemputte, M., Vangerven, L., and Hespel, P., Long-term creatine intake is beneficial to muscle performance during resistance training, *J. Appl. Physiol.*, 83, 2055, 1997.

35. Krieder, R. B., Klesges, R., Harmon, K., Grindstaff, P., Ramsey, L., Bullen, D., Wood, L., Li, Y., and Almada, A., Effects of ingesting supplements designed to promote lean tissue accretion on body composition during resistance training, *Int. J. Sport Nutr.*, 6, 234, 1996.

36. Bermon, S. P., Venembre, Sachet, C., Valour, S., and Dolisi, C., Effects of creatine monohydrate ingestion in sedentary and weight-trained older adults, *Acta Physiol. Scand.*, 164, 147, 1998.

37. Grindstaff, P. D., Krieder, R., Bishop, R., Wilson, M., Wood, L., Alexander, C., and Almada, A., Effects of creatine supplementation on repetitive sprint performance and body composition in competitive swimmers, *Int. J. Sport Nutr.*, 7, 330, 1997.

38. Leenders, N., Sherman, W. M., Lamb, D. R., and Nelson, T. E., Creatine supplementation and swimming performance, *Int. J. Sport Nutr.*, 9, 251, 1999.

39. Rawson, E. S., Wehnert, M. L., and Clarkson, P. M., Effects of 30 days of creatine ingestion in older men, *Eur. J. Appl. Physiol.*, 80, 139, 1999.

40. Ingwall, J. S., Morales, M. F., and Stockdale, F. E., Creatine and the control of myosin synthesis in differentiating skeletal muscle, *Proc. Nat. Acad. Sci.*, 69, 2250, 1972.

41. Haussinger, D., Roth, E., Lang, F., and Gerok, W., Cellular hydration state: an important determinant of protein catabolism in health and disease, *Lancet*, 341, 1330, 1993.

42. Volek, J. S., Boetes, M., Bush, J. A., and Kraemer, W. J., Testosterone and cortisol response to high-intensity resistance exercise following creatine monohydrate supplementation, *J. Str. Cond. Res.*, 11, 182, 1997.

43. Peyrebrune, M. C., Nevill, M. E., Donaldson, F. J., and Cosford, D. J., The effects of oral creatine supplementation on performance in single and repeated sprint swimming, *J. Sports Sci.*, 16, 271, 1998.

44. Stroud, M. A., Holliman, D., Bell, D., Green, A. L., MacDonald, I. A., and Greenhaff, P. L., Effect of oral creatine supplementation on respiratory gas exchange and blood lactate accumulation during steady-state incremental treadmill exercise and recovery in man, *Clin. Sci.*, 87, 707, 1994.

45. Volek, J. S., Mazzetti, S. A., Farquhar, W. B., Barnes, B. R., Gómez, A. L., and Kraemer W. J., Physiological responses to exercise in the heat after creatine supplementation, *Med. Sci. Sports Exerc.*, in review.

46. Peeters, B. M., Lantz, C. D., and Mayhew, J. L., Effect of oral creatine monohydrate and creatine phosphate supplementation on maximal strength indices, body composition, and blood pressure, *J. Str. Cond. Res.*, 13, 3, 1999.

47. Earnest, C. P., Almada, A., and Mitchell, T. L., High-performance capillary electrophoresis-pure creatine monohydrate reduces blood lipids in men and women, *Clin. Sci.*, 91, 113, 1996.

48. Kreider, R. B., Ferreira, M., Wilson, M., Grindstaff, P. A., Plisk, S., Reinardy, J., Cantler, E., and Alamada, A. L., Effects of creatine supplementation on body composition, strength, and sprint performance, *Med. Sci. Sports Exerc.*, 30, 73, 1998.

49. Volek, J. S., Duncan, N. D., Mazzetti, S. A., Putukian, M., Gómez, A. L., and Kraemer, W. J., No effect of heavy resistance training and creatine supplementation on blood lipids, *Int. J. Sports Exerc. Metab.,* 10, 144, 2000.

50. Poortmans, J. R., Auquier, H., Renaut, V., Durassel, A., Saugy, M., and Brisson, G. R., Effect of short-term creatine supplementation on renal responses in men, *Eur. J. Appl. Physiol.,* 76, 566, 1997.

51. Kamber, M., Koster, K., Kreis, R., Walker, G., Boesch, C., and Hoppler H., Creatine supplementation—Part I: performance, clinical chemistry, and muscle volume, *Med. Sci. Sports Exerc.,* 31, 1763, 1999.

52. Poortmans, J. R. and Francaux, M., Long-term oral creatine supplementation does not impair renal function in healthy athletes, *Med. Sci. Sports Exerc.,* 31, 1108, 1999.

53. Walker, J. B., Metabolic control of creatine biosynthesis. Restoration of transamidinase activity following creatine repression, *J. Biol. Chem.,* 236, 493, 1961.

54. Becque, M. D., Lochmann, J. D., and Melrose, D. R., Effects of oral creatine supplementation on muscular strength and body composition, *Med. Sci. Sports Exerc.,* 32, 654, 2000.

55. Earnest, C. P., Snell, P. G., Rodriguez, R., Almada, A. L., and Mitchell, T. L., The effect of creatine monohydrate ingestion on anaerobic power indices, muscular strength and body composition, *Acta Physiol. Scand.,* 153, 207, 1995.

56. Kelly, V. G. and Jenkins, D. G., Effect of oral creatine supplementation on nearmaximal strength and repeated sets of high-intensity bench press exercise, *J. Str. Cond. Res.,* 12, 109, 1998.

57. Kirksey, K. B., Stone, M. H., Warren, B. J., Johnson, R. L., Stone, M., Haff, G. G., Williams, F. E., and Proulx, C., The effects of 6 weeks of creatine monohydrate supplementation on performance measures and body composition in collegiate track and field athletes, *J. Str. Cond. Res.,* 13, 148, 1999.

58. Noonan, D., Berg, K., Latin, R. W., Wagner, J. C., and Reimers, K., Effects of varying dosages of oral creatine relative to fat free body mass on strength and body composition, *J. Str. Cond. Res.,* 12:104, 1998.

59. Pearson, D. R., Hamby, D. G., Russel, W., and Harris, T., Long-term effects of creatine monohydrate on strength and power, *J. Str. Cond. Res.,* 13, 187, 1999.

60. Stone, M. H., Sanborn, K., Smith, L. L., O'Bryant, H. S., Hoke, T., Utter, A. C., Johnson, R. L., Boros, R., Hruby, J., Pierce, K. C., Stone, M. E., and Garner, B., Effects of in-season (5 weeks) creatine and pyruvate supplementation on anaerobic performance and body composition in American football players, *Int. J. Sport Nutr.,* 9, 140, 1999.

9

Supporting the Immune System: Nutritional Considerations for the Strength Athlete

Shawn R. Simonson

CONTENTS

9.1 Introduction

The human body is a complex interaction of multiple systems, all working together to maintain homeostasis. It is impossible to discuss a single organ or organ system without considering its impact on other physiological systems. This is especially true for the effects of nutrition and strength training. Much of the impact of strength training is mediated through the endocrine and nervous systems, which are intricately linked with the immune system. It has been suggested that a single term, neuroendocrineimmunology, be used to show the essential integration of the three disciplines.[1] The immune cells are affected by many hormones, such as cortisol and epinephrine, and produce their own class of hormones, the cytokines. Some hormones, including those that have an immunological impact, also serve as neurotransmitters (i.e., norepinephrine). The immune system also plays a critical role in the adaptive response to strength training, specifically in the healing and recovery process after strenuous exercise.

The immune system is also quite responsive to nutrition, as all organ systems are. Strength training can be a stressful activity and perhaps dietary intervention can reduce the impact of this stress on the body's defense mechanisms. Thus, a discussion of the nutritional considerations for strength training is incomplete if the immune system is not mentioned.

9.2 Immune Response to Resistance Conditioning

9.2.1 Role of the Immune System

The immune system plays a significant role in the adaptation to exercise. Exercise-induced muscle damage must be repaired, and it is the immune cells (leukocytes) that handle this detail. Neutrophils arrive at the injured tissue first and clean up the damaged area by phagocytosing cellular debris and releasing cytokines and free radicals.[2–4] Macrophages are slower to arrive and assist in the clean-up process and attract and stimulate, by releasing chemotactants and growth factors, muscle precursor cells to initiate reconstruction.[2,4–6] Without macrophage infiltration, healing and reversal of the degenerative process do not occur.[2] Lymphocytes will eventually migrate to the damaged area and provide additional free radicals, cytokines, and growth factors.[5]

Unfortunately, the leukocytes can be overzealous and break down neighboring healthy tissue and create local inflammation.[2,4,5] It has been hypothesized that overuse injuries, such as those seen in repeated bouts of strength training, may be a result of insufficient healing time, leading to chronic inflammation and tissue degradation.[5] The healing process can require several days,[7] and participation in intense activities too soon after initial damage can delay recovery and adaptation. Regular exercise participation reduces the severity of exercise-induced muscle damage and the subsequent need for immune intervention for repair.[2,8] Thus, the immune system is responsible for many exercise-induced adaptations. A reduction in immune function from using nonsteroidal antiinflammatories or excessive antioxidants may not be desired when trying to heal from and adapt to resistance exercise.

9.2.2 Studies Linking Immune Function and Physical Activity

The number of studies of the relationship between physical activity and immune function has quadrupled in the last 10 years.[9] Aerobic exercise and aerobic conditioning have been the focus of most of these and have allowed the modeling of the effect of aerobic conditioning as a J-curve. Moderate levels of chronic aerobic activity provide increased resistance to infectious episodes, while severe levels of chronic aerobic conditioning increase the incidence of infection beyond that of nonactive individuals.[9,10]

The immune response to resistance exercise and conditioning is not as clear as that to aerobic exercise and conditioning. Fewer than a dozen studies have been published in this area.[11–14] The immune response to these different types of exercise may be dissimilar because of their different physiological demands. Resistance conditioning does not have a significant impact on hemodynamic and cardiorespiratory variables,[15–17] and these variables do not typically reach the same levels during resistance and aerobic activities.[15,16,18,19] Additionally, the energy systems and muscle fibers recruited are dissimilar[18,20,21] as are the secretion rates and actions of hormones released during each activity.[22,23] Therefore, a review of resistance exercise and conditioning studies is warranted.

9.2.3 Studies of the Immune Response to Resistance Exercise

The acute immune cell response to resistance exercise is a generalized leukocytosis, with the lymphocytes and neutrophils increasing the most, and does not appear to differ based on training level.[24-26] All major cell subpopulations, except the basophils, participate in this leukocytosis.[25,26] The cell numbers begin to decline within the first 15 minutes after cessation of exercise, with the lymphocytes recovering more quickly than the phages.[26] The phages probably recover more slowly because they are moving into the exercised muscles to initiate and maintain the repair process.[6]

Humoral immunosurveillance appears to be unaltered, as there was no exercise-induced change in salivary IgA.[27] Cellular immunosurveillance results are mixed in resistance-trained individuals. Lymphocyte proliferation was unaffected by resistance exercise, but total NK cell activity is reduced even when increases in NK cell number are considered.[25] Thus, an acute bout of strength training causes a similar generalized leukocytosis and functional alteration as a bout of high-intensity endurance or aerobic exercise.[25,26]

Resting total leukocyte and immune cell subpopulation numbers do not change with resistance conditioning.[24,26-31] Chronic strength training over a period of years does not alter resting immune parameters.[32,33] The CD4+/CD8+ ratio, an indicator of immunosurveillance,[34] is unchanged.[26,28,30,31] Humoral and cellular immune cell function (immunoglobulin and cytokine production, proliferative responses, and delayed type hypersensitivity, [DTH]) remains constant as well.[22,27,29,30,32,33] Unlike long-term aerobic training, there do not appear to be any long-term alterations in immune cell numbers or function as a result of strength training by young or old persons.[24,26-33,35]

Steroid use during bodybuilding, however, does impact immunosurveillance. Immunoglobulin production was decreased even though B cell proliferation was unaltered.[32] The response to a *Staphylococcus aureus* challenge was greater than the control's as was natural killer cell activity, but whether this is advantageous or injurious is unclear.[32] Increased immunosurveillance may result in improved resistance to infection or in a level of surveillance that can lead to autoimmune disorders.[32]

With these studies in mind, it is still difficult to make global statements concerning the immune response to resistance exercise. Individual variability, nutritional status, stress level, seasonal variation, and level of current immunochallenge will have a more significant impact than the resistance exercise.[26,27,30,36]

Surveys of the peripheral immune system are valuable and instructive, but the real question is, does physical activity improve the participant's resistance to infectious episodes? This is a difficult response to assess. For example, while resistance to upper respiratory tract infections appears to be improved in moderately aerobically conditioned individuals, the mechanisms for this have not been identified.[10] Additional work is still needed in this area.

9.3   Nutrition for the Immune System

9.3.1   General Considerations

The human immune system is highly responsive to dietary manipulation; simple caloric restriction to micronutrient supplementation can have profound effects. It is just this responsiveness that makes studying this relationship so challenging because it is difficult to determine *in vitro* or *in vivo* if it is the presence or absence of a particular nutrient, some other nutrient not currently being considered, or some combination of various macro and micronutrients which causes alterations. What follows is a review of pertinent nutrients, limited for the most part to human *in vivo* studies.

9.3.2 Macronutrients

9.3.2.1 Carbohydrate

Carbohydrates are essential as an energy source, especially for nervous tissue. It is the brain's need for glucose that drives much of our behavior and homeostatic mechanisms. Carbohydrate, or portions of the sugar molecule, is used in virtually all of the structures and functions of the human organism, such as enzymes, structural components, and hormones. Although carbohydrate is the most difficult macronutrient to supply in the diet, carbohydrate intake, as a significant portion of dietary intake, is not typically a problem; most athletes understand that without carbohydrate, there is no athletic performance.

9.3.2.2 Lipids

Lipids, or fats, are essential as components of cell membranes, neuron insulation, hormones (testosterone, for example), storage sites, and as energy sources. The American public typically consumes too much fat. Excess dietary fat is associated with increased cell membrane cholesterol content, which results in a reduced fluidity of the membrane and ease of transmembrane transport.[37] This may be the cause of the observed reduction of phagocytosis and inflammatory reactions, which in turn result in an increased incidence of infection.[37]

Decreasing fat intake from 40% of total calories to 25% enhances lymphocyte proliferation and NK cell activity, but does not impact the DTH reaction.[38-40] A further reduction below 25%, characterized as a fat deficiency, decreases the immunoglobulin response to a challenge such as DTH or vaccination.[37,41] This is a concern for athletes because they may have a tendency to consume too little fat.

Fatty acid supplementation has also grown in popularity. Fish oils are often used as a polyunsaturated fatty acid supplement for the protective effect they may provide for some aspects of cardiovascular disease. What is the impact of polyunsaturated fatty acid intake on immune function? Unfortunately, it appears that what is beneficial to the heart may be detrimental to immunity. Individuals consuming a normal or low-fat diet who supplement with polyunsaturated fatty acids experience a wide distribution of immunosuppression. Lymphocyte cytokine production and proliferation are reduced[41,42] as is the DTH response.[37] Additionally, there is an increased percentage of $T_{suppressor}$ cells, the downregulating cells of the immune system.[41] The phages are also compromised as monocyte/macrophage eicosanoid (inflammatory agents) and cytokine production are reduced, as is neutrophil phagocytosis.[37,41-43] The macrophage interaction with specific immunity is also inhibited as their antigen-presenting capability declines.[44] This all adds up to a reduced defense against invading pathogens. However, there is an up side to this downregulation of the immune system with polyunsaturated fatty acid supplementation; it lessens the severity of autoimmune diseases, inflammation, and transplant rejection while improving transplant function.[41,45]

9.3.2.3 Protein

Protein (amino acids) is essential as a building block of cell membranes, enzymes, and hormones, and as a potential energy source. Some have even suggested that the immune cells prefer the amino acid glutamine to carbohydrate as a fuel source. Protein deficiency is not a typical problem for strength athletes, but is a concern for those consuming a vegetarian diet. Protein deficiencies result in lymphoid tissue atrophy.[46] There is a reduction in the number of circulating lymphocytes, and these exhibit inhibited proliferation and DNA synthesis.[46] Humoral immunity is impaired via a reduction in cell numbers and immunoglobulin secretion that leads to a lower DTH response.[37,46] This altered immunoglobulin response to a viral or DTH challenge does yield mixed results as it is complicated by other deficiencies.[46] T cell function and numbers are also influenced as the number of mature T cells declines.[46] The CD4+ cells fall markedly while CD8+ are only mildly reduced. This results in a greatly reduced CD4+/CD8+ ratio (indicative of immunosuppression).[46] T cells also exhibit a reduced responsiveness to cytokines and production of IL-1, IL-2, and IFN-γ.[46] The phagocytes are also negatively impacted as general phagocytosis declines. Complement levels are reduced, as is bactericidal activity.[46]

Vegetarian diets, when care is taken to ensure adequate intake of all macro and micronutrients, do not impact immune function.[47,48]

Glutamine supplementation has been suggested as a method to augment potentially diminished immune function. It is a nonessential amino acid manufactured by the body and is the most abundant in muscle and plasma, allowing it to serve as an amino acid reserve.[40] Immune cells use glutamine as an energy source and for carbon and nitrogen precursors for RNA, DNA, and protein synthesis.[40,49] Optimum plasma levels improve macrophage phagocytosis and IL-1 production.[50] Plasma glutamine and muscle synthesis fall after exhaustive exercise, and it has been suggested that this may explain the observed exercise-induced immunosuppression.[51] However, little experimental data exist to confirm this theory, and what is available suggests that there is no, or very little, effect of glutamine supplementation on immune function.[40,52] The supplementation of branched chain amino acids (BCAA) leads to increases of some amino acids in plasma, but there is no effect on T-cell proliferation or production of IL-1 and IL-6.[53]

9.3.2.4 Energy Intake Restriction of Macronutrients

Severe caloric restriction, however, can cause problems. Insufficient caloric intake results in increased incidence of infection. This may be due to inadequate energy for metabolism and/or to insufficient micronutrients for the support of normal immune function.

Moderate caloric restriction (1250 Kcal/d intake) without exercise, which results in weight loss, a lower body mass index, and a reduction in body fat, does not affect the majority of immune parameters.[54] However, a larger caloric deficit (950 Kcal/d intake) decreases many of the immune variables, although they may remain within clinically normal levels.[55] Moderate caloric restriction appears to reduce only the lymphocyte responses to mitogens, while more severe reductions decrease the total leukocyte count, circulating neutrophil numbers, and NK cell activity (by 50%).[54,55] Nieman et al.[54] also found no alteration in the incidence of upper respiratory tract infections during 12 weeks of a 12,500 Kcal/d diet. Thus it appears that moderate caloric restriction does not overtly impact the immune response but that the immune system is more severely affected with greater dietary insufficiencies.

9.3.3 Micronutrients

9.3.3.1 Coenzyme Q_{10}

Coenzyme Q_{10} is involved in energy production and as an antioxidant. Supplementation of Coenzyme Q_{10} has been suggested and may lead to immunoenhancement as the concentration of IgG increases in the blood. The CD4+ count also increases, while the CD8+ count is unaffected, resulting in an increased CD4+/CD8+ ratio (immunoenhancement).[56] The addition of vitamin B_6 to the supplement does not alter this effect.

9.3.3.2 Minerals

9.3.3.2.1 Iron

Iron is essential for oxygen transport, some enzymatic processes, and is used by lymphocytes during proliferation and by macrophages and NK cells for cytotoxicity.[46,57] Iron levels are of particular concern for female athletes, not necessarily because of athletic participation (low iron levels are not more prevalent in athletes than in the general population), but because iron deficiency is rather high in the general female population.[57,58] Of additional concern is that immune cells will respond to an iron deficiency that is too small to be manifested as anemia.[37] An actual iron-deficiency anemia results in an increased incidence of infection and tumor growth via lymphoid atrophy and reduced phagocytic activity, lymphocyte proliferation, immunoglobulin production, and NK cell activity.[37,46,59,60] The up side to low iron levels is that they also reduce microorganism growth rate, but not enough to warrant the other detrimental effects and not enough to reduce the rate of infection.[46,57]

As with the majority of other nutrients, if a deficiency is bad, then an excess is not necessarily good. High dietary levels of iron do not reduce macrophage fungicidal effectiveness,[61] but do reduce neutrophil phagocytosis and the CD4+/CD8+ ratio.[57,62] They also affect other systems as the uptake of other trace elements falls and organ damage and coronary artery disease increase.[57] Excess iron also increases microorganism growth.[37]

9.3.3.2.2   Magnesium

Magnesium affects the mitochondria, enzymes, membrane receptors, and protein, lipid, and carbohydrate synthesis.[57] Serum levels of magnesium are elevated during high-intensity anaerobic exercise such as that found in strength training. Loss occurs via sweat and urine.[57] Low levels result in muscle weakness, fasciculation (spasm of motor nerves leading to muscle spasm), cramps, myoclonus (muscle spasm), and muscle sarcoplasmic reticulum and mitochondrial damage.[57] The immunologic effects of low levels are increases in circulating cytokine and histamine levels (inflammation) and a decline in the immunoglobulin response to a challenge.[37,57] There is little evidence documenting low magnesium levels as problematic in athletes.[57]

9.3.3.2.3   Selenium

Selenium modulates the synthesis of prostaglandins[63] and is integral to the synthesis of glutathione peroxidase (an antioxidant), which helps protect phages from autodigesting themselves.[64] Supplementation does not impact plasma levels of vitamin E,[65] but does enhance the immunoglobulin response to a viral or DTH challenge and T cell responsiveness to IL-2.[37,64]

9.3.3.2.4   Zinc

Zinc regulates several enzymatic reactions in energy release, enhances activity of hormones such as growth hormone, and regulates antioxidant defense.[57] A zinc deficiency is of concern because approximately 30% of Americans are zinc deficient, especially those with caloric or energy intake restriction and those who participate in regular intense exercise.[57] This can result in lymphoid atrophy, reduced lymphocyte function (DTH and proliferative responses and cytotoxic activity), and decreased phagocytosis.[37,46] Supplementation will restore impaired immune function and lower free radical damage to membrane-bound lipids and proteins,[37,57] but the mechanisms for this are not clear because there is no impact on resting neutrophil reactive oxygen species release or T-cell proliferation.[66] As with other nutrients, excess zinc can suppress immune function.[37,57]

9.3.3.3   Vitamins

9.3.3.3.1   B Group Vitamins

9.3.3.3.1.1   Folate

Folate is essential to cellular metabolism as a component of the energy transfer process during construction of cellular components. Folate deficiencies manifest themselves much as other micronutrient deficiencies do with lymphoid atrophy, a reduced total leukocyte count, and a hampered immunoglobulin response to a DTH or viral challenge.[37] Low folate levels result in increased opportunities for cell mutation in many cell types, especially the lymphocytes and erythrocytes, as the ability to repair DNA damage in impaired and lymphocyte growth slows.[67] Females appear to be more responsive to low folate levels than males.[47] Supplementation has no impact on normal leukocyte counts.[68]

9.3.3.3.1.2 *Vitamin B₆ (pyridoxine)*

Vitamin B_6 is essential for carbohydrate, fat, hemoglobin, and protein synthesis. Deficiencies are rare but manifest as impaired DNA and protein synthesis, which results in lymphoid atrophy, reduced lymphocyte proliferation, immunoglobulin production and response to a challenge, and T cell cytotoxicity.[37,46] Supplementation decreased protein degradation, increased protein synthesis in neutrophils,[69] increased peripheral CD4+ count, and had no effect on CD8+, which resulted in an increased CD4+/CD8+ ratio.[56]

9.3.3.3.1.3 *Vitamin B₁₂ (cobalamin)*

Vitamin B_{12} is important for the nervous system and is essential for carbohydrate, fat, hemoglobin, and protein metabolism. A vitamin B_{12} deficiency leads to increased DNA damage in lymphocytes and reduces phage bactericidal and phagocytic abilities.[37,47,70]

9.3.3.3.2 *Vitamin D*

Vitamin D, produced when the body is exposed to ultraviolet light, plays a role in calcium and phosphorus metabolism. Low levels decrease IL-2.[71]

9.3.3.3.3 *Antioxidants*

Antioxidants such as vitamins A, C, and E have received much attention because they play key roles in the body's defenses. Antioxidants scavenge or neutralize free radicals, which are reactive oxygen or nitrogen species produced during cellular metabolism. Immune cells also generate oxygen free radicals in doing their job to attack bacteria, viruses, and damaged and infected cells. Excess free radicals affect membrane integrity (lipids), enzymes (proteins), DNA (nucleic acids) and this increases susceptibility to and/or progression of diseases such as cancer, inflammatory responses, arteriosclerosis, and neurological impairments. Exercise augments the generation of free radicals via the activities of the mitochondria, vascular endothelium, neutrophils, monocytes/macrophages, and eosinophils.[8,72] This process undergoes a conditioning effect just as much of the rest of the organism does as exercise training reduces exercise-induced oxidative stress.[8]

The antioxidant status is the balance between antioxidants and oxidants and is a determinant of immune cell function or how well membrane lipids, cellular proteins, and nucleic acids will be maintained and control signal transduction and gene expression.[73] In general, antioxidant supplementation retards the aging process and reduces the incidence of cancer.[64,74] However, supplementation, as a means of reducing exercise-induced oxidative stress is not necessary because regular training reduces free radical generation and enhances antioxidant mechanisms.[8]

9.3.3.3.3.1 Fat-Soluble Antioxidant Vitamins

9.3.3.3.3.1.1 Vitamin A (retinol, retinoic acid, beta-carotene). Vitamin A maintains cell membranes and is integral to night vision.[37] It is fat-soluble and must be consumed with dietary fat for absorption to occur.[75] A deficiency of vitamin A leads to an increased incidence of infection because of reduced immunosurveillance, because T cell numbers are lower as is their mitogen proliferative response and the production of immunoglobulins by B cells.[37,46] Supplementation increases resistance to infection and inhibits cancer growth.[37,76,77] This is due to increases in immunoglobulin synthesis, IL-6 production (although there is some disagreement concerning this concept), IL-1β production, NK cell activity, T cell proliferation, and membrane-bound activation markers.[76,78-81] The CD4+/CD8+ ratio also increases as CD4+ numbers go up and CD8+ decline.[82] TNF-α cytolytic activity drops,[83] while IL-2, IL-4, and IL-10 are unchanged.[76] IFN-γ production modulation is unclear as a decrease or no impact has been noted.[76,78] Again, excessive doses are not appropriate because high intakes of vitamin A inhibit DNA synthesis.[80]

9.3.3.3.3.1.2 Vitamin E (α-tocopherol). Vitamin E is the most abundant and most effective lipophilic antioxidant.[84] A vitamin E deficiency negatively impacts the lymphocytes by reducing the proliferation and DTH responses and immunoglobulin synthesis when faced with a viral challenge and the basophils by decreasing histamine release.[37,46,77] Supplementation up to a normal intake will increase resistance to infection and increase the DTH response.[37] Additional supplementation, up to 100 mg/day has no effect on DTH or on IL-2, IL-4, and IFN-γ production.[85] Increasing the dose to 300 mg/day still does not affect DTH, but will decrease IL-2, IL-4, IL-6, and IFN-γ release.[63,71,86] Four hundred mg/day will initially increase IL-1β and TNF-α, but these return to baseline with continued supplementation.[87] Further increasing vitamin E augmentation to 1 g/day temporarily decreases lipid peroxidation and PGE$_2$ production, but both return to normal levels with long-term high intake levels.[87] Continued megadoses reduce monocyte adhesion, which in turn reduces their ability to leave vascular space to perform immunosurveillance within the extravascular spaces[88] and inhibits immunity and increases incidence of infection.[37]

9.3.3.3.3.2 Water-Soluble Antioxidant Vitamins

9.3.3.3.3.2.1 Vitamin C (ascorbic acid). Vitamin C is the major water-soluble antioxidant and is part of the first line of defense against free radicals in whole blood and plasma.[84,89] Deficiencies reduce DTH and phage bactericidal activity.[37,46] Supplementation reverses this and improves phagocytosis and cell migration.[37] Two hundred mg/day supplementation increases total leukocyte, neutrophil, and lymphocyte counts, while decreasing monocyte and eosinophil numbers.[90] Increasing supplemental vitamin C intake to 1 g/day temporarily decreases lipid peroxidation and increases IL-1β and TNF-α, but these return to baseline with long-term augmentation.[87] Natural killer cell activity will increase 8 to 24 hours post ingestion and can be maintained with continued administration.[91] Like other nutrients however, if a little is good then more is better does not hold true because excess vitamin C can increase cellular oxidative damage.[92]

Combining vitamins C and E does have a greater effect than either alone, but the combination is not synergistic because the effect is less than the sum of both would be, and it appears to be short-term just as it is with either alone.[87] A general multivitamin can reverse age-associated increases in DTH.[93]

9.3.3.4 Summary of the Micronutrient Effects on Immunity

Chandra[46] made five observations concerning the micronutrients and immunity: (1) the immune system responds quickly to changes in micronutrient balance, (2) immune impairment depends on micronutrient levels, the interaction with other nutrients, and the health and age of the individual, (3) micronutrient abnormalities predict the end result such as the type of infection, (4) excessive micronutrient intake results in immune impairment, and (5) individual testing is beneficial if a deficiency is suspected. Thus a healthy diet that ensures adequate micronutrient intake is recommended. The supplementation of the micronutrients beyond normal dietary requirements does not enhance, and may even impair, immune function.

9.4 Immune Response to Common Nutritional Ergogenic Aids

Very little research has been done on the immune response to the ergogenic aids commonly used in strength training. In fact, the research into many of the nutritional ergogenic aids frequently used to enhance strength and muscle mass is insufficient in general. Inferences about the immune response must be made from the supplement's impact on other systems, such as known endocrine responses. The role of β-endorphin is not clear, but it does not appear to play a major role in modulating immune function.[94] The catecholamines tend to increase peripheral leukocyte numbers (with the exception of the neutrophils) and NK cell activity.[94] Growth hormone has the opposite effect and increases circulating neutrophil numbers but does not affect the other leukocytes.[94] Cortisol and the other corticosteroids are immunosuppressive and may be responsible for resequestration of the leukocytes and the decreased peripheral numbers associated with exercise recovery.[94] Prolactin generally enhances immunosurveillance.[95] Testosterone at physiologic levels enhances immune function,[96] but suppresses it at supra-physiologic levels.[32]

What inferences can be drawn from the effects of various ergogenic aids on the endocrine response to resistance exercise? Ergogenic aids that affect β-endorphin probably do not significantly impact immune function. Those that reduce the catecholamine response will probably reduce exercise-induced leukocytosis and attenuate NK cell activity, such as increased carbohydrate consumption before, during, and after exercise.[97] Modulators of growth hormone may then impact the exercise-induced increase in circulating neutrophils, but not the majority of the leukocytes. Thus carbohydrate, ginseng, and carbohydrate with ginseng probably do not impact the neutrophils via growth hormone as there is no impact on growth hormone, while carbohydrate with protein may increase the peripheral neutrophil count as it increased the growth hormone response to resistance exercise.[98,99] Those supplements that reduce the cortisol response to exercise may also reduce post-exercise immunosuppression. Carbohydrate and carbohydrate with protein may attenuate this immunosuppression by decreasing cortisol release,[97,99] while ginseng will not affect cortisol levels.[100] The prolactin picture is not as clear because carbohydrate with protein may reduce its responsiveness and perhaps reduce immunoenhancement.[99] Ergogenic aids that typically decrease testosterone, carbohydrate and protein may reduce immunosurveillance.[98-100] However, it has been suggested that testosterone production does not decrease, rather uptake is increased, as the luteinizing hormone levels do not change.[98] Supplementing androstenedione, boron, fat, and ginseng do not impact testosterone levels.[100-103] It has been suggested that β-hydroxy β-methylbutyrate (HMB) augmentation may increase lymphocyte proliferation and macrophage numbers, but that high doses will reduce proliferation and total peripheral leukocytes.[104] Thus the effect of ergogenic aids on the immune response is difficult to predict and more studies need to be completed in this area.

9.5   Immune Response to Conditioning with Dietary Intervention

The majority of studies that have measured the immune response to exercise and dietary intervention involve aerobic rather than strength training. General trends from these studies indicate that caloric or energy restriction with moderate aerobic training tends not to overtly impact immunosurveillance.[54,55] However, strenuous prolonged exercise and insufficient energy intake (Army Ranger training) tend to be immunosuppressive.[105-107] A gradient exists in that greater energy deficiencies result in greater immunosuppression.[55,107] Varying the dietary fat levels of runners resulted in the same general modulation of the immune response as altering dietary fat intake without exercise. Reduced fat enhanced immune function up to a point and then very low levels hindered it.[108] Insufficient iron intake during basic training increased indicators of a generalized stress response but did not generally affect immune cell numbers or function.[109] Modifying the diet of aerobic exercisers appears to have the same general affects as modifying the diet of non-exercisers.

The beginning of a strength-training program is often the most stressful stage, with the greatest amount of tissue damage and delayed onset muscle soreness. It is at this time that carbohydrate and protein supplementation may enhance the immune system's ability to repair muscle damage.[7] Increased carbohydrate intake will help offset the reduced glycogen synthesis associated with eccentric exercise and increased protein intake may enhance muscle mass gains, although it does not appear to affect strength.[7] Adequate dietary intake and recovery time are especially important during training program initiation.

The immunological impact of supplementing the diet with minerals is poorly understood. Increasing iron levels in those who are deficient does improve oxygen transport and availability but has no measurable impact on those with normal iron levels.[57] The temporary exercise-induced decline in iron may actually prove to be beneficial to immunosurveillance because it increases the activity of the macrophage-produced cytokines.[57] Magnesium levels decline when muscle damage is present, but no causative relationship has been established.[57] Strenuous exercise may impact magnesium levels and play a role in the post-exercise increase in circulating cytokines.[57] Selenium augmentation enhances muscle glutathione peroxidase (antioxidant) activity after acute exercise and may provide some protection against exercise-induced oxidative damage.[65] Zinc supplementation does not demonstrate an ergogenic effect,[57] but it does magnify the exercise-induced neutrophil increase while minimizing the exercise-induced neutrophil oxidant release.[66] No effect on exercise-induced suppressed T-cell proliferation or on cortisol release has been measured with increased dietary zinc.[66]

Antioxidant supplementation after exercise has little impact on physical performance; lactate production, creatine kinase release, and maximal strength are not altered, but vitamin C may slow the onset of fatigue and improve the initial recovery rate.[110] Efflux of antioxidants into the plasma is unaffected by post-exercise intake, thus the reduction of free radicals is unaltered.[110] Additional vitamin C intake does reduce the incidence of upper respiratory tract infections in athletes, but the mechanism for this has not been elucidated.[111] Supplementation of vitamin E before, during, and after exercise does not impact the exercise-induced creatine kinase release or the increase in circulating neutrophils, but does decrease lipid peroxidation activity during exercise.[7,112] Older athletes can reverse the aging-associated decrements in the exercise-induced creatine kinase release and the increase in circulating neutrophils with additional vitamin E.[7]

A balanced (67% CHO, 29% fat, 14% PRO) ovo-lacto vegetarian diet does not impact T cell, CD4+, CD8+, NK, or monocyte numbers, monocyte proliferation, or the NK cell activity of athletes and is acceptable from an immunologic viewpoint.[48]

9.6 Summary and Conclusions

The old sage advice about the recommended diet where food, not supplements, is the source of macro and micronutrients holds true for the immune system. A moderate, well-rounded diet is best; deficiencies or excesses are not suggested. No dietary intervention is required when a nutritionally and calorically balanced diet is consumed. Excessive supplementation of immunomodulating nutrients may be counterproductive, as an overabundance can reduce the immune system's performance. Additionally, high levels of antioxidants may reduce immune function with free radical formation to such a level as to be detrimental to the healing and adaptive processes.

References

1. Brines, R., NeuroendocrineImmunologytoday, *Immunol. Today*, 15, 503, 1994.
2. Evans, W. J. and Gannon, J. G., The metabolic effects of exercise-induced muscle damage in *Exercise and Sport Science Reviews*, Holloszy, J. O. (Ed.), Williams and Wilkins, Baltimore, MD, 1991, vol. 19, p. 99.
3. Fielding, R. A., Manfredi, T. J., Ding, W., Fiatarone, M. A., Evans, W. J., and Gannon, J. G., Acute phase response in exercise: III. Neutrophil and IL-1β accumulation in skeletal muscle, *Am. J. Physiol.*, 265, R166, 1993.
4. Tidball, J. G., Inflammatory cell response to acute muscle injury, *Med. Sci. Sports Exerc.*, 27, 1022, 1995.
5. Northoff, H., Enkel, S., and Weinstock, C., Exercise, injury, and immune function, *Exerc. Immunol. Rev.*, 1, 1, 1995.
6. Robertson, T. A., Maley, M. A. L., Grounds, M. D., and Papadimitriou, J. M., The role of macrophages in skeletal muscle regeneration with particular reference to chemotaxis, *Exp. Cell. Res.*, 207, 321, 1993.
7. Evans, W. J., Muscle damage: nutritional considerations, *Int. J. Sport Nutr.*, 1, 214, 1991.
8. Niess, A. M., Dickhuth, H.-H., Northoff, H., and Fehrenbach, E., Free radicals and oxidative stress in exercise-immunological aspects, *Exerc. Immunol. Rev.*, 5, 22, 1999.
9. Nieman, D. C., Exercise immunology: practical applications, *Int. J. Sports Med.*, 18, S91, 1997.
10. Nieman, D. C., Exercise, infection, and immunity, *Int. J. Sports Med.*, 15, S131, 1994.

11. Boros, R. L., Koch, A., and Nieman, D. C., Compendium of the exercise immunology literature, 1995-1997 (June), *Abstract Compendium,* International Society of Exercise Immunology, Paderborn, 1997.

12. Hardesty, A. J., Greenleaf, J. E., Simonson, S. R., Hu, A., and Jackson, C. G. R., Exercise, exercise training, and the immune system: a compendium of research (1902-1991), *Abstract Compendium, NASA TM 108778,* NASA Ames Research Center, Moffett Field, 1993.

13. Hjertman, J. M. E. and Nieman, D. C., Compendium of the exercise immunology literature 1997 (June) – 1999 (April), *Abstract Compendium,* International Society of Exercise and Immunology, Paderborn, 1999.

14. Rainwater, M. K., Nieman, D. C., and Thomas, S. A., Compendium of the exercise immunology literature, 1991–1995 (June), *Abstract Compendium,* International Society of Exercise and Immunology, Paderborn, 1995.

15. Allen, E. T., Byrd, R. J., and Smith, D. P., Hemodynamic consequences of circuit weight training, *Res. Q.,* 47, 299, 1976.

16. Hickson, R. C., Rosenkoetter, M. A., and Brown, M. M., Strength training effects on aerobic power and short-term endurance, *Med. Sci. Sports Exerc.,* 12, 336, 1980.

17. Hurley, B. F., Seals, D. R., Ehsani, A. A., Cartier, L. J., Dalsky, G. P., Hagberg, J. M., and Holloszy, J. O., Effects of high-intensity strength training on cardiovascular function, *Med. Sci. Sports Exerc.,* 16, 483, 1984.

18. Keul, J., Haralambie, G., Bruder, M., and Gottstein, H.-J., The effect of weight lifting exercise on heart rate and metabolism in experienced weight lifters, *Med. Sci. Sports,* 10, 13, 1978.

19. MacDougall, J. D., Tuxen, D., Sale, D. G., Moroz, J. R., and Sutton, J. R., Arterial blood pressure response to heavy resistance exercise, *J. Appl. Physiol.,* 58, 785, 1985.

20. Gollnick, P. D., Armstrong, R. B., Saubert, C. W., IV, Piehl, K., and Saltin, B., Enzyme activity and fiber composition in skeletal muscle of untrained and trained men, *J. Appl. Physiol.,* 33, 312, 1972.

21. MacDougall, J. D., Sale, D. G., Moroz, J. R., Elder, G. C. B., Sutton, J. R., and Howald, H., Mitochondrial volume density in human skeletal muscle following heavy resistance training, *Med. Sci. Sports,* 11, 164, 1979.

22. Horne, L., Bell, G., Fisher, B., Warren, S., and Janowska-Wieczorek, A., Interaction between cortisol and tumor necrosis factor with concurrent resistance and endurance training, *Clin. J. Sport Med.,* 7, 247, 1997.

23. Kraemer, W. J., Neuroendocrine responses to resistance exercise, in *Essentials of Strength Training and Conditioning,* Baechle, T. R. (Ed.), Human Kinetics, Champaign, IL, 1994 p. 86.

24. Flynn, M. G., Fahlman, M., Braun, W. A., Lambert, C. P., Bouillon, L. E., Brolinson, P. G., and Armstrong, C. W., Effects of resistance training on selected indexes of immune function in elderly women, *J. Appl. Physiol.,* 86, 1905, 1999.

25. Nieman, D. C., Henson, D. A., Sampson, C. S., Hering, J. L., Suttles, J., Conley, M., Stone, M. H., Butterworth, D. E., and Davis, J. M., The acute immune response to exhaustive resistance exercise, *Int. J. Sports Med.,* 16, 322, 1995.

26. Simonson, S. R., The effects of acute and chronic weight training by moderately conditioned and weight trained individuals on selected immune parameters, doctoral dissertation, University of Northern Colorado, Greeley, 1998.

27. McDowell, S. L., Weir, J. P., Eckerson, J. M., Wagner, L. L., Housh, T. J., and Johnson, G. O., A preliminary investigation of the effect of weight training on salivary immunoglobulin A, *Res. Q. Exerc. Sport*, 64, 348, 1993.
28. Bermon, S., Phillip, P., Ferrari, P., Candito, M., and Dolisi, C., Effects of a short-term strength training program on lymphocyte subsets at rest in elderly humans, *Eur. J. Appl. Physiol.*, 79, 336, 1999.
29. Rall, L. C., Rosen, C. J., Dolnikowski, G., Hartman, W. J., Lundgren, N., Abad, L. W., Dinarello, C. A., and Roubenoff, R., Protein metabolism in rheumatoid arthritis and aging: Effects of muscle strength training and tumor necrosis factor α, *Arthritis Rheum.*, 39, 1115, 1996.
30. Rall, L. C., Roubenoff, R., Cannon, J. G., Abad, L. W., Dinarello, C. A., and Meydani, S. N., Effects of progressive resistance training on immune response in aging and chronic inflammation, *Med. Sci. Sports Exerc.*, 28, 1356, 1996.
31. Weiss, C., Kinscherf, R., Roth, S., Friedman, B., Fischbach, T., Reus, J., Droge, W., and Bartsch, P., Lymphocyte subpopulations and concentrations of soluble CD8 and CD4 antigen after anaerobic training, *Int. J. Sports Med.*, 16, 117, 1995.
32. Calabrese, L. H., Kleiner, S. M., Barna, B. P., Skibinski, C. I., Kirkendall, D. T., Lahita, R. G., and Lombardo, J. A., The effects of anabolic steroids and strength training on the human immune response, *Med. Sci. Sports Exerc.*, 21, 386, 1989.
33. Nieman, D. C., Henson, D. A., Herring, J., Sampson, C., Suttles, J., Conley, M., and Stone, M. H., Natural killer cell cytotoxic activity in weight trainers and sedentary controls, *J. Strength Cond. Res.*, 8, 241, 1994.
34. Keast, D. and Morton, A. R., Long-term exercise and immune functions, in *Exercise and Disease*, Watson, R. R. and Eisinger, M. (Eds.), CRC Press, Boca Raton, 1992, p. 89.
35. Eberhardt, A., Influence of motor activity on some serologic mechanisms of nonspecific immunity of the organism, *Acta Physiol. Pol.*, 22, 201, 1971.
36. Cannon, J. G., Exercise and resistance to infection, *J. Appl. Physiol.*, 74, 973, 1993.
37. Beisel, W. R., Edelman, R., Nauss, K., and Suskind, R. M., Single-nutrient effects on immunologic functions, *JAMA*, 245, 53, 1981.
38. Hebert, J. R., Barone, J., Reddy, M. M., and Backlund, J.-Y. C., Natural killer cell activity in a longitudinal dietary fat intervention trial, *Clin. Immunol. Immunopathol.*, 54, 103, 1990.
39. Kelley, D. S., Dougherty, R. M., Branch, L. B., Taylore, P. C., and Iacono, J. M., Concentration of dietary n-6 polyunsaturated fatty acids and the human immune system, *Clin. Immunol. Immunopathol.*, 62, 240, 1992.
40. Shephard, R. J. and Shek, P. N., Immunological hazards from nutritional imbalance in athletes, *Exerc. Immunol. Rev.*, 4, 22, 1998.
41. Meydani, S. N., Lichtenstein, A. H., Cornwall, S., Meydani, M., Goldin, B. R., Rasmussen, H., Dinarello, C., and Schaefer, E. J., Immunologic effects of national cholesterol education panel step-2 diets with and without fish-derived n-3 fatty acid enrichment, *J. Clin. Invest.*, 92, 105, 1993.
42. Meydani, S. N., Endres, S., Woods, M. M., Goldin, B. R., Soo, C., Morrill-Labrode, A., Dinarello, C. A., and Gorbach, S. L., Oral (n-3) fatty acid supplementation suppresses cytokine production and lymphocyte proliferation: comparison between young and older women, *J. Nutr.*, 121, 547, 1991.
43. Calder, P. C., Effects of fatty acids and dietary lipids on cells of the immune system, *Proc. Nutr. Soc.*, 55, 127, 1996.

44. Hughes, D. A., Pinder, A. C., Piper, Z., Johnson, I. T., and Lund, E. K., Fish oil supplementation inhibits the expression of major histocompatibility complex class II molecules and adhesion molecules on human monocytes, *Am. J. Clin. Nutr.*, 63, 267, 1996.

45. Calder, P. C., Dietary fatty acids and the immune system, *Nutr. Rev.*, 56, S70, 1998.

46. Chandra, R. K., 1990 McCollum award lecture. Nutrition and immunity: lessons from the past and new insights into the future, *Am. J. Clin. Nutr.*, 53, 1087, 1991.

47. Fenech, M., Important variables that influence base-line micronucleus frequency in cytokinesis-blocked lymphocytes — a biomarker for DNA damage in human populations, *Mutat. Res.*, 404, 155, 1998.

48. Richter, E. A., Kiens, B., Raben, A., Tvede, N., and Pedersen, B. K., Immune parameters in male athletes after a lacto-ovo vegetarian diet and a mixed western diet, *Med. Sci. Sports Exerc.*, 23, 517, 1991.

49. Walsh, N. P., Blannin, A. K., Robson, P. J., and Gleeson, M., Glutamine, exercise and immune function, *Sports Med.*, 26, 177, 1998.

50. Wallace, C. and Keast, D., Glutamine and macrophage function, *Metabolism*, 41, 1016, 1992.

51. Newsholme, E. A., Biochemical mechanisms to explain immunosuppression in well-trained and overtrained athletes, *Int. J. Sports Med.*, 15, S142, 1994.

52. Rohde, T., MacLean, D. A., and Pedersen, B. K., Effect of glutamine supplementation on changes in the immune system induced by repeated exercise, *Med. Sci. Sports Exerc.*, 30, 856, 1998.

53. Parry-Billings, M., Budgett, R., Koutedakis, Y., Blomstrand, E., Brooks, S., Williams, C., Calder, P. C., Pilling, S., Baigrie, R., and Newsholme, E. A., Plasma amino acid concentrations in the overtraining syndrome: possible effects on the immune system, *Med. Sci. Sports Exerc.*, 24, 1353, 1992.

54. Nieman, D. C., Nehlsen-Cannarella, S. L., Henson, D. A., Koch, A. J., Butterworth, D. E., Fagoaga, O., and Utter, A., Immune response to exercise training and/or energy restriction in obese women, *Med. Sci. Sports Exerc.*, 30, 679, 1998.

55. Scanga, C. B., Verde, T. J., Paolone, A. M., Andersen, R. E., and Wadden, T. A., Effects of weight loss and exercise training on natural killer cell activity in obese women, *Med. Sci. Sports Exerc.*, 30, 1666, 1998.

56. Folkers, K., Morita, M., and McRee, J., Jr., The activities of coenzyme Q_{10} and vitamin B_6 for immune responses, *Biochem. Biophys. Res. Commun.*, 193, 88, 1993.

57. Konig, D., Weinstock, C., Keul, J., Northoff, H., and Berg, A., Zinc, iron, and magnesium status in athletes — influence on the regulation of exercise-induced stress and immune function, *Exerc. Immunol. Rev.*, 4, 2, 1998.

58. Risser, W. L., Lee, E. J., Poindexter, H. B. W., West, M. S., Pivarnik, J. M., Risser, J. M. H., and Hickson, J. F., Iron deficiency in female athletes: its prevalence and impact on performance, *Med. Sci. Sports Exerc.*, 20, 116, 1988.

59. Kinik, S. T., Tuncer, A. M., and Altay, C., Transferrin receptor on peripheral blood lymphocytes in iron deficiency anemia, *Br. J. Haematol.*, 104, 494, 1999.

60. Spear, A. T. and Sherman, A. R., Iron deficiency alters DMBA-induced tumor burden and natural killer cell cytotoxicity in rats, *J. Nutr.*, 122, 46, 1992.

61. Minn, Y., Brummer, E., and Stevens, D. A., Effect of iron on fluconazole activity against *Candida albicans* in presence of human serum or monocyte-derived macrophages, *Mycopathologia*, 138, 29, 1997.

62. van Asbek, B. S., Marx, J. J. M., Struyvenberg, A., van Kats, J. H., and Verhoef, J., Effect of iron (III) in the presence of various ligands on the phagocytic and metabolic activity of human polymorphonuclear leukocytes, *J. Immunol.*, 132, 851, 1984.

63. Shephard, R. J. and Shek, P. N., Heavy exercise, nutrition and immune function: is there a connection, *Int. J. Sports Med.*, 16, 491, 1995.

64. Hughes, D. A., Effects of dietary antioxidants on the immune function of middle-aged adults, *Proc. Nutr. Soc.*, 58, 79, 1999.

65. Tessier, F., Hida, H., Favier, A., and Marconnet, P., Muscle GSH-Px activity after prolonged exercise, training, and selenium supplementation, *Biol. Trace. Elem. Res.*, 47, 279, 1995.

66. Singh, A., Failla, M. K., and Deuster, P. A., Exercise-induced changes in immune function: effects of zinc supplementation, *J. Appl. Physiol.*, 76, 2298, 1994.

67. Duthie, S. J. and Hawdon, A., DNA instability (strand breakage, uracil misincorporation, and defective repair) is increased by folic acid depletion in human lymphocytes *in vitro*, *FASEB J.*, 12, 1491, 1998.

68. Morgan, S. L., Baggott, J. E., Vaughn, W. H., Austin, J. S., Veitch, T. A., Lee, J. Y., Koopman, W. J., Krumdieck, C. L., and Alarcon, G. S., Supplementation with folic acid during methotrexate therapy for rheumatoid arthritis, *Ann. Intern. Med.*, 121, 833, 1994.

69. Stern, F., Berner, Y. N., Polyak, Z., Komarnitsky, M., Sela, B.-A., and Dror, Y., Effect of vitamin B_6 supplementation on degradation rates of short-lived proteins in human neutrophils, *J. Nutr. Biochem.*, 10, 467, 1999.

70. Fenech, M., Micronucleus frequency in human lymphocytes is related to plasma vitamin B_{12} and homocysteine, *Mutat. Res.*, 428, 299, 1999.

71. Payette, H., Rola-Pleszcynski, M., and Ghadirian, P., Nutrition factors in relation to cellular and regulatory immune variables in a free-living elderly population, *Am. J. Clin. Nutr.*, 52, 927, 1990.

72. Roberts, C. K., Barnard, R. J., Jasman, A., and Balon, T., Acute exercise increases nitric oxide synthase activity in skeletal muscle, *Am. J. Physiol.*, 277, E390, 1999.

73. De la Fuente, M., Ferrandez, M. D., Burgos, M. S., Soler, A., Prieto, A., and Miquel, J., Immune function in aged women is improved by ingestion of vitamins C and E, *Can. J. Physiol. Pharmacol.*, 76, 373, 1998.

74. Meydani, M., Lipman, R. D., Han, S. N., Wu, D., Beharka, A., Martin, K. R., Bronson, R., Cao, G., Smith, D., and Meydani, S. N., The effect of long-term dietary supplementation with antioxidants, *Ann. N. Y. Acad. Sci.*, 854, 352, 1998.

75. Blomhoff, R., Green, M. H., Green, J. B., Berg, T., and Norum, K. R., Vitamin A metabolism: new perspectives on absorption, transport, and storage, *Physiol. Rev.*, 71, 951, 1991.

76. Allende, L. M., Corell, A., Madrono, A., Gongora, R., Rodriguez-Gallego, C., Lopez-Goyanes, A., Rosal, M., and Arnaiz-Villena, A., Retinol (vitamin A) is a cofactor in CD3-induced human T-lymphocyte activation, *Immunology*, 90, 388, 1997.

77. Gibbs, B. F., Wolff, H. H., and Grabbe, J., Effects of free radical scavengers on histamine release from human basophils stimulated by immunological and non-immunological secretagogues, *Inflamm. Res.*, 1, S13, 1999.

78. Ballow, M., Wang, W., and Xiang, S., Modulation of B-cell immunoglobulin synthesis by retinoic acid, *Clin. Immunol. Immunopathol.*, 80, S73, 1996.

79. Ballow, M., Xiang, S., Wang, W., and Brodsky, L., The effects of retinoic acid on immunoglobulin synthesis: role of interleukin 6, *J. Clin. Immunol.,* 16, 171, 1996.
80. Blomhoff, H. K., Smeland, E. B., Erikstein, B., Rasmussen, A. M., Skrede, B., Skjonsberg, C., and Blomhoff, R., Vitamin A is a key regulator for cell growth, cytokine production, and differentiation in normal B cells, *J. Biol. Chem.,* 267, 23988, 1992.
81. Garbe, A., Buck, J., and Hammerling, U., Retinoids are important cofactors in T cell activation, *J. Exp. Med.,* 176, 109, 1992.
82. Semba, R. D., Muhilal, Ward, B. J., Griffin, D. E., Scott, A. L., Natadisastra, G., West, K. P., Jr., and Sommer, A., Abnormal T-cell subset proportions in vitamin A-deficient children, *Lancet,* 341, 5, 1993.
83. Hughes, T. K. and Fulep, E., Effects of retinoic acid (vitamin A) on tumor necrosis factor cytolytic action, *Biochem. Biophys. Res. Commun.,* 206, 223, 1995.
84. Niki, E., Yamamoto, Y., Takahashi, M., Yamamoto, K., Yamamoto, Y., Komuro, E., Miki, M., Yasuda, H., and Mino, M., Free radical-mediated damage of blood and its inhibition by antioxidants, *J. Nutr. Sci. Vitaminol.,* 34, 507, 1988.
85. Pallast, E. G., Schouten, E. G., de Waart, F. G., Fonk, H. C., Doekes, G., von Blomberg, B. M., and Kok, F. J., Effect of 50- and 100-mg vitamin E supplements on cellular immune function in noninstitutionalized elderly persons, *Am. J. Clin. Nutr.,* 69, 1273, 1999.
86. Prasad, J. S., Effect of vitamin E supplementation on leukocyte function, *Am. J. Clin. Nutr.,* 33, 606, 1980.
87. Jeng, K.-C. G., Yang, C.-S., Siu, W.-Y., Tsai, Y.-S., Liao, W.-J., and Kuo, J.-S., Supplementation with vitamins C and E enhance cytokine production by peripheral blood mononuclear cells in healthy adults, *Am. J. Clin. Nutr.,* 64, 960, 1996.
88. Williams, J. C., Forster, L. A., Tull, S. P., and Ferns, G. A. A., Effects of vitamin E on human platelet and mononuclear cell responses *in vitro, Int. J. Exp. Path.,* 80, 227, 1999.
89. Frei, B., England, L., and Ames, B. N., Ascorbate is an outstanding antioxidant in human blood plasma, *Proc. Natl. Acad. Sci. USA.,* 86, 6377, 1989.
90. Jayachandran, M. and Panneerselvam, C., Cellular immune responses to vitamin C supplementation in ageing humans assessed by the *in vitro* leucocyte migration inhibition test, *Med. Sci. Res.,* 26, 227, 1998.
91. Vojdani, A. and Namatalla, G., Enhancement of human natural killer cytotoxic activity by Vitamin C in pure and augmented formulations, *J. Nutr. Environ. Med.,* 7, 187, 1997.
92. Anderson, D. and Phillips, B. J., Comparative *in vitro* and *in vivo* effects of antioxidants, *Food and Chem. Toxicol.,* 37, 1015, 1999.
93. Buzina-Suboticanec, K., Buzina, R., Stavljenic, A., Farley, T. M. M., Haller, J., Bergman-Markovic, B., and Gorajscan, M., Ageing, nutritional status and immune response, *Int. J. Vit. Nutr. Res.,* 68, 133, 1998.
94. Pedersen, B. K., Bruunsgaard, H., Klokker, M., Kappel, M., MacLean, D. A., Nielsen, H. B., Rohde, T., Ullum, H., and Zacho, M., Exercise-induced immunomodulation — possible roles of neuroendocrine and metabolic factors, *Int. J. Sports Med.,* 18, S2, 1997.
95. Gala, R. R., Prolactin and growth hormone in the regulation of the immune system, *Proc. Soc. Exp. Biol. Med.,* 198, 513, 1991.

96. Grossman, C. J., Interactions between the gonadal steroids and the immune system, *Science*, 227, 257, 1985.
97. Nieman, D. C., Influence of carbohydrate on the immune response to intensive, prolonged exercise, *Exerc. Immunol. Rev.*, 4, 64, 1998.
98. Chandler, R. M., Byrne, H. K., Patterson, J. G., and Ivy, J. L., Dietary supplements affect the anabolic hormones after weight-training exercise, *J. Appl. Physiol.*, 76, 839, 1994.
99. Kraemer, W. J., Volek, J. S., Bush, J. A., Putukian, M., and Sebastianelli, W. J., Hormonal responses to consecutive days of heavy-resistance exercise with or without nutritional supplementation, *J. Appl. Physiol.*, 85, 1544, 1998.
100. Kang, H. Y., Endogenous anabolic hormonal and growth factor responses to resistance exercise in carbohydrate and/or ginseng consumption, *Med. Sci. Sports Exerc.*, 31, S125, 1999.
101. Ferrando, A. A. and Green, N. R., The effect of boron supplementation on lean body mass, plasma testosterone levels, and strength in male bodybuilders, *Int. J. Sport Nutr.*, 3, 140, 1993.
102. King, D. S., Sharp, R. L., Vukovich, M. D., Brown, G. A., Reigenrath, T. A., Uhl, N. L., and Parsons, K. A., Effect of oral androstenedione on serum testosterone and adaptations to resistance training in young men: a randomized controlled trial, *JAMA*, 281, 2020, 1999.
103. Volek, J. S., Kraemer, W. J., Bush, J. A., Incledon, T., and Boetes, M., Testosterone and cortisol in relationship to dietary nutrients and resistance exercise, *J. Appl. Physiol.*, 82, 49, 1997.
104. Nissen, S. L. and Abumrad, N. L., Nutritional role of the leucine metabolite β-hydroxy β-methylbutyrate (HMB), *Nutr. Biochem.*, 8, 300, 1997.
105. Montain, S. J., Shipee, R. L., Tharion, W. J., and Kramer, T. R., Carbohydrate-electrolyte solution during military training: effect on physical performance, mood state and immune function, *Technical Report, T95-13*, US Army Research Institute of Environmental Medicine, Natick, MA, 1995.
106. Moore, R. J., Friedl, K. E., Kramer, T. R., Martinez-Lopez, K. E., Hoyt, R. W., Tulley, R. E., DeLany, J. P., Askew, E. W., and Vogel, J. A., Changes in soldier nutritional status and immune function during the ranger training course, *Technical Report, T13-92*, US Army Research Institute of Environmental Medicine, Natick, MA, 1992.
107. Shipee, R., Friedl, K., Kramer, T., Mays, M., Popp, K., Askew, W., Fairbrother, B., Hoyt, R., Vogel, J., Marchitelli, L., Frykman, P., Martinez-Lopez, L., Bernton, E., Kramer, M., Tulley, R., Rood, J., Delany, J., Jezior, D., and Arsenault, J., Nutritional and immunological assessment of ranger students with increased caloric intake, *Technical Report, T95-5*, US Army Research Institute of Environmental Medicine, Natick, MA, 1994.
108. Venkatraman, J. T., Rowland, J. A., Denardin, E., Horvath, P. J., and Pendergast, D., Influence of the level of dietary lipid intake and maximal exercise on the immune status in runners, *Med. Sci. Sports Exerc.*, 29, 333, 1997.
109. Westphal, K. A., Friedl, K. E., Sharp, M. A., King, N., Kramer, T. R., Reynolds, K. L., and Marchitelli, L. J., Health, performance, and nutritional status of U.S. Army women during basic combat training, *Technical Reports, T96-2*, US Army Research Institute of Environmental Medicine, Natick, MA, 1995.
110. Jakeman, P. and Maxwell, S., Effect of antioxidant vitamin supplementation on muscle function after eccentric exercise, *Eur. J. Appl. Physiol.*, 67, 426, 1993.

111. Hemila, H., Vitamin C and common cold incidence: a review of studies with subjects under heavy physical stress, *Int. J. Sports Med.*, 17, 379, 1996.
112. Dillard, C. J., Litov, R. E., Savin, W. M., Dumelin, E. E., and Tappel, A. L., Effects of exercise, vitamin E and ozone on pulmonary function and lipid peroxidation, *J. Appl. Physiol.*, 45, 927, 1978.

10

Hydration and the Strength Athlete

Michael G. Coles

CONTENT

10.1   Introduction

Successful and safe strength training, irrespective of whether it is being done competitively or exclusively for its health benefits, is dependent on a multitude of factors. These include following a sound training program and being well nourished. Both of these factors have received a great deal of attention and are covered in detail elsewhere in this book. Hydration status is also an important factor to consider with regard to strength training and conditioning. While the relationship between hydration and successful endurance performance has been well documented,[1-8] much less has been written about fluid balance and its potential influence on strength training and indices of strength. The purpose of this chapter is to review what is known about the influence of hydration on strength training and measures of muscular strength. A discussion of the relationship between weightlifting and shifts in body water, specifically plasma volume, will be presented. In addition, a brief review concerning the relationship of hydration to protein supplementation, amino-acid supplementation, and creatine monohydrate supplementation will be provided. Last, recommendations for fluid replacement and monitoring water balance will be reviewed.

10.2   Water

It has been estimated that over 70% of the Earth's surface is made up of water. In addition to other countless global functions, water supports aquatic life forms, regulates environmental climates, and even generates hydroelectric power. This unique molecule, composed of two hydrogen atoms and one oxygen atom, is also the most abundant inorganic substance in the human body. It is a vital nutrient to life even though it has no caloric value. Individuals can survive and function near normal for extended periods of time without food, but without water physiological function becomes compromised almost immediately and death is certain within days. Simply stated, life, as it is known, could not exist without water.

The average human has approximately 40 L of total body water. This constitutes about 60 to 65% of total body mass. Total body water can be theoretically divided into two major compartments. There is water that is found in membrane-bound cells, known as intracellular volume, and there is water found outside the cell, known as extracellular volume. The extracellular volume can be further subdivided into water that is found outside the cells but within the confines of the vascular system, termed plasma volume, and that which is found outside of both the membrane bound cells and the vascular system, termed interstitial volume. Of compartments identified, the intracellular volume is the largest. It contains approximately 24 of the 40 L, or 60%, of total body water. The extracellular volume contains about 16 L of water, or 40%, of which approximately 10 L (25%), resides within the interstitial space and 3 L (7.5%) are found in the plasma. The remaining 3 liters are considered to be transcellular water and are found in places such as the gastrointestinal and urinary tracts. Under homeostatic conditions these volumes of water are maintained within a narrow range, but the water itself is not stagnant. It is in a constant state of dynamic flux between compartments, and it plays a major role in many physiological functions.

The many roles of water in the body include its actions as a solvent, a suspending medium to carry nutrients and waste products, a participant in both catabolic and anabolic chemical reactions, and a lubricating agent, while it also participates in the regulation and control of body heat via the evaporative cooling of sweat.[9] Because some individuals may lose as much as 1 to 2.5 L water in the form of sweat per hour during strenuous activity,[8] the maintenance of proper fluid balance by matching fluid losses with fluid intake before, during, and after exercise is extremely important.

10.3 Body Hydration Terminology

The term hydration refers to the general state of body fluid balance. As shown in Figure 10.1, the term euhydration refers to normal fluctuations in daily hydration state. Euhydration variability due to temperature conditions is approximately ±0.165L (±0.22% body weight). Euhydration variability, due to heat and exercise is about ±0.382L (±0.48% body weight).[10] Hyperhydration and hypohydration are steady-state conditions associated with an overall increase or reduction in body water content, respectively. The commonly used term "dehydrate" refers to the process of losing water from either a hyperhydrated down to an euhydrated state or from a euhydrated state down to a hypohydrated state. Likewise, the term rehydrate refers to the process of gaining water from a hypohydrated state toward a euhydrated condition.[10] Superhydrate refers to the process of increasing body water volume above euhydrated conditions without having been previously hypohydrated.

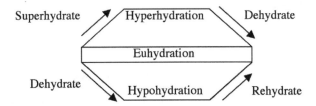

FIGURE 10.1
Hydration terminology. (Adapted from Greenleaf, J. E., Problem: thirst, drinking behavior, and involuntary dehydration. *Med. Sci. Sports Exerc.*, 24(6), 645, 1992.)

10.4 Water Balance

Water balance is achieved when water output is matched by water input. Under normal conditions adults metabolize between 2.2 and 2.9 L of water each day in an attempt to maintain this balance. Traditionally, there are thought to be three sources of water input. First, water is provided in the form of various drinks. This represents approximately 1200 to 1500 ml/day or about 60% of total water input. Second, water is provided by the fluid contained in foods consumed. Food ingestion can contribute approximately 750 to 1000 ml/day or approximately 30% of total water input. Finally, 250 to 350 ml/day, or 10% of total body water input, is provided via the metabolic water produced from the oxidation of food (100 g of fat, carbohydrate, or protein is equivalent to the generation of approximately 107, 55, and 100 g of metabolic water, respectively).[11] It should be noted that for each gram of glycogen that is metabolized as fuel an additional 2.7 grams of water become available for use by the body.[11]

Water output is primarily in the form of urinary excretion. This loss is equivalent to approximately 1250 to 1500 ml/day, or 60% or total water output. Other major sources of water output are in the form of insensible water loss through the skin and lungs, that amounts to 700 ml/day, or 28% of total water output, and sweat loss, which represents approximately 200 ml/day, or 8% total water output under average environmental conditions. An additional 100 ml/day, or approximately 4%, of daily water loss is in the form of fecal elimination. Balancing this appreciable volume of water turnover presents a considerable daily physiological challenge. The everyday challenge is heightened during exercise due to the added demands of both thermoregulation, representing the potential for an additional 4000 ml of sweat loss, and the concomitant shifting of fluid within the body fluid compartments. Shifting of fluids is due largely to changes in hydrostatic pressure within the vascular system.

10.5   Plasma Volume Shifts

10.5.1   Plasma Volume Shifts and Endurance Exercise

Conditions associated with dehydration or hyperhydration can cause drastic changes in plasma volume and subsequent plasma osmolality. If this is left uncompensated, severe consequences such as coma and death could result.[12] Sawka and Greenleaf[13] reported that plasma osmolality can increase from about 283 to over 300 mOsm/kg when going from a euhydrated state to that of hypohydration. Exercise has the potential to dramatically contribute to a change in hydration state and plasma osmolality, especially when activity is done in environmental extremes. Ironically, the ability to optimally perform endurance exercise itself becomes challenged when a change in exercise-induced hypertonic hypovolemia (increased plasma tonicity caused by a reduced plasma volume) of the magnitude reported by Sawka and Greenleaf[13] develops. Nadel et al.[14] reported that the probable reason that body water loss equivalent to 2% of pre-exercise body weight, leading to hypovolemia, can cause endurance performance impairment is because of an associated decreased cardiac output, increased heart rate, and increased core body temperature. Therefore, maintaining optimal plasma volume is essential for optimizing endurance performance.

10.5.2   Plasma Volume Shifts, Hydrostatic Pressure, and Strength Training

Although Convertino and associates[15] concluded and confirmed that there is a compensatory expansion of blood volume following exercise training, the maintenance of plasma volume during exercise is a relatively large challenge. Keeping plasma volume maximal during exercise is a greater challenge than maintaining normal volumes of water in the other compartments because it is lost at a much greater rate than volumes from the other compartments.[16] The initial loss of plasma volume during the early stages of exercise, due largely to increased intravascular hydrostatic pressure, can result in a substantial loss of plasma volume (5 to 10%) with little effect on total body water loss.[16] The loss seems to be largely dependent on exercise intensity (percentage of VO_2max) and is in direct proportion to increased mean arterial pressure.[17-19] Most studies which have investigated the effects of weightlifting on plasma volume shifts have reported results similar to low-resistance, short-term, dynamic exercise such as arm and leg cycling. In a study designed to specifically examine the relationship of plasma volume change and exercise intensity, Collins et al.[20] concluded that plasma volume decreased linearly in relation to intensity as measured by a percentage of 1 repetition maximum of weightlifting. These investigators reported that their findings were similar to those reported in other weightlifting and low-resistance cycling or running exercise studies.

10.6   Measures of Muscular Strength and Endurance

It is common for individuals who perform muscular work in hot environments to have a 2 to 8% reduction in body mass at the end of the activity.[21] This reduction is generally associated with dehydration. The dehydration results primarily from situations in which fluid ingestion does not match sweat rate. The inability to keep up with sweat loss often occurs despite the availability of rehydrating fluids. In many instances dehydration is taken to extremes by athletes who attempt to lose weight rapidly in order to qualify for competition in lower weight classifications. For an excellent review related to the topic of weight categories in weight-controlled sports, the reader is referred to the work of Wilmore.[22]

Although the unfavorable effects of hypohydration on aerobic endurance performance are well documented (Sawka et al.[23]), studies that have assessed the effects of hypohydration on muscular strength and endurance have produced inconsistent and confounding results. Furthermore, most measures of muscular performance have had either isometric muscular strength and/or endurance as dependent variables, which leaves the impact of hydration status on dynamic strength (maximal expression of torque throughout a range of motion), a more functional measure of muscular performance, unmeasured and unresolved.

Current research regarding the effects of hydration status, specifically hypohydration, on maximal strength has been inconsistent. Ahlman and Karvonen[24] reported no change in back leg lift strength in wrestlers dehydrated 2 kg of body weight by means of a sauna combined with exercise regimen. These results are consistent with those Saltin,[7] in whose study reported no change in elbow flexion and knee extension strength in men dehydrated 3% of body weight. Likewise, Singer and Weiss[25] showed no strength change in wrestlers dehydrated 7% of body weight. Furthermore, Mnatzakian and Vaccaro[26] reported no change in isokinetic strength or endurance following 4% dehydration, and Serfass et al.[27] showed that strength and endurance of hand grip muscles of college wrestlers were not affected by a rapid dehydration equivalent to 5% of body weight. In a more recent study, Greiwe et al.[28] reported no effects of hypohydration on isometric strength (peak torque) and endurance (the length of time before dropping below 50% of peak torque for 5 seconds) on seven healthy, unacclimated men. An experimental group dehydrated 4% of body weight by sauna exposure were compared to controls. The controls also experienced sauna exposure but were rehydrated with fluid intake in a quantity equal to weight loss. The results indicated no significant difference between the groups. In fact, although nonsignificant, there was a trend for improved performance in the hypohydrated group. Others have reported no change in isometric strength following varying degrees of dehydration.[21,29-31]

In contrast to the aforementioned studies, Bosco et al.[32] suggested that there is a general trend of decreased strength with increased dehydration. They reported a significant decrease in elbow flexion of 10.7% when subjects were hypohydrated 3.1% of body weight. Similar results were reported in a subsequent study by Bosco et al.[33] Likewise, Greenleaf et al.[34] found that maximal isometric strength in women was reduced to 19% following an acute 3% hypohydration. More recently, Webster et al.[35] reported a 7% reduction in shoulder and chest strength following a 5% exercise and sauna-induced dehydration. Interestingly, the same researchers also reported no change in leg strength in the same study of college wrestlers. Houston et al.[36] reported an 11% reduction in isokinetic strength following a fluid restricted 8% dehydration.

The effects of hydration on isometric and isotonic endurance have also been specifically studied. For example, Torranin et al.[37] compared isometric and isotonic endurance in 20 healthy men who had been dehydrated 4% of body weight, by means of a sauna exposure, to euhydrated conditions. Four muscle groups were tested by means of hand grip contraction, one-arm curl, bench press, and leg press exercises. Isometric endurance was assessed as the length of time a muscle group could maintain a force of 75% of maximal voluntary contraction (MVC). Isotonic endurance was assessed as the length of time that repetitions could be continued, at a rate of 30/minute, with a weight that was 75% MVC. The results suggested that isometric and isotonic endurance were reduced by almost 30% when the men were hypohydrated. It is not clear, however, if the results were associated with hypohydration alone or if they were due to the combined effects of hypohydration and heat exposure.

Care must be taken when comparing and interpreting the results of hypohydration studies on muscular strength and endurance because many different dehydration procedures are used. Experimental procedures range from exercise in the heat (or sauna),[7,24,29,35] to heat alone (sauna exposure),[7,35,37,38] and to fluid restriction.[30,33,36] Viitasalo et al.[39] emphasized the importance of accounting for the effects of heat alone in studies which assess muscular strength and hydration. The researchers[39] found that although a 3.4% loss of body weight by sauna exposure contributed to a 7.8% decrease in maximal isometric strength, dehydration of 2.5% of body weight by diuretics, without heat exposure, did not affect muscular strength.

It has been suggested that electrolyte shifts, in addition to water loss, may explain the reductions in strength associated with a number of the dehydration studies.[33] Additional support of this possible mechanism is offered by Greiwe et al.[28] These authors speculate that the lack of significant change in isometric muscular strength and endurance seen in their study was associated with a restoration of predehydrated serum Na^+ and K^+ concentrations.

10.7 Supplements and Hydration

10.7.1 Protein and Fluid Balance

Although it is widely believed in strength training circles that an increased protein intake, above the recommended dietary allowance (RDA) of 0.8 grams per kilogram of body weight per day, is of physiological benefit to athletes, supplementation is probably not necessary for the vast majority of these individuals.[11] The RDA for protein can usually be obtained by consuming a balanced diet which contains a total energy intake of 2500 to 5000 kcals/day for sedentary and highly active people, respectively. In fact, many Americans consume more than twice their protein needs, and, due to the considerable quantity of food that resistive-trained athletes consume, their diet may contain three or more times the requirement. Supplementation is probably only needed during periods of rapid growth and development and in individuals who have extremely poor dietary habits. Despite these facts, and as a result of unfounded and grandiose advertising campaigns claiming increased strength gains or muscle mass following protein supplementation, many strength athletes continue to consume excessive quantities of this nutrient. Fortunately, it does not appear that diets high in protein are a health hazard, despite the potential additional demands placed on the kidneys to excrete the nitrogen load associated with protein metabolism, provided the athlete is well hydrated. Therefore, it is clear that optimal hydration for strength-training athletes is important, especially if excessive protein is consumed.

It should also be mentioned that the consumption of high-protein diets is sometimes used to further potentiate dehydration in athletes attempting to lose weight for weight classification. A suspected mechanism for water loss during periods of high protein consumption is probably due to the diuretic effect of ketone body formation. Ketosis is associated with increased fat metabolism due to a lack of adequate carbohydrate availability.

10.7.2   Amino Acid Supplements and Fluid Balance

Another common practice among weightlifters is to ingest megadoses of individual amino acids. Despite considerable investigation, there are few documented studies that suggest any ergogenic benefit in amino acid supplementation.[40–46] In addition, this practice also increases the likelihood of developing a variety of complications.[47,48] Adverse effects include cramping, bowel irritation, and diarrhea. The side effects result from the ability of concentrated amino acid solutions to draw water out of the vascular, interstitial, and intracellular spaces and into the intestines. An ultimate consequence of this is, among other things, a compromise in water balance within the body and a concomitant increased risk of dehydration. As a result, it is recommended that these supplements be avoided.

10.7.3   Creatine Monohydrate

Creatine monohydrate supplementation has become very popular among strength athletes to boost short-term anaerobic performance, enhance recovery, and induce muscular hypertrophy. The energy needed for strength and resistance types of activity comes from the dephosphorylation of adenosine triphosphate (ATP) to adenosine diphosphate (ADP), the immediate resynthesis of which is dependent on degradation of phosphocreatine (PCr).[49,50] Thus, the availability of PCr seems to be one of the limiting factors for high-intensity, short-term muscle work.[51] It has been shown that an increase in intramuscular total creatine (Cr) concentration increased the intramuscular PCr content.[52] It has been suggested, therefore, that a delay in the onset of muscle fatigue, during high-intensity muscle work, may be possible if an athlete follows a regime of creatine supplementation.[53]

Creatine supplementation of 20 g/day for 5 consecutive days has been shown to increase the total Cr concentration in human skeletal muscle by 20 to 25%.[54-57] The increased Cr, and subsequent PCr, concentration is thought to be causally related to an increase in anaerobic muscular performance.[58] As with any other form of dietary supplementation, care must be taken to avoid potential health risks associated with consumption of a supplement. Although there have been anecdotal reports linking Cr supplementation to muscle cramping and potential kidney damage,[49,57] especially if consumed when the individual is exposed to heat stress, there is little empirical data to support this. However, because of this potential risk, it would be prudent for strength athletes to remain well hydrated if they choose to consume chronic high doses of creatine supplements.

10.8   Maintaining Fluid Balance

As has been suggested, there are many consequences of strength training in a hypohydrated state. Some of these may be performance related, while others are health consequences. Regardless of the concern, it is essential that fluid balance be maintained as completely as possible before, during, and after strength training. During endurance performance, the opportunities for fluid replacement may be limited. In this type of activity, post-exercise rehydration may be the most appropriate means of restoring fluid balance. This is not generally the case during strength training. Because there is no physical limitation associated with fluid intake during strength training, maintaining fluid balance does not present a tremendous challenge to the strength athlete provided it is done with some fundamental knowledge of the factors that influence hydration.

The primary factors that influence the hydration process are the volume and composition of the fluid consumed. Four distinct types of beverages have traditionally been used in hydration studies. Formulas most often tested are plain water, carbohydrate, carbohydrate electrolyte (frequently sodium based), and plain electrolyte (sodium) solutions.

Plain, hypotonic water has been suggested as a hydrating agent, but research has established that it may not be the ideal beverage. Shirreffs[59] has done an excellent review of several studies comparing plain water with other rehydrating beverage compositions and has summarized the results. For example, it was demonstrated by Costill and Sparks[60] that ingestion of plain water as a rehydration beverage resulted in a large fall in serum osmolality. This, in turn, resulted in an additional urinary water loss leading to a subsequent creation of a negative fluid balance over a 4-hour study. In addition, it was also reported that when an electrolyte-containing solution (106 g/L carbohydrate, 22 mmol/L Na+, 2.6 mmol/L K+, 17.2 mmol/L Cl-) was used as a rehydrating beverage post-exercise, urine output was reduced and net water balance was returned closer to the pre-exercise level. In a similar study, Nose et al.[61] rehydrated subjects with either plain water or a weak saline solution, (0.45% sodium), following voluntary dehydration by an exercise and heat protocol. After 3 hours of recovery, the researchers determined that plasma volume and total body water were restored to a greater extent with saline than with water. Likewise, Shirreffs and associates[62] found that drinking a volume of water equivalent to one half to twice the volume of sweat lost during exercise was not sufficient to achieve complete rehydration unless accompanied by sodium. The authors concluded that, unless the sodium content of the beverage is sufficiently high and similar to that found in sweat (between 23 mmol/L and 61 mmol/L), ingestion of a volume of fluid necessary to restore fluid balance will merely result in an increased urinary output without restoring hydration to pre-exercise levels. The results reported by Nielsen et al.[63] also support the importance of sodium. They suggested that recovery from exercise-induced dehydration was best when sodium, at a concentration of 43 and 128 mmol/L, was added to a carbohydrate solution. These authors go on to say that the observed plasma volume increase was greater than that seen when drinks containing additional potassium, at a concentration of 51 mmol/L, or less electrolytes and more carbohydrate were consumed. Additional confirmation of sodium's fundamental role in rehydration comes from the work of Gonzalez-Alonso et al.[64] in which they report that a dilute carbohydrate electrolyte solution (60 g/L carbohydrate, 20 mmol/L Na+, 3 mmol/L K+, 20 mmol/L Cl-) was significantly more effective in restoring weight loss (which was used as a index of rehydration) than a caffeinated diet cola or plain water.

The aforementioned studies establish that fluid balance was better maintained when electrolytes were present in the fluid ingested, and it seemed likely that this effect was due primarily to the presence of sodium in the drinks. Recent investigations by Greenleaf et al.[65] have confirmed the importance of sodium in stabilization and expansion of plasma volume. Shirreffs[59] justifies the addition of sodium to rehydration beverages based on two mechanistic factors. First, it was suggested that because sodium can stimulate glucose absorption in the small intestine[66] and create a large osmotic gradient to drive the passive process of water absorption from the intestinal lumen, the rate of absorption and thus rehydration is potentially greater for glucose-sodium chloride solutions than plain water. A second mechanism discussed by Shirreffs[59] centers on the potential to dilute the plasma and reduce its osmolality if sweat loss is replaced by large quantities of hypotonic water. It was suggested that this can reduce the drive to drink, stimulate greater urine output,[61] and lead to a more pronounced negative fluid balance. For a comprehensive summary of fluid replacement and exercise, the reader is encouraged to review the American College of Sports Medicine's (ACSM) Position Stand on Exercise and Fluid Replacement, (Appendix K),[67] as well as a current review of the topic by Armstrong and Epstein.[68]

The ACSM position stand emphasizes the following recommendations regarding the prevention of dehydration:

1. Ingest at least 500 ml (about 17 oz) of fluid in the form of water, fruit juice, or sports drinks about 2 hours before exercise. This will allow enough time for urine excretion, which can provide an excellent indication of hydration status. This is discussed in more detail in the next section.

2. Athletes should continue to consume water at a rate sufficient to replace all the water lost through sweating during the exercise session. Change in body weight can be used as a measure of fluid loss.

3. Fluids ingested should be cooler than room temperature (between 15 and 22°C or 59 to 72°F) and flavored to enhance palatability.

4. Fluids should be readily available and convenient to consume.

5. Carbohydrate (30 to 60 g/hr) and sodium (0.5 to 0.7 g/L of water) should be consumed during periods of exercise longer than 1 hour in duration.

10.9   Indices of Hydration

The most obvious stimulus for fluid replacement is thirst. Greenleaf[10] defined thirst, among other ways, as a desire to drink resulting from a water deficit. It appears that thirst itself, as an indicator of hydration status, is adequate in normal, healthy people. If, however, physiological and/or psychological stress is introduced, thirst no longer provides an adequate stimulus for fluid replacement. As a result, individuals are likely to drink yet still create a self-imposed, involuntary water debt. This phenomenon is called involuntary dehydration.[10] For a more complete discussion on the topic of thirst, readers should consult the reviews of Fitzsimons[69] and Greenleaf.[10] Because water intake, as stimulated by a complex interaction of thirst mechanisms, is often incomplete, athletes should carefully monitor additional indices of hydration status.

Aside from thirst, monitoring urinary indices of hydration can provide another practical means of tracking body fluid balance and have been used extensively by wrestlers, soldiers, and children.[70,71] The most commonly used index of urine concentration is specific gravity. A euhydrated individual is defined as having a urine specific gravity between 1.013 and 1.029. Likewise, urine osmolality is also frequently used as an indicator. It is suggested that a euhydrated individual has a urine osmolality in the range of 442 to 1052 mOsm/kg.[72] In providing some guidelines for using urinary indices of hydration, Armstrong et al.[72] suggest that direct measurements of urinary specific gravity and osmolality are more sensitive indicators of hydration status and should be used in laboratory settings when possible. They go on to point out that urine color may, however, provide a practical and meaningful index in "real-world" settings. It is recommended that an athlete's urine color be "very pale yellow," "pale yellow," or "straw colored." At these colors, urine osmolality and specific gravity will be less than 520 mOsm/kg and 1.014, respectively. However, it cannot be emphasized enough that athletes who participate in strenuous activity should also monitor their rate of weight loss for optimal hydration and thus performance.[73]

10.10 Summary

Although successful and safe strength training depends on many factors, the importance of hydration should not be overlooked. Water may be the most important nutrient to life even though it contains no caloric value. The approximate 40 L of total body water, stored in the two major compartments, intracellular and extracellular, is constantly in a state of flux. The compartments function in many capacities including helping to regulate body heat via the evaporative cooling of sweat. Sweat loss, which can potentially be over 4000 ml during exercise in warm environments, along with the added shifting of fluid out of the vascular space and into the interstitial space due to the increased hydrostatic pressure associated with resistance exercise, can cause dramatic changes in fluid balance. In the most severe cases, and if left uncompensated, these changes can lead to dehydration, which can progress to death.

There is ample evidence to support the important role adequate hydration plays in long-duration, moderate-intensity exercise. It has been reported that even a 2% reduction of body weight, leading to a reduction in plasma volume, can impair endurance performance. It has been suggested that this is due largely to cardiovascular and thermoregulatory compromise. Strength athletes have a great potential to dehydrate during exercise due to thermal stress being combined with a concomitant increase in hydrostatic pressure that is associated with resistance exercise. This increase in hydrostatic pressure, leading to a reduction in plasma volume, has been shown to be inversely proportional to the exercise intensity as measured by a percentage of a 1 repetition maximum lift. This value is similar to the results seen during other short-term dynamic exercises such as cycling.

The performance-related consequences of dehydration, although inconsistent, have been documented. The results range from no change to a significant change occurring in measures of elbow flexion or knee extension, isometric grip strength, isokinetic strength, and isometric endurance. Interpretation of these results should include careful analysis of the dehydration procedure employed. It has been suggested that the method used to dehydrate individuals might contribute to the inconsistency of the results of these studies. Electrolyte shifts, in addition to pure water loss, might help explain reductions in strength that are associated with dehydration studies.

The health concerns of being hypohydrated are similar for all athletes. These concerns are often magnified for the strength athlete if protein and/or creatine are supplemented in the diet. It is recommended that athletes hydrate with water, fruit juice, or a sports drink before, during, and after exercise. It is suggested that the fluid be slightly cooler than ambient conditions, flavored, abundant, and easily accessible. It is also recommended that carbohydrate and sodium be added to the beverage. For practical purposes, changes in body weight and analysis of urine color can be used as indicators of athlete hydration status.

References

1. Armstrong, L. E., Costill, D. L., and Fink, W. J., Influence of diuretic-induced dehydration on competitive running performance, *Med. Sci. Sports Exerc.*, 17(4), 456, 1985.
2. Burge, C. M., Carey, M. F., and Payne, W. R., Rowing performance, fluid balance, and metabolic function following dehydration and rehydration, *Med. Sci. Sports Exerc.*, 25(12), 1358, 1993.
3. Buskirk, E. R., Iampietro, P. F., and Bass, D. E., Work performance after dehydration: Effects of physical conditioning and heat acclimatization, *J. Appl. Physiol.*, 12, 189, 1958.
4. Caldwell, J. E., Ahonen, E., and Nousiainen, U., Differential effects of sauna-, diuretic-, and exercise-induced hypohydration, *J. Appl. Physiol.*, 57(4), 1018, 1984.
5. Craig, E. N. and Cummings, E. G., Dehydration and muscular work, *J. Appl. Physiol.*, 21(2), 670, 1966.
6. Luetkemeier, M. J. and Thomas, E. L., Hypervolemia and cycling time trial performance, *Med. Sci. Sports Exerc.*, 26(4), 503, 1994.
7. Saltin, B., Aerobic and anaerobic work capacity after dehydration, *J. Appl. Physiol.*, 19, 1114, 1964.
8. Sawka, M. N. and Pandolf, K. B., Effects of body water loss on exercise performance and physiological functions, in *Fluid Homeostasis During Exercise*, Gisolfi, C. V. and Lamb, D. R. (Eds.), Benchmark Press, Indianapolis, 1990, 1.
9. Tortora, G. J. and Evans, R. L., *Principles of Human Physiology*, 2nd ed., Harper & Row Publishers, New York, 1986.
10. Greenleaf, J. E., Problem: thirst, drinking behavior, and involuntary dehydration, *Med. Sci. Sports Exerc.*, 24(6), 645, 1992.

11. McArdle, W. D., Katch, F. I., and Katch, V. L., *Exercise Physiology: Energy Nutrition, and Human Performance*, 4th ed., Williams and Wilkins, Baltimore, 1996, chap. 2.

12. Ganong, W. F., *Review of Medical Physiology*, 17th ed., Appleton & Lang, Norwalk, CT, 1995.

13. Sawka, M. N. and Greenleaf, J. E., Current concepts concerning thirst, dehydration, and fluid replacement: overview, *Med. Sci. Sports Exerc.*, 24(6), 643, 1992.

14. Nadel, E. R., Fortney, S. M., and Wenger, C. B., Effect of hydration state on circulatory and thermal regulation, *J. Appl. Physiol.*, 49, 715, 1980.

15. Convertino, V. A., Mack, G. W., and Nadel, E. R., Elevated central venous pressure: a consequence of exercise training-induced hypervolemia?, *Am. J. Physiol.*, 260(2 Pt 2), R273, 1991.

16. Senay, L. C., Effects of exercise in the heat on body fluid distribution, *Med. Sci. Sports Exerc.*, 11, 42, 1979.

17. Convertino, V. A., Keil, L. C., Bernauer, E. M., and Greenleaf, J. E., Plasma volume, osmolality, vasopressin, and renin activity during graded exercise in man, *J. Appl. Physiol.*, 50(1), 123, 1981.

18. Miles, D. S., Sawka, M. N., Glaser, R. M., and Petrofsky, J. S., Plasma volume shifts during progressive arm and leg exercise, *J. Appl. Physiol.*, 54(2), 491, 1983.

19. Senay, L. C., Jr., Rogers, G., and Jooste, P., Changes in blood plasma during progressive treadmill and cycle exercise, *J. Appl. Physiol.*, 49(1), 59, 1980.

20. Collins, M. A., Cureton, K. J., Hill, D. W., and Ray, C. A., Relation of plasma volume change to intensity of weight lifting, *Med. Sci. Sports Exerc.*, 21(2), 178, 1989.

21. Greenleaf, J. E. and Castle, B. L., Exercise temperature regulation in man during hypohydration and hyperhydration, *J. Appl. Physiol.*, 30(6), 847, 1971.

22. Wilmore, J. H., Weight category sports, in *Nutrition in Sport*, Malden, R. J. (Ed.), Blackwell Science, Malden, MA., 2000, chap. 49.

23. Sawka, M. N., Young, A. J., Cadarette, B. S., Levine, L., and Pandolf, K. B., Influence of heat stress and acclimation on maximal aerobic power, *Eur. J. Appl. Physiol.*, 53(4), 294, 1985.

24. Ahlman, K. and Karvonen, M. J., Weight reduction by sweating in wrestlers, and its effect on physical fitness, *J. Sports Med. Phys. Fitness*, 1, 58, 1961.

25. Singer, R. N. and Weiss, S. A., Effects of weight reduction on several anthropometric, physical, and performance measures of wrestlers, *Res. Q. Exer. Sport*, 39, 361, 1968.

26. Mnatzakian, P. A. and Vaccaro, P., Effects of 4% dehydration and rehydration on hematological profiles, urinary profiles, and muscular endurance of college wrestlers, *Med. Sci. Sports Exerc.*, 14, 117, 1982.

27. Serfass, R. C., Stull, G. A., Alexander, J. F., and Ewing, J. L., The effects of rapid weight loss and attempted rehydration on strength and endurance of the hand-gripping muscles in college wrestlers, *Res. Q. Exer. Sport*, 55, 46, 1968.

28. Greiwe, J. S., Staffey, K. S., Melrose, D. R., Narve, M. D., and Knowlton, R. G., Effects of dehydration on isometric muscular strength and endurance, *Med. Sci. Sports Exerc.*, 30(2), 284, 1998.

29. Tuttle, W. W., The effect of weight loss by dehydration and the withholding of food on the physiological responses of wrestlers, *Res. Q. Exerc. Sport*, 14, 159, 1943.

30. Greenleaf, J. E., Matter, Jr., M., Bosco, J. S., Douglas, L. G., and Averkin, E. G., Effects of hypohydration on work performance and tolerance to +Gz acceleration in man, *Aerosp. Med.*, 37(1), 34, 1966.
31. Bijlani, R. L. and Sharma, K. N., Effect of dehydration and a few regimes of rehydration on human performance, *Indian J. Physiol. Pharmacol.*, 24(4), 255, 1980.
32. Bosco, J. S., Terjung, R. L., and Greenleaf, J. E., Effects of progressive hypohydration on maximal isometric muscular strength, *J. Sports Med. Phys. Fitness*, 8(2), 81, 1968.
33. Bosco, J. S., Greenleaf, J. E., Bernauer, E. M., and Card, D. H., Effects of acute dehydration and starvation on muscular strength and endurance, *Acta Physiol. Pol.*, 25(5), 411, 1974.
34. Greenleaf, J. E., Prange, E. M., and Averkin, E. G., Physical performance of women following heat-exercise hypohydration, *J. Appl. Physiol.*, 22(1), 55, 1967.
35. Webster, S., Rutt, R., and Weltman, A., Physiological effects of a weight loss regimen practiced by college wrestlers, *Med. Sci. Sports Exerc.*, 22(2), 229, 1990.
36. Houston, M. E., Marrin, D. A., Green, H. J., and Thomson, J. A., The effect of rapid weight loss on physiological functions in wrestlers, *Physician Sportsmed.*, 9, 73, 1981.
37. Torranin, C., Smith, D. P., and Byrd, R. J., The effect of acute thermal dehydration and rapid rehydration on isometric and isotonic endurance, *J. Sports Med. Phys. Fitness*, 19(1), 1, 1979.
38. Jacobs, I., The effects of thermal dehydration on performance of the Wingate Anaerobic Test., *Int. J. Sports Med.*, 1, 21, 1980.
39. Viitasalo, J. T., Kyrolainen, H., Bosco, C., and Alen, M., Effects of rapid weight reduction on force production and vertical jumping height, *Int. J. Sports Med.*, 8(4), 281, 1987.
40. Bigard, A. X., Lavier, P., Ullmann, L., Legrand, H., Douce, P., and Guezennec, C. Y., Branched-chain amino acid supplementation during repeated prolonged skiing exercises at altitude, *Int. J. Sport Nutr.*, 6(3), 295, 1996.
41. Fogelholm, G. M., Naveri, H. K., Kiilavuori, K. T., and Harkonen, M. H., Low-dose amino acid supplementation: no effects on serum human growth hormone and insulin in male weightlifters, *Int. J. Sport Nutr.*, 3(3), 290, 1993.
42. Isidori, A., Lo Monaco, A., and Cappa, M., A study of growth hormone release in man after oral administration of amino acids, *Curr. Med. Res. Opin.*, 7(7), 475, 1981.
43. Kasai, K., Kobayashi, M., and Shimoda, S. I., Stimulatory effect of glycine on human growth hormone secretion, *Metabolism*, 27(2), 201, 1978.
44. Maughan, R. J. and Sadler, D. J., The effects of oral administration of salts of aspartic acid on the metabolic response to prolonged exhausting exercise in man, *Int. J. Sports Med.*, 4(2), 119, 1983.
45. Segura, R. and Ventura, J. L., Effect of L-tryptophan supplementation on exercise performance, *Int. J. Sports Med.*, 9(5), 301, 1988.
46. Suminski, R. R., Robertson, R. J., Goss, F. L., Arslanian, S., Kang, J., DaSilva, S., Utter, A. C., and Metz, F., Acute effect of amino acid ingestion and resistance exercise on plasma growth hormone concentration in young men, *Int. J. Sport Nutr.*, 7(1), 48, 1997.
47. Benevenga, N. J. and Steele, R. D., Adverse effects of excessive consumption of amino acids, *Ann. Rev. Nutr.*, 4, 157, 1984.

48. Harper, A. E., Benevenga, N. J., and Wohlhueter, R. M., Effects of ingestion of disproportionate amounts of amino acids, *Physiol. Rev.*, 50(3), 428, 1970.

49. Brooks, G. A., Fahey, T. D., White, T. P., and Baldwin, K. M., *Exercise Physiology: Human Bioenergetics and Its Applications*, 3rd ed., Mayfield Publishing Company, Mountain View, CA, 2000.

50. Jackson, C. G. R., Overview: nutrition in exercise and sport, in *Nutrition in Exercise and Sport*, 3rd ed., Wolinsky, I. (Ed.), CRC Press, Boca Raton, FL, 1998, chap. 2.

51. Hultman, E., Greenhaff, P. L., Ren, J. M., and Soderlund, K., Energy metabolism and fatigue during intense muscle contraction, *Biochem. Soc. Trans.*, 19(2), 347, 1991.

52. Francaux, M., Demeure, R., Goudemant, J. F., and Poortmans, J. R., Effect of exogenous creatine supplementation on muscle PCr metabolism, *Int. J. Sports Med.*, 21(2), 139, 2000.

53. Greenhaff, P. L., Casey, A., Short, A. H., Harris, R., Soderlund, K., and Hultman, E., Influence of oral creatine supplementation of muscle torque during repeated bouts of maximal voluntary exercise in man, *Clin. Sci.*, 84(5), 565, 1993.

54. Balsom, P. D., Soderlund, K., and Ekblom, B., Creatine in humans with special reference to creatine supplementation, *Sports Med.*, 18(4), 268, 1994.

55. Greenhaff, P. L., Creatine and its application as an ergogenic aid, *Int. J. Sport Nutr.*, 5 Suppl., S100, 1995.

56. Harris, R. C., Soderlund, K., and Hultman, E., Elevation of creatine in resting and exercised muscle of normal subjects by creatine supplementation, *Clin. Sci.*, 83(3), 367, 1992.

57. Maughan, R. J., Creatine supplementation and exercise performance, *Int. J. Sport Nutr.*, 5(2), 94, 1995.

58. Kreider, R. B., Ferreira, M., Wilson, M., Grindstaff, P., Plisk, S., Reinardy, J., Cantler, E., and Almada, A. L., Effects of creatine supplementation on body composition, strength, and sprint performance, *Med. Sci. Sports Exerc.*, 30(1), 73, 1998.

59. Shirreffs, S. M., Rehydration and recovery after exercise, in *Nutrition in Sport*, Malden, R. J. (Ed.), Blackwell Science, Malden, MA, 2000, chap. 19.

60. Costill, D. L. and Sparks, K. E., Rapid fluid replacement following thermal dehydration, *J. Appl. Physiol.*, 34(3), 299, 1973.

61. Nose, H., Mack, G. W., Shi, X., and Nadel, E. R., Shifts in body fluid compartments after dehydration in humans, *J. Appl. Physiol.*, 65, 318, 1988.

62. Shirreffs, S. M., Taylor, A. J., Leiper, J. B., and Maughan, R. J., Post-exercise rehydration in man: effects of volume consumed and drink sodium content, *Med. Sci. Sports Exerc.*, 28(10), 1260, 1996.

63. Nielsen, B., Sjogaard, G., Ugelvig, J., Knudsen, B., and Dohlmann, B., Fluid balance in exercise dehydration and rehydration with different glucose-electrolyte drinks, *Eur. J. Appl. Physiol.*, 55(3), 318, 1986.

64. Gonzalez-Alonso, J., Heaps, C. L., and Coyle, E. F., Rehydration after exercise with common beverages and water, *Int. J. Sports Med.*, 13(5), 399, 1992.

65. Greenleaf, J. E., Jackson, C. G. R., Geelen, G., Keil, L. H., Hinghofer-Szalkay, H., and Whittam J. H., Plasma volume expansion with oral fluids in hypohydrated men at rest and during exercise, *Aviat. Space Environ. Med.*, 69(9), 837, 1998.

66. Olsen, W. A. and Ingelfinger, F. J., The role of sodium in intestinal glucose absorption in man, *J. Clin. Invest.*, 47(5), 1133, 1968.

67. Convertino, V. A., Armstrong, L. E., Coyle, E. F., Mack, G. W., Sawka, M. N., Senary, Jr., L. C., and Sherman, W. M., American College of Sports Medicine position stand. Exercise and fluid replacement, *Med. Sci. Sports Exerc.*, 28(1), i, 1996.

68. Armstrong, L. E. and Epstein, Y., Fluid-electrolyte balance during labor and exercise: concepts and misconceptions, *Int. J. Sport Nutr.*, 9(1), 1, 1999.

69. Fitzsimons, J. T., The physiology of thirst and sodium appetite, *Monogr. Physiol. Soc.*, 35, 1, 1979.

70. Ballauff, A., Rascher, W., Tolle, H. G., Wember, T., and Manz, F., Circadian rhythms of urine osmolality and renal excretion rates of solutes influencing water metabolism in 21 healthy children, *Miner. Electrolyte Metab.*, 17(6), 377, 1991.

71. Francesconi, R. P., Hubbard, R. W., Szlyk, P. C., Schnakenberg, D., Carlson, D., Leva, N., Sils, I., Hubbard, L., Pease, V., Young, J. et al., Urinary and hematologic indexes of hypohydration, *J. Appl. Physiol.*, 62(3), 1271, 1987.

72. Armstrong, L. E., Maresh, C. M., Castellani, J. W., Bergeron, M. F., Kenefick, R. W., LaGasse, K. E., and Riebe, D., Urinary indices of hydration status, *Int. J. Sport Nutr.*, 4(3), 265, 1994.

73. Senay, Jr., L. C., Water and electrolytes during physical activity, in *Nutrition in Exercise and Sport*, 3rd ed., Wolinsky, I. (Ed.), CRC Press, Boca Raton, FL, 1998, chap. 11.

11

Nutritional Concerns of Women Who Resistance Train

Ann C. Snyder

CONTENTS

11.1   Women and Physical Activity

Women have become much more involved in exercise activities in the last 20 years. In 1995, it was projected that approximately 40% of all American women over the age of 18 performed some type of physical activity.[1] While exercise walking (37%) represented the greatest single percentage of the activities reported, resistance training also became much more popular during this time. The enhanced interest in resistance training for women has a great range. One end of the range involves the health and fitness level; the 1998 American College of Sports Medicine's position stand recommends that resistance training be performed by all adults to enhance muscular strength and endurance and ensure overall fitness.[2] At the other end of the range is the inclusion of women's weightlifting as a world championship event in 1987, and as an Olympic event at the summer games in Sydney in 2000, with weight classes of 48, 53, 59, 63, 75, and 75+ kg.[3] Therefore, this chapter will deal with defining resistance training, especially with regard to women, adaptations that occur following resistance training, and finally, nutritional needs and concerns of women who perform resistance training.

In examining the performance of resistance training by women and the nutritional needs of these individuals, we must first remember that while women have been involved in organized sport for a long time (they indeed participated in the 1900 Olympic games), it has only been "recently" that their performance in sport has been recognized. As such, much of the research literature has used college-aged males as the subject population. In this chapter I will cite what is known specifically concerning the female athlete, but I have had to draw on the scientific literature in general to present the entire picture. I do so knowing that further research might show that, with respect to certain physiological functions, women will respond and adapt to exercise and training differently than men.

11.2   Resistance Training for Women

11.2.1   Types of Resistance Training

For the most part, four different types of exercises make up resistance training: isometric training, external resistance training (also called isotonic training), variable resistance training, and isokinetic training. The main differences among the four types of exercises have to do with the resistance, whether or not the resistance is constant or variable, and whether or not the forces generated by the contracting muscles are greater than the resistance or not.

Isometric training is performed when the resistance is constant and the resistance is greater than the muscular forces produced. An example of this type of contraction would be an arm curl (or arm flexion) performed against an immovable counter. Since isometric contractions involve no movement through a range of motion, they should be performed at various joint angles, with each contraction held for 3 to 5 seconds and repeated at least 15 to 20 times per session. Isometric training should be performed daily.

Similar to isometric training, with external resistance training the resistance is constant; however, with external resistance training, the resistance is less than the muscular forces produced, therefore movement of the muscle occurs and motor performance enhancements occur. While the number of repetitions and sets will depend on the needs of the individual, a minimum of one set for each of the major muscle groups is recommended if general fitness is the goal.[2] To achieve greater strength gains, however, an athlete may need to perform multiple sets of the exercises. Generally, 8 to 12 repetitions are recommended per set to enhance muscular strength and endurance. However, a lower number of repetitions (6 to 8) with greater resistance may result in greater gains in muscular strength. Two to three training sessions per week for each major muscle group are recommended for those interested in enhancing fitness, while a minimum of three training sessions per week are recommended to ensure optimal strength gains for athletes. The performance of two exercise sessions in a single day has now become more common, and due to the recovery allowed, two half sessions may indeed elicit greater strength gains than one complete session.[4] External resistance training exercises can be separated into two components: a concentric component, which is generally performed in opposition to the force of gravity, thus the joint angle decreases and the muscle shortens, and an eccentric component, which is generally performed in the direction of gravity, thus the joint angle increases and the muscle lengthens. Since eccentric contractions move in the direction of gravity, greater work can generally be performed. However, eccentric training alone has not been shown to result in any greater gains than when both eccentric and concentric components are combined, and performance of eccentric training alone will probably lead to the development of delayed-onset muscle soreness and will also require assistance to perform.[4] Therefore, eccentric only training is not recommended.

With variable resistance training, similar to external resistance training, the resistance is less than the muscular force produced; however, due to the use of lever arms, cams, or pulley systems, the resistance is altered to match the force production of the muscle. Motor performance increases similar to those of external resistance training will occur, but greater strength gains can be obtained due to the muscle being equally stressed through the range of motion. The number of repetitions, sets, and sessions necessary to enhance muscular strength are similar to that of external resistance training.

Finally, isokinetic training can be performed when using equipment that allows the muscle to contract at a constant angular velocity. Because the contraction is controlled by the angular velocity of the movement, there is in essence no resistance. With isokinetic training it is possible for the muscle to exert a maximal force throughout the full range of motion of a movement. Most isokinetic training devices allow for concentric-only muscle contractions; thus, the incidence of delayed muscle soreness is greatly reduced. As with both external and variable resistance training, motor performance enhancements occur with isokinetic training due to the movement of the joint through a range of motion. Generally, sets of 1 to 15 contractions at various velocities of contraction are needed to optimally increase muscular strength.

Other types of activities, such as plyometrics, have been used to enhance muscular strength and endurance. Greater details on these, and all resistance training programs, may be found in Chapter 1.

11.2.2   Adaptations to Resistance Training

In general, a woman has approximately 64% of the total body strength of a man.[5,6] The absolute strength of the upper body of a woman is about 52 to 56% that of a man, while the lower-body strength is about 66 to 72% that of a man.[5–7] However, when relative strength is examined, that is, corrected for body weight, lower-body strength is generally more similar for the two genders, while upper-body strength is still greater for men.[4,6–8] Like muscular strength, maximal anaerobic power outputs of women are only about 54 to 66% that of men, and correcting for differences of body composition, physique, strength, or neuromuscular difference did not remove the significant difference between the genders.[9] When muscular endurance was examined by the number of contractions to fatigue at 60% of 1 repetition maximum (1 RM), women performed significantly more elbow flexion repetitions than did the men; however, there was no difference between the genders in the number of knee extension contractions performed.[6]

Even though there are indeed anatomical differences between men and women, such as height, weight, muscle fiber size, and hip to shoulder and body fat to body weight proportions that lead to the absolute difference in muscular strength, research to date has shown that resistance training is as beneficial for women as it is for men, if not more so.[4,7,8] Gains in strength can occur at a similar rate, and, while absolute gains in strength are probably greater for men, relative gains are similar for men and women. In general, resistance training by women can lead not only to gains in muscular strength, but also muscular, metabolic, and body composition adaptations, with few changes in cardiovascular function. These adaptations occur in both young and aged women, and for the most part are dependent on total exercise volume.[10]

11.2.2.1 Exercise Performance Adaptations to Resistance Training

Increases in muscular strength are almost a universal adaptation to resistance training, independent of age[11,12] and body composition.[4,8,10,13–22] Likewise, anaerobic power and capacity are also increased with resistance training.[14] Little agreement in the literature occurs concerning the influence of resistance training on aerobic ability (oxygen uptake) where increases[4,14,17] or no change[19] has been demonstrated. The conflict more than likely is due to the initial ability or fitness level of the subjects in the studies and the intensity and duration of the resistance training exercises.

11.2.2.2 Muscular and Bone Adaptations to Resistance Training

Even though the muscle fiber size and cross-sectional area of the average woman is only about 70% that of man's,[6,8,23] resistance training in women has been shown to increase muscle fiber size of the Type I (slow) and Type IIA and IIAB (fast) fibers.[4,16,20,21,24,25] This increase in muscle fiber size has led to an increase[26] or no change[21] in muscle girth. The metabolic enzyme levels in the different muscle fiber types are similar in women and men; however, women have greater amounts of intramuscular fat.[6,23] Resistance training has induced a significant increase in the activity of the enzymes cytochrome oxidase and hexokinase, but no changes were observed in the activity of the enzymes creatine kinase, citrate synthase, phosphofructokinase, glyceraldehyde phosphate dehydrogenase, and hydroxyacyl CoA dehydrogenase.[25] Resistance training did not cause a change in the capillary density, nor in the capillary/fiber ratio.[25] Training-induced conversions of myosin heavy chains and enhanced metabolic levels have resulted in conversions of muscle fibers from Type IIB (II AB) to IIA fibers.[4,8,20,21,25]

Performance of resistance training is associated with an increase in bone mineral density, possibly the most important adaptation to resistance training other than increases in muscular strength.[27,28] As bone density in women is generally less than that of men, and because bone density decreases rapidly immediately postmenopause and then slowly thereafter, the performance of resistance training may be critical to bone health in women. Other types of exercises have also been shown to enhance bone density, such as aerobic exercise and weight-bearing activities; however, resistance training activities have the greatest impact on bone density, especially to those bones attached to the active muscles utilized.[27] (See Reference 28 for a further review of the effects of physical activity and nutrition on bone health.)

11.2.2.3 Body Weight and Composition Adaptations to Resistance Training

Numerous studies have investigated the effects of resistance training on body weight and composition, with much interest in the decrease in body

weight and fat in the obese individual.[16-19,26] In general, with resistance training alone, body weight has been shown not to change significantly[21,22] or
increase slightly,[7,8] while percent body fat decreases[4,7,20-22,29] and fat-free mass
increases.[4,7,20-22,29] The magnitude of the decrease in body fat and the increase
in fat-free mass is similar to that in comparably trained men.[4] When a caloric
restriction program is added to a resistance training program, obese women
have been shown to conserve a greater percentage of their fat-free mass when
weight loss occurs, through minimal loss,[10,16] maintenance[17,19] or an
increase[16,26] in muscle mass, primarily through hypertrophy of the Type I and
II fibers.[16,26]

11.2.2.4 Serum Lipid Adaptations to Resistance Training

In men, resistance training has been shown to decrease LDL-C levels and
increase HDL-C levels in individuals at low risk of cardiovascular disease.[30]
Few studies have been performed on women that examine the serum lipid
adaptations following a resistance training program; therefore, little conclusive information may be given. The three investigations that used a resistance
training program on women for 12 to 20 weeks observed conflicting results;
one showed decreased levels of cholesterol and LDL-C, with increased levels
of HDL-C,[29] while the other two observed no change in cholesterol, HDL-C,
and LDL-C levels.[18,22] In a population at risk for cardiovascular disease, resistance training did not significantly alter the lipoprotein levels.[31] Similarly,
two cross-sectional investigations that examined women who had been resistance training for a period of time (minimum of 9 to 36 months) observed
conflicting results. One of these investigations noted that HDL-C levels and
the total cholesterol:HDL-C ratio were greater in the resistance-trained
women than in the controls, while total cholesterol, triglycerides, and LDL-C
levels and the LDL:HDL ratio were similar for the two populations of subjects.[32] The second investigation observed that the HDL-C levels for the
resistance-trained athletes were similar to those of the controls, but less than
those of the runners, while total cholesterol and triglyceride levels were similar for all three groups.[33] The conflicting results concerning the serum lipid
adaptations to resistance training in women are probably due to differences
in intensity, rest duration, and total exercise volume between the studies
and/or to factors other than exercise training which influence serum lipid
levels that were not controlled sufficiently with these studies. More work in
this area using women as the population is definitely warranted.

11.2.2.5 Neuroendocrine Adaptations to Resistance Training

Women generally have about one tenth the circulating levels of testosterone
as men.[4] Therefore, women tend to have higher pre-exercise growth hormone
levels, while men tend to have higher pre-exercise testosterone levels.[8,34] With
moderate-intensity/short-duration rest resistance exercise, greater increases

in circulating levels of growth hormone were observed in women[34,35] than in men.[34] However, following high-intensity/long-duration rest resistance exercise, minimal increases in growth hormone were observed in both men[34] and women.[34,35] With both types of exercise (moderate-intensity/short-duration rest and high intensity/long duration rest), circulating testosterone levels were not increased in the women,[34,35] while they were greatly increased in men.[34] Moderate-intensity/short-duration rest resistance exercise also resulted in elevated levels of serum cortisol[35] and somatomedin-C[34] in women. In another series of experiments, 2 months of resistance training resulted in significantly increased resting serum testosterone levels in women.[36] Following a single bout of resistance exercise (3 sets of 10 reps with each set to failure of 6 different exercises), testosterone and cortisol increased in relation to time and lactate levels.[36] However, others have observed no difference in resting testosterone and cortisol in women following 9 weeks of resistance training.[8] More than likely, the differences in these results are again associated with the initial fitness levels of the subjects and the resistance training program used.

In response to a survey, a group of resistance-trained athletes (n = 61) reported a greater incidence of menstrual dysfunction (30%, defined as those with oligomenorrhea or amenorrhea) than did a control population (13%, n=56).[37] In a subset of the resistance-trained women who had performed in bodybuilding competitions (n=7), 86% of the women (n=6) were classified as having menstrual dysfunctions.[37] Amenorrhea in athletes has been associated with many factors, such as body weight, body fat, exercise intensity and duration, and food quantity and quality/type.[38] More than likely, menstrual dysfunction in athletes is an individual problem per athlete that involves multiple factors, with no one factor contributing significantly for all athletes.[38]

11.3 Nutritional Needs of Resistance Training for Women

Nutrient intake is important for overall health, but also for the full benefits of a resistance training program to occur for women. Everyday food or energy intake and that associated with the performance of exercise are therefore both important.

11.3.1 Proper Nutrition During Training

As most individuals perform exercise bouts for the sake of training, rather than for competition, nutrition during the training phase is extremely important for the performance of future exercise bouts and the training adaptations, and thus ultimately to performance in competition. The typical person consumes a diet of approximately 40 to 45% carbohydrates; however, the recommended intake is about 55 to 60%, as would occur if the food guide pyramid (Figure 11.1) were followed. As recommended from the food guide pyramid, carbohydrate (from bread, cereal, rice, pasta group; vegetable group; and fruit group) would make up the largest percentage of macronutrients, followed by fats (about 25%) and proteins (about 15%). Since, for the most part, carbohydrates are the preferred fuel during exercise, athletes should consume at least the minimal amounts of carbohydrates, especially during periods of resistance training.

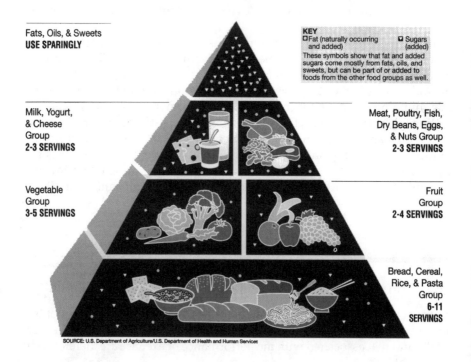

FIGURE 11.1
Food guide pyramid.

11.3.1.1 Carbohydrate Utilization and Intake

The body has very limited stores of carbohydrates, as glycogen is stored only in the muscle (approximately 1600 kcal for 70-kg or 150-lb person) and liver (approximately 280 kcal for a 70-kg person).[39] Glucose in the blood (approximately 80 kcal for a 70-kg person) provides the only other readily available source of carbohydrate in the body, though indeed protein can be converted to carbohydrates.[39] However, once glucose enters the muscle it cannot leave the muscle and can only be used for energy in that muscle; the available carbohydrate stores in the body are much smaller than the total glycogen stores. That is, carbohydrates stored in the arm cannot be utilized for energy during exercise involving only the legs.

Due to the limited carbohydrate stores and the usage of carbohydrates during physical activity, body carbohydrates must be replaced with dietary carbohydrates. In general, physical activities performed at moderate intensity (70% maximal oxygen uptake, approximately 80% maximal heart rate) for less than 75 to 90 minutes should not deplete muscle glycogen levels if the athlete started the activity with normal resting levels of muscle glycogen.[40] Activities of higher intensity, such as resistance exercise, and activities lasting a longer duration could indeed lead to depleted carbohydrate stores.[41–43] In trained athletes both complex and simple carbohydrates have been shown to be equally effective in replenishing muscle and liver glycogen during the first 24 hours post exercise.[44] However, complex carbohydrates resulted in more muscle glycogen stored 48 hours post exercise.[44] Thus, for 24-hour concerns either type of carbohydrate is appropriate, but for longer-term glycogen synthesis, complex carbohydrates should be consumed. Table 11.1 lists some food choices that are high and low in carbohydrate content, while also indicating if they contain complex and/or simple carbohydrates.

11.3.1.2 *Protein Utilization and Intake*

The goal of most people who perform resistance training is to increase muscular strength and muscle mass. While many individuals try to increase muscle mass by overeating (that is, increasing caloric or energy intake), only 30 to 40% of the weight gained with overeating is fat-free mass, with most of the weight gained being in the form of fat mass.[45] In order to increase muscle mass athletes must be in a state of positive nitrogen balance and have all of the essential amino acids available to them.

There are 20 amino acids that make up the proteins in the body; 8 amino acids are essential. That is, they must be consumed in the diet (Table 11.2). Protein can be complete, containing all of the essential amino acids, or incomplete, lacking in at least one of the amino acids. Protein can be obtained from animal and plant sources, with incomplete proteins usually coming from plant sources (Table 11.3). Individuals who consume animal food generally have no problems obtaining all of the essential amino acids, while people who do not consume food from an animal source can obtain all of the essential amino acids if they choose their food wisely. All of the essential amino acids can be obtained from plant foods as long as the proper combinations of foods are consumed. The amino acids methionine and lysine are the two amino acids most deficient in plant foods, with methionine found only in vegetables and legumes and lysine found only in grains, nuts, and seeds. Therefore, to

TABLE 11.1

Examples of Foods High and Low in Carbohydrates (CHO) Composed of
Simple and Complex Carbohydrates

	% CHO	Simple	Complex
High Carbohydrate Foods			
Bananas	91	X	X
Apple juice	100	X	X
Baked potato	91		X
Spaghetti with marinara sauce	75		X
Cheerios	71		X
Nondiet soda	100	X	
Jelly beans	100	X	
Vegetable stir fry	64	X	
Vegetarian baked beans	78		X
Oatmeal	69		X
Pancakes (buttermilk)	79		X
Plain popcorn (air popped)	83		X
Low Carbohydrate Foods			
Cheddar cheese	1		
Sliced turkey	3		
Spaghetti with Alfredo sauce	44		
Scrambled eggs	9		
Croissant	44		
Sausage pizza	40		
Quiche Lorraine	30		
Baked beans with beef	54		
Cheese manicotti	40		
Cream of broccoli soup	39		
Guacamole dip	23		
Tofu	12		

Source: Reprinted, by permission, from Snyder, A. C., Welsh, R. S., and Hanisch, R. J.,
Nutritional concerns of recreational athletes who cross-train, in *Nutrition for the Recreational Athlete,* Jackson, C. G. R. (Ed.), CRC Press, Boca Raton, FL, 1994, chap. 5.

obtain all of the essential amino acids, vegetarians should combine grains and
legumes, or legumes, nuts and/or seeds. As many women athletes are either
vegetarian or consume very few animal products,[46,47] proper combining of
food is critical for optimal muscle development.

While the recommended intake for sedentary individuals is 0.8 g pro-
tein/kg body weight/day or approximately 12 to 15% of their nutrient
intake, a more appropriate intake for individuals performing resistance training and who want to increase muscle mass would seem to be 1.7 to 1.8 g pro-
tein/kg body weight/day.[48] Further, no evidence has been found that
consuming greater than 2.0 g protein/kg body weight/day would enhance
muscle mass to a greater extent; in fact, excess protein has been shown to be
oxidized and excreted and not stored as lean tissue/muscle mass.[48]

TABLE 11.2

Essential and Nonessential Amino Acids

Essential Amino Acids (must be consumed)

Isoleucine	Phenylalanine
Leucine	Threonine
Lysine	Trytophan
Methionine	Valine

Nonessential Amino Acids (can be produced by body)

Alanine	Glutamine
Arginine	Glycine
Asparagine	Histidine
Aspartic acid	Proline
Cysteine	Serine
Cystine	Tyrosine
Glutamic acid	

TABLE 11.3

Examples of Complete and Incomplete Protein Food Sources

Complete Protein Foods	Incomplete Protein Foods
Chicken	Nuts
Fish	Soybeans
Turkey	Rice
Beef	Kidney beans
Eggs	Corn
Dairy Products	
Rice and beans	
Tofu	

Source: Reprinted, by permission, from Snyder, A. C., Welsh, R. S., and Hanisch, R. J., Nutritional concerns of recreational athletes who cross-train, in *Nutrition for the Recreational Athlete,* Jackson, C. G. R. (Ed.), CRC Press, Boca Raton, FL, 1994, chap 5.

Although the recommended protein intake for those performing resistance training is greater (at 1.7 to 1.8 g protein/kg body weight/day) than for those who are sedentary, most athletes already consume this increased amount. A women weighing 65 kg (143 lbs) who consumed a total of 3000 kcals/day, of which 15% was protein, would be consuming 450 kcals as protein, or 112.5 g of protein, or 1.7 g protein/kg body weight/day.

The secretion of numerous hormones, including growth hormone, insulin and the somatomedins, all anabolic hormones which promote muscular growth, has been shown to be increased by the consumption of amino acids. Supplemental amino acids are readily available on the worldwide web, with hundreds of thousands of sites for amino acids, most of them offering the opportunity to purchase amino acid supplements costing from $0.10 to $3.50 per supplement. However, very little information is known about the affects of supplemental amino acids on women. Please refer to Chapter 6 for a general discussion of amino acid supplements and resistance training.

The literature does appear clear that both protein (at 1.7 to 1.8 g protein/kg body weight/day or approximately 15% of nutrient intake) and carbohydrates (at 60% of nutrient intake) are necessary to maximize muscle growth. With sufficient levels of energy (carbohydrates) the consumed protein can be used to synthesize protein and enhance muscle mass within the body. The sufficient carbohydrate levels should also lead to elevated insulin levels that will promote the synthesis of protein. In men, further support for this ratio of protein:carbohydrate intake can be obtained from resting testosterone levels, which are greatest when the ratio of protein to carbohydrate is 1:4 (or 15 to 60%). Increasing the ratio by either increasing protein intake or decreasing carbohydrate intake results in reducing testosterone levels.[49] Similar information is not available for women.

11.3.1.3 *Problems Associated with Excess Protein Consumption*

Excess protein intake can be detrimental to an athlete's health and should be avoided whenever possible. Numerous actions are required by the body when excess protein is consumed. Increased water loss due to excess protein occurs because proteins require more water to be broken down than either fat or carbohydrates due to the need to rid the body of the nitrogen attached to the amino acid. This excess loss of fluid could lead to dehydration. Greater kidney activity caused by the need to get rid of the nitrogen could result in increased urinary calcium loss.[50] Since most women are already more prone to osteoporosis than men because of lack of calcium intake and low bone density, consuming a diet with excess protein could exacerbate this problem. Consumption of high-protein foods can also easily lead to the consumption of high amounts of fat, because high-protein foods tend to contain high amounts of fats. Therefore, consumption of excess protein may also increase the risk of coronary artery disease. Thus, excess protein should not be consumed because it is not beneficial in enhancing muscle mass, as pointed out above, and it could be detrimental to one's health.

Two problems emerge from the literature pertaining to protein intake and resistance training. The first is that almost all of the research has been performed on men, and therefore, inferences to women are only extrapolated. The accuracy of this extrapolation will not be known until further research is performed which includes women in the subject population. The second problem is that while many studies have shown enhanced muscle mass and muscular strength, very few studies have shown that exercise performance, other than muscular strength, has been enhanced. Again, further work is needed in this area.

11.3.1.4 *Vitamins and Minerals*

Following the food guide pyramid and consuming a diet of 60% carbohydrates, 25% fat, and 15% protein will generally provide all of the vitamins and minerals in the proper amount needed. However, the majority of women fail to consume the recommended quantities of the vitamins — vitamin B_6, vitamin A, and folacin — along with the minerals — iron, calcium, magnesium, and zinc.[51] Two of these minerals, iron and calcium, require special attention in women.

Iron is a component of hemoglobin and myoglobin and as such is important for the transportation of oxygen from the lungs to the exercising muscle. Unfortunately, iron intake is closely tied to the amount of energy and the types of foods consumed. There are roughly 6 mg of iron in every 1000 kcal consumed of a balanced diet. As many women athletes consume only 2000 to 2500 kcal (or roughly 12 to 15 mg iron), their iron intake is frequently less than the recommended intake of 15 mg of iron.[38,52] The type of iron is also important, as heme iron, found in animal products, is absorbed to a much greater extent (23%) than is nonheme iron (5%), found in foods from plant origin.[53] Consuming heme iron with nonheme iron will enhance the absorption of the nonheme iron, as will the consumption of ascorbic acid (vitamin C).[53] Conversely, dietary fiber, tannins (found in tea), and high amounts of calcium supplements will inhibit the absorption of iron. As many athletes are known to consume little heme iron in their diet,[46,47,52,54] mild cases of iron deficiency, as shown by low serum ferritin levels, may result.[47]

Calcium is another extremely important mineral for women in general, and women athletes in particular. Calcium is used in the body in the transmission of nerve impulses and in the contraction of muscle fibers, but most important, calcium is stored in the body in the bones, making them dense and strong. Dairy products (milk, cheese, yogurt, ice cream) are the primary sources of dietary calcium, but calcium can also be obtained by consuming certain vegetables (broccoli) and some types of fish (oysters, salmon, and sardines). Many women, both athletes and sedentary individuals, fail to consume sufficient quantities of calcium.[52] As chronic low calcium intake can lead to reduced bone growth, women who are at risk of having low bone density, postmenopausal and secondary amenorrheic women, are at greater risk of reduced bone density and bone fractures. Two to three servings of dairy products daily are recommended to ensure proper intake of calcium.

11.3.2 Nutritional Needs of Resistance Exercise for Women

If an appropriate and balanced food intake program is followed, as described above, resistance exercise should not be limited by the diet. However, to ensure that the athlete is always prepared for the exercise bout, a few suggestions are offered.

Resistance exercise has been shown to utilize great amounts of muscle glycogen in men (Figure 11.2),[41–43] with women having a comparable rate of decline in glycogen concentration during exercise.[55] Therefore, replenishment of this form of carbohydrate is required before the next exercise bout takes place. Likewise, depending on the time of day when an athlete performs his/her resistance exercise, he/she could already be slightly glycogen depleted. Therefore, if the resistance exercise is to be performed in the early morning, after an overnight fast, a high-carbohydrate dinner and/or bedtime snack should be consumed, because just an overnight fast will deplete body glycogen stores to some extent. A high-carbohydrate snack (bagel and juice) or liquid meal (Instant Breakfast®, GatorPro®) should be consumed in the morning to ensure that body glycogen levels are as high as possible. If the exercise is to be performed at noon or later, high carbohydrate meals and snacks should be consumed to ensure that the athlete is not hungry during the resistance exercise and has sufficient body glycogen levels.

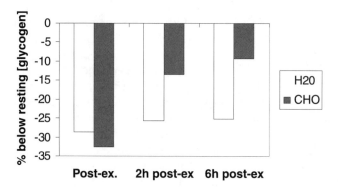

FIGURE 11.2
Percent change in muscle glycogen level following exercise with either water or carbohydrate consumption. (Adapted from data in Pascoe, D. D., Costill, D. L., Fink, W. L., Robergs, R. A., and Zachwieja, J. J., Glycogen resynthesis in skeletal muscle following resistive exercise, *Med. Sci. Sports Exerc.*, 25, 349, 1993.)

When performing resistance exercise programs that last more than 60 minutes, one should consume carbohydrates, either liquid or solid, during the exercise to maintain energy supply.[56–59] Fluids that have a carbohydrate concentration of about 6% are great sources of carbohydrates during an exercise bout, as they are readily absorbed by the body and provide energy.[40] Soft drinks and fruit juices contain approximately 10 to 12% carbohydrates and therefore need to be diluted for optimal absorption during exercise.[60] Chilled fluids are absorbed faster than fluids that are warm, so slightly chilled fluids should be consumed whenever possible.[60] As consumption of glucose just before or during resistance exercise increases circulating levels of insulin (an anabolic hormone), consumption of glucose may also protect muscle from damage by decreasing the rate of protein breakdown.[61] Consumption of carbohydrates immediately and 1 hour after resistance exercise has also been shown to decrease the rate of protein breakdown, and thus maintains or increases a positive body protein balance.[62,63]

While carbohydrate, or glycogen, loading has been shown to be effective in men, whether or not it works in women is now being questioned. Tarnopolsky and co-workers[48] increased the carbohydrate intake of men and women from 55 to 60% to 75% for 4 days and then exercised the subjects. While the men increased both muscle glycogen concentration (41%) and exercise time (45%), the women had no change in muscle glycogen (0%) and a very small increase in exercise time (5%). In place of greater amounts of carbohydrate, the women oxidized more lipids and proteins and less carbohydrates during the 75% $VO_{2\,max}$ exercise than did the men as was evident by their lower RER values.[55] The greater response in the men may have been due to the fact that they consumed a greater absolute amount of carbohydrate than the women, though the same relative amount, and possibly an absolute threshold amount of carbohydrate is necessary to enhance muscle glycogen levels and thus exercise performance.

Post exercise, muscle glycogen synthesis has been found to be greatest when a small amount (300 kcal) of carbohydrate and protein is consumed within the first 2 hours after exercise, though just the consumption of carbohydrates will enhance synthesis somewhat.[42,43,64–66] More than likely, the greater enhancement of glycogen storage with carbohydrate and protein consumption is due to the greater circulating insulin concentrations, because both carbohydrates and protein cause insulin release.[43] While most of these investigations were performed on men, women have been found to have a similar rate of post-exercise muscle glycogen synthesis following both resistance exercise and aerobic endurance exercise.[64] Consumption of just protein following an exercise bout resulted in much lower rates of muscle glycogen synthesis than did consumption of carbohydrate and protein, or just carbohydrate.[66]

Finally, the greatest rate of protein synthesis in women following exercise occurred when resistance training and swimming training were combined; but, both swimming alone and resistance exercise alone increased the post-exercise rate of protein synthesis. The increase, however, was not statistically significant (Figure 11.3).[67] These subjects did not consume any carbohydrates or carbohydrates with protein following the exercise bout, which may have led to different results. Future studies will have to examine the impact of carbohydrate and protein consumption on glycogen and protein synthesis post exercise.

11.4 Summary

In recent years resistance training has become more popular with women. Many beneficial adaptations occur with resistance training, including an

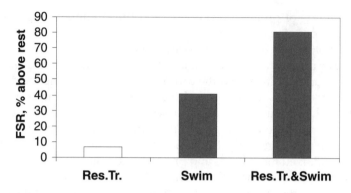

FIGURE 11.3

Percent increase in rate of protein synthesis following resistance training, swimming, and resistance training plus swimming. (Adapted from data in Tipton, K. D., Ferrando, A. A., Williams, B. D., and Wolfe, R. R., Muscle protein metabolism in female swimmers after a combination of resistance and endurance exercise, *J. Appl. Physiol.*, 81, 2034, 1996.)

increase in muscular strength, along with an increase in muscle mass and bone density. Body weight and composition may also be affected by resistance training, but varied results have occurred. Nutritionally, proper overall food or energy intake, by following the food guide pyramid, is important to ensure the muscular adaptations. That is, a carbohydrate intake of approximately 60% of the calories and a protein intake of about 15% of the calories (or 1.7 to 1.8 g protein/kg body weight/day) will maximize muscular gains. Consumption of excess protein does not lead to greater muscular adaptations and could be detrimental to health. Most women fail to consume the minerals calcium and iron in proper amounts; thus, care must be taken to ensure that appropriate intake occurs.

Acknowledgment

The author thanks Mark Parmenter for his valuable assistance and comments on this manuscript.

References

1. Jackson, C. G. R., Nutritional concerns of the female recreational athlete, in *Nutritional Concerns of Women*, Wolinsky, I. and Klimis-Tavantzis, D. (Eds.), CRC Press, Boca Raton, FL, 1996, 234.

2. American College of Sports Medicine Position Stand, The recommended quantity and quality of exercise for developing and maintaining cardiorespiratory and muscular fitness, and flexibility in healthy adults, *Med. Sci. Sports Exerc.*, 30, 975, 1998.

3. Stone, M. H. and Kirksey, K. B., Physiology of weightlifting, in *Exercise and Sport Science*, Garrett, W. E. and Kirkendall, D. T. (Eds.), Lippincott Williams & Wilkins, Philadelphia, 2000, chap 60.

4. Fleck, S. J. and Kramer, W. J., *Designing Resistance Training Programs*, 2nd ed., Human Kinetics Publishers, Champaign, IL, 1997.

5. Laubach. L. L., Comparative muscular strength of men and women: a review of the literature, *Aviat. Space Environ. Med.*, 47, 534, 1976.

6. Miller, A. E. J., MacDougall, J. D., Tarnopolsky, M. A., and Sale, D. G., Gender differences in strength and muscle fiber characteristics, *Eur. J. Appl. Physiol.*, 66, 254, 1993.

7. Holloway, J. B. and Baechle, T. R., Strength training for female athletes: a review of selected aspects, *Sports Med.*, 9, 216, 1990.

8. Staron, R. S., Karapondo, D. L., Kraemer, W., Fry, A. C., Gordon, S. E., Faldek, J. E., Hagerman, F. C., and Hikida, R. S., Skeletal muscle adaptations during early phase of heavy-resistance training in men and women, *J. Appl. Physiol.*, 76, 1247, 1994.

9. Mayhew, J. L. and Salm, P. C., Gender differences in anaerobic power tests, *Eur. J. Appl. Physiol.*, 60, 133, 1990.

10. Fielding, R. A., The role of progressive resistance training and nutrition in the preservation of lean body mass in the elderly, *J. Am. College Nutr.*, 14, 587, 1995.

11. Campbell, W. W., Crim, M. C., Young, V. R., and Evan, W. J., Increased energy requirements and changes in body composition with resistance training in older adults, *Am. J. Clin. Nutr.*, 60, 167, 1994.

12. Campbell, W. W., Crim, M. C., Young, V. R., Joseph, L. J., and Evans, W. J., Effects of resistance training and dietary protein intake on protein metabolism in older adults, *Am. J. Physiol.*, 268, E1143, 1995.

13. Forbes, G. B., Exercise and body composition, *J. Appl. Physiol.*, 70, 994, 1991.

14. Gravelle, B. L. and Blessing, D. L., Physiological adaptation in women concurrently training for strength and endurance, *J. Strength Cond. Res.*, 14, 5, 2000.

15. Bishop, D., Jenkins, D. G., Mackinnon, L. T., McEniery, M., and Carey, M. F., The effects of strength training on endurance performance and muscle characteristics, *Med. Sci. Sports Exerc.*, 31, 886, 1999.

16. Donnelly, J. E., Sharp, T., Houmard, J., Carlson, M. G., Hill, J. O., Whatley, J. E., and Israel, R. G., Muscle hypertrophy with large-scale weight loss and resistance training, *Am. J. Clin. Nutr.*, 58, 561, 1993.

17. Kraemer, W. J., Volek, J. S., Clark, K. L., Gordon, S. E., Incledon, T., Puhl, S. M., Triplett-McBride, N. T., McBride, J. M., Putukian, M., and Sebastianelli, W. J., Physiological adaptations to a weight-loss dietary regimen and exercise programs in women, *J. Appl. Physiol.*, 83, 270, 1997.

18. Manning, J. M., Dooly-Manning, C. R., White, K., Kampa, I., Silas, S., Kesselhaut, M., and Ruoff, M., Effects of a resistive training program on lipoprotein — lipid levels in obese women, *Med. Sci. Sports Exerc.*, 23, 1222, 1991.

19. Marks, B. L., Ward, A., Moris, D. H., Castellani, J., and Rippe, J. M., Fat-free mass is maintained in women following a moderate diet and exercise program, *Med. Sci. Sports Exerc.*, 27, 1243, 1995.

20. Staron, R. S., Leonardi, M. J., Karapondo, D. L., Malicky, E. S., Falkel, J. E., Hagerman, F. C., and Hikida, R. S., Strength and skeletal muscle adaptations in heavy-resistance-trained women after detraining and retraining, *J. Appl. Physiol.*, 70, 631, 1991.

21. Staron, R. S., Malicky, E. S., Leonardi, M. J., Falkel, J. E., Hagerman, F. C., and Dudley, G. A., Muscle hypertrophy and fast fiber type conversions in heavy resistance-trained women, *Eur. J. Appl. Physiol.*, 60, 71, 1989.

22. Staron, R. S., Murray, T. E., Gilders, R. M., Hagerman, F. C., Hikida, R. S., and Ragg, K. E., Influence of resistance training on serum lipid and lipoprotein concentrations in young men and women, *J. Strength Cond. Res.*, 14, 37, 2000.

23. Drinkwater, B. L., Women and exercise: physiological aspects, in *Exercise and Sport Sciences Reviews, Vol. 12*, Terjung, R. L. (Ed.), The Collamore Press, Lexington, MA, 1984, chap. 2.

24. Staron, R. S. and Johnson, P., Myosin polymorphism and differential expression in adult human skeletal muscle, *Comp. Biochem. Physiol. B. Comp. Biochem.*, 106, 463, 1993.

25. Wang, N., Hikida, R. S., Staron, R. S., and Simoneau, J. A., Muscle fiber types of women after resistance training — qualitative ultrastructure and enzyme activity, *Pflugers Arch.*, 424, 494, 1993.

26. Ballor, D. L., Katch, V. L., Becque, M. D., and Marks, C. R., Resistance weight training during caloric restriction enhances lean body weight maintenance, *Am. J. Clin. Nutr.*, 47, 19, 1988.

27. Layne, J. E. and Nelson, M. E., The effects of progressive resistance training on bone density: a review, *Med. Sci. Sports Exerc.*, 31, 25, 1999.

28. Lewis, R. D. and Modlesky, C. M., Nutrition, physical activity, and bone health in women, *Int. J. Sport Nutr.*, 8, 250, 1998.

29. Boyden, T. W., Parmenter, R. W., Going, S. B., Lohman, T. G., Hall, M. C., Houtkooper, L. B., Bunt, J. C., Titenbaugh, C., and Aickin, M., Resistance exercise training is associated with decreases in serum low-density lipoprotein cholesterol levels in premenopausal women, *Arch. Intern. Med.*, 153, 97, 1993.

30. Hurley, B. F., Hagberg, J. M., Goldberg, A. P., Seals, D. R., Ehsani, A. A., Brennan, R. E., and Holloszy, J. O., Resistance training can reduce coronary risk factors without altering $VO_{2\,max}$ or percent body fat, *Med. Sci. Sports Exerc.*, 20, 150, 1988.

31. Hurley, B. F., Effects of resistance training on lipoprotein-lipids profiles: a comparison to aerobic exercise training, *Med. Sci. Sports Exerc.*, 21, 6, 1989.

32. Moffatt, R. J., Wallace, M. B., and Sady, S. P., Effects of anabolic steroids on lipoprotein profiles of female weight lifters, *Phys. Sportsmed.*, 18, 106, 1990.

33. Morgan, D. W., Cruise, R. J., Girardin, B. W., Lutz-Schneider, V., Girardin, B. W., Morgan, D. H., and Qi, W. M., HDL-C concentrations in weight-trained, endurance-trained, and sedentary females, *Phys. Sportsmed.*, 14, 166, 1986.

34. Kraemer, W. J., Gordon, S. E., Fleck, S. J., Marchitelli, L. J., Mello, R., Dziados, J. E., Friedl, K., Harman, E., Maresh, C., and Fry, A. C., Endogenous anabolic hormonal and growth factor responses to heavy resistance exercise in males and females, *Int. J. Sports Med.*, 12, 228, 1991.

35. Kraemer, W. J., Fleck, S. J., Dziados, J. E., Harman, E. A., Marchitelli, L. J., Gordon, S. E., Mello, R., Frykman, P. N., Koziris, L. P., and Triplett, N. T., Changes in hormonal concentrations after different heavy-resistance exercise protocols in women, *J. Appl. Physiol.*, 75, 594, 1993.

36. Cumming, D. C., Wall, S. R., Galbraith, M. A., and Belcastro, A. N., Reproductive hormone responses to resistance exercise, *Med. Sci. Sports Exerc.*, 19, 234, 1987.
37. Walberg, J. L. and Johnston, C. S., Menstrual function and eating behavior in female recreational weight lifters and competitive body builders, *Med. Sci. Sports Exerc.*, 23, 20, 1991.
38. Snyder, A. C., Naik, J., and Welsh, R., A multi-factorial approach to the mechanism of athletic amenorrhea, *Med. Sci. Sports Exerc.*, 29, S70, 1997.
39. Cahill, G. F., Aoki, T. T., and Rossini, A. A., Metabolism in obesity and anorexia nervosa, *Nutr. Brain*, 3, 1, 1979.
40. Sherman, W. M. and Lamb, D. R., Nutrition and prolonged exercise, in *Perspectives in Exercise Science and Sports Medicine, Volume 1: Prolonged Exercise*, Lamb, D. R. and Murray, R. (Eds.), Benchmark Press, Indianapolis, IN, 1988, 213.
41. Pascoe, D. D., Costill, D. L., Fink, W. L., Robergs, R. A., and Zachwieja, J. J., Glycogen resynthesis in skeletal muscle following resistive exercise, *Med. Sci. Sports Exerc.*, 25, 349, 1993.
42. Robergs, R. A., Pearson, D. R., Costill, D. L., Fink, W. J., Pascoe, D. D., Benedict, M. A., Lambert, C. P., and Zachweija, J. J., Muscle glycogenolysis during differing intensities of weight-resistance exercise, *J. Appl. Physiol.*, 70, 1700, 1991.
43. Roy, B. D. and Tarnopolsky, M. A., Influence of differing macronutrient intakes on muscle glycogen resynthesis after resistance exercise, *J. Appl. Physiol.*, 84, 890, 1998.
44. Costill, D. L., Sherman, W. M., Fink, W. J., Maresh, C., Witten, M., and Miller, J. M., The role of dietary carbohydrates in muscle glycogen resynthesis after strenuous running, *Am. J. Clin. Nutr.*, 34, 1831, 1981.
45. Kreider, R. B., Dietary supplements and the promotion of muscle growth with resistance exercise, *Sports Med.*, 27, 97, 1999.
46. Brooks, S. M., Sanborn, C. F., Albrecht, B. H., and Wagner, W. W., Diet in athletic amenorrhea, *Lancet*, 1, 559, 1984.
47. Snyder, A. C., Dvorac, L. L., and Roepke, J. B., Influence of dietary iron source on measures of iron status among female runners, *Med. Sci. Sports Exerc.*, 21, 7, 1989.
48. Tarnopolsky, M. A., Atkinson, S. A., MacDougall, J. D., Chesley, A., Phillips, S., and Schwarcz, H. P., Evaluation of protein requirements for trained strength athletes, *J. Appl. Physiol.*, 73, 1986, 1992.
49. Volek, J., Kraemer, W., Bush, J., Incledon, T., and Boestes, M., Testosterone and cortisol in relationship to dietary nutrients and resistance exercise, *J. Appl. Physiol.*, 82, 49, 1997.
50. Allen, L., Oddoye, E., and Margen, S., Protein-induced hypercalciuria: a longer term study, *Am. J. Clin. Nutr.*, 32, 741, 1979.
51. Welsh, S. and Guthrie, J. F., Changing American diets, in *Micronutrients in Health and Disease Prevention*, Bendich, A. and Butterworth, C. E. (Eds.), Marcel Dekker, New York, 1991.
52. Kaiserauer, S., Snyder, A. C., Sleeper, M., and Zeirath, J., Nutritional and physiological influences on menstrual function of distance runners, *Med. Sci. Sports Exerc.*, 21, 120, 1989.
53. Monsen, E. R., Hallberg, L., Layrisse, M., Hegsted, D. M., Cook, J. D., Mertz, W., and Finch, C. A., Estimation of available dietary iron, *Am. J. Clin. Nutr.*, 31, 134, 1978.

54. Snyder, A. C. and Clark, N., Stress fractures of male distance runners: lack of association with nutritional practices, *Nutr. Res.*, 13, 995, 1993.
55. Tarnopolsky, M. A., Atkinson, S. A., Phillips, S. M., and MacDougall, J. D., Carbohydrate loading and metabolism during exercise in men and women, *J. Appl. Physiol.*, 78, 1360, 1995.
56. Snyder, A. C., Lamb, D. R., Baur, T., Connors, D., and Brodowicz, G., Malto-dextrin feedings immediately before prolonged cycling at 62% $VO_{2\,max}$ increases time to exhaustion, *Med. Sci. Sports Exerc.*, 13, 126, 1983.
57. Snyder, A. C., Moorhead, K., Luedtke, J., and Small, M., Carbohydrate consumption prior to repeated bouts of high intensity exercise, *Eur. J. Appl. Physiol.*, 66, 141, 1993.
58. Coyle, E. F., Coggan, A. R., Hemmert, M. K., and Ivy, J. L., Muscle glycogen utilization during prolonged strenuous exercise when fed carbohydrates, *J. Appl. Physiol.*, 61, 165, 1986.
59. Coggan, A. R. and Coyle, E. F., Reversal of fatigue during prolonged exercise by carbohydrate infusion or ingestion, *J. Appl. Physiol.*, 63, 2388, 1987.
60. Gisolfi, C. V. and Duchman, S. M., Guidelines for optimal replacement of beverages for different athletic events, *Med. Sci. Sports Exerc.*, 24, 679, 1992.
61. Cade, J. R., Reese, R. H., Privette, R. M., Hommen, N. M., Rogers, J. L., and Fregly, M. J., Dietary intervention and training in swimmers, *Eur. J. Appl. Physiol.*, 63, 210, 1991.
62. Roy, B. D., Tarnopolsky, M. A., MacDougall, J. D., Fowles, J., and Yarasheski, K. E., Effect of glucose supplement timing on protein metabolism after resistance training, *J. Appl. Physiol.*, 82, 1882, 1997.
63. Walberg, J. L., Leidy, M. K., Sturgill, D. J., Hinkle, D. E., Ritchey, S. J., and Sebolt, D. R., Macronutrient needs in weight lifters during caloric restriction, *Med. Sci. Sports Exerc.*, 19, S70, 1987.
64. Tarnopolsky, M. A., Bosman, M., MacDonald, J. R., Vandeputte, D., Martin, J., and Roy, B. D., Postexercise protein-carbohydrate and carbohydrate supplements increase muscle glycogen in men and women, *J. Appl. Physiol.*, 83, 1877, 1997.
65. Ivy, J. L., Lee, M. C., Brozinick, J. T., and Reed, M. J., Muscle glycogen storage after different amounts of carbohydrate ingestion, *J. Appl. Physiol.*, 65, 2018, 1988.
66. Zawadzki, K. M., Yaspelkis, B. B., and Ivy, J. L., Carbohydrate-protein complex increases the rate of muscle glycogen storage after exercise, *J. Appl. Physiol.*, 72, 1854, 1992.
67. Tipton, K. D., Ferrando, A. A., Williams, B. D., and Wolfe, R. R., Muscle protein metabolism in female swimmers after a combination of resistance and endurance exercise, *J. Appl. Physiol.*, 81, 2034, 1996.

12

Nutritional Concerns of Strength Athletes with an Emphasis on Tennis

Tracey A. Richers

CONTENTS

0-8493-8198-3/01/$0.00+$.50
© 2001 by CRC Press LLC

12.1 Introduction

Tennis is a popular sport played worldwide and year round by boys, girls, men, and women. Formats include singles, doubles (same-sex pairs), mixed doubles (mixed-sex pairs), father–son, father–daughter, mother–son, and mother–daughter doubles. Tennis is one of the few sports that players can continue to compete in as they get older. Variables involved in how the game is played are: different court surfaces (hard court, clay, and grass), indoor vs. outdoor facilities, and high altitude vs. low altitude.

Tennis has changed over the past 20 years and dramatically within the last decade due to advances in equipment and the physical conditioning of tennis players. Tennis is emerging as a strength sport. The sport has moved from slow, long rallies with wood racquets to powerful and explosive short rallies with racquets manufactured with stiffer materials made out of fiberglass, graphite, boron, titanium, and kevlar. Recent technology has given tennis players longer racquets, larger racquet heads, wider and lighter frames, and bigger sweet spots. These new racquet materials and designs have brought on an ever-increasing power game.[1]

In the 1980s, tennis pros Martina Navratilova and Ivan Lendl took advantage of research in sports training, conditioning, and nutrition to enhance their games.[2,3] Since then, tennis players have incorporated strength, flexibility, endurance, speed, aerobic conditioning, agility, and nutrition into their regular training routines. Players are stronger, quicker, more agile, and can hit the ball harder than ever before. Physical training and conditioning programs for tennis players help to improve stroke technique, achieve better positioning and movement,[4] prevent injuries, rehabilitate injuries faster, delay fatigue, and recover more rapidly between matches.

Modern technology and highly conditioned athletes have made tennis a game of power. The components of power are speed and strength. More specifically, "power is speed applied to strength."[5] Scientific measurement of these variables starts with the calculation of work. Work is defined as the amount of force that can be applied over a distance(d): Work = $F \times d$. Power (P) is defined as the amount of work (W) per unit of time (t): $P = W/t$. Therefore, $P = (F \times d)/t$ or W/t. A high level of power and strength corresponds to a greater ability to accelerate the body and external objects.[6] The elements of power and muscular strength allow players to accelerate their bodies across the court and hit the ball with maximum impact.[7] Since tennis is increasingly becoming more of a strength-related sport,[8] players must have the ability to exert muscular forces at high rates of speed; thus, they need more power. In recent years, a greater emphasis has been placed on strength- and speed-training programs for recreation and competition.[9,10–12]

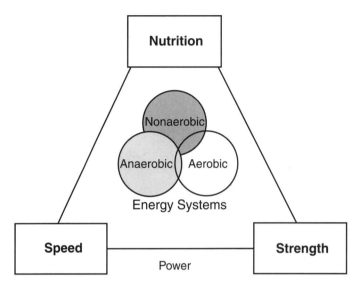

FIGURE 12.1
The interrelationships among energy systems and performance factors in tennis.

12.1.1 Energy Systems

Nutrient utilization for sport activities depends upon which energy systems are stressed during the activity (Figure 12.1). All of the macronutrient substrates for utilization which come from carbohydrates, fats, and protein are used in producing the ATP molecule.[13] Time and intensity establish which systems predominate during activity.

Tennis involves short-term, highly intense, stopping and starting movements interspersed with periods of rest.[14] Individual points may require 1 to 25 intense short bursts of energy with periods of submaximal effort between the intense exertions. During a singles tennis match, a player may exert between 200 and 600 explosive movements. While the ball is in play, players are continually accelerating and decelerating. During a point, energy is provided via the nonaerobic and anaerobic systems.[14–18] During high-intensity intermittent sports, such as tennis, hockey, football, sprinting, interval training, and strength training, the breakdown of adenosine triphosphate (ATP) and creatine phosphate (CP) and the degradation of glycogen are the predominant energy-yielding pathways. At high intensity, if tennis points are less than 10 seconds, the primary energy system utilized is the nonaerobic (ATP–CP) system. If the point continues from 10 seconds to 2 or 3 minutes, the glycolytic/lactic acid system predominates during the tennis rally. The glycolytic/lactic acid system and the oxygen system aid in ATP resynthesis between points. Tennis matches usually last from 30 minutes to 2 hours.

Some can last as long as 4 hours, with few rare matches lasting as long as 6 hours. Certain men's professional tournaments are played with the best of three sets out of five and can commonly last 2 to 4 hours or longer. Thus, tennis can be classified as activity which is primarily anaerobic and which can benefit from strength training.

12.1.2 General Requirements for Tennis

Tennis requires power, speed, strength, agility, stamina, and skill. The value of appropriate nutrition is to sustain high levels of moderate to intense training and competition. Proper nutrition for tennis has the following benefits:

- It allows players to operate within the nonaerobic and anaerobic energy systems more comfortably and efficiently
- Players are capable of competing at high intensity for longer periods of time if the match is extended (nonaerobic and anaerobic endurance)
- Players will be able to recover more quickly and adequately between training and competition — which is especially important if the player has matches on consecutive days
- Dehydration and fatigue are delayed
- Players may achieve and maintain peak performance more quickly and efficiently.

12.2 Calculation of Energy Costs

Caloric expenditure varies among individuals and depends on body size, level of training or conditioning, gender, and age. The intensity of a particular exercise or sport can be calculated from a person's metabolic capacity as measured in METS. One MET (**M**etabolic **E**quivalen**T**) is defined as the amount of oxygen that is required per minute under quiet resting conditions and is equal to 3.5 ml of oxygen consumed per kilogram of body weight per minute (ml/kg-min).[15] An exercise that requires 7.0 METS means that the oxygen cost of the activity is 7.0 times 3.5 or 24.5 ml/kg-min. MET values have been identified to estimate calories or energy utilized per hour and have been calculated for tennis. Tennis in general is listed at 7.0 METS, doubles tennis at 6.0 METS, and singles tennis at 8.0 METS.[19] The American College of Sports Medicine has listed tennis at an average of 6.5 METS with a range of 4.0 to 9.0+ METS.[20] Energy costs in Calories (kilocalories) per hour can be determined by multiplying the MET value by kilograms of individual body weight. In one particular investigation, two different weight individuals were compared for approximate kilocalories used during moderate and vigorous singles tennis.[21] One individual weighed 125 lb and the other 205 lb. For moderate tennis activity, the 125-lb individual expended 347 kilocalories, and the 205-lb person expended 565 kilocalories per hour. For vigorous activity, the kilocalories used for the 125-lb and the 205-lb individuals were 488 and 797 kilocalories, respectively.

12.3 Training and Competition Diet

The macronutrients carbohydrate, fat, and protein are utilized for energy during rest and exercise. Time and intensity of the exercise or event will dictate which macronutrients are used. For activities of high intensity and short duration involving the anaerobic energy system, blood glucose and muscle glycogen are the primary energy sources. Glycogen is stored in the muscle and liver. For activities of low intensity and continuous long duration (aerobic), fat is the principal fuel used. Plasma fatty acids and intramuscular triglycerides are the forms of fat that are used for energy. Protein is not used as a primary source of energy during activity as its main role in the body is tissue synthesis. Amino acids, which are the building blocks of protein, can provide small amounts of energy in certain situations. However, carbohydrates and fats are more efficient, and they spare protein from being used as energy.

12.3.1 Carbohydrate

12.3.1.1 Description of Types

Carbohydrate is the most important fuel for strength athletes[22] and for highly intense physical activities.[23,24] The principal role of carbohydrate in human nutrition is to provide energy. There are two main categories of carbohydrates: simple and complex. Simple carbohydrates are sugars that can be further divided into two major groups: monosaccharides (single sugar molecules) and disaccharides (two monosaccharides combined). The three major monosaccharides are glucose, galactose, and fructose. Polysaccharides (complex carbohydrates) are known as starches and are formed when three or more glucose molecules are linked together.[24] Blood glucose and intramuscular stores of glycogen are the two forms of carbohydrates used for ATP production.

12.3.1.2 Carbohydrate Measurement in Tennis

Singles tennis is classified as essentially utilizing the nonaerobic energy system (ATP–CP) followed closely by the anaerobic system. During exercise, muscle glycogen and blood glucose are substantial fuels for ATP resynthesis within contracting skeletal muscle.[25] Players in tennis matches which lasted less than 2 hours exhibited increases in blood glucose levels. One study of Division I college players, reported blood glucose increased at the beginning of play; then levels remained steady and slightly above the pre-exercise value throughout play.[26] The glucose level declined slightly after 30 minutes of play but still remained above the pre-exercise value. The players in this study competed for 85 minutes, which included time for changeovers and data collection. Average time of each point was not calculated. In another study, two groups of female players, young (15 to 30 years old) and veteran (40 to 51 years old), competed for 120 minutes.[27] The average time of each point, when the ball was in play, was 12 ± 1 seconds vs. out of play for 17 ± 1 seconds. Blood glucose values for both groups increased from pre-exercise to post-exercise. In another study, eight nationally ranked tennis players competed for 4 hours.[18] Pre-match vs. post-match values showed that blood glucose levels dropped by an average of 18 mg/dl. The study only took pre- and post-samples and did not indicate the time at which blood glucose levels began to decrease.

12.3.1.3 Recommendations

In general, athletes should consume 55 to 70% carbohydrates in the diet. Some recommend that carbohydrate intake for athletes should minimally be 60%.[23] Recommendations for athletes involved in heavy endurance-training programs such as long distance running have been as high as 70%.[28] Tennis players who compete on a frequent basis should ingest between 60 and 65% carbohydrates. Grandjean reported nutrient intake data for 9 female tennis Olympic athletes.[29] The players consumed 279 grams per day (g/d) and 4.8 grams per kilogram of body weight (g/kg), which was 54% of total energy. This amount of carbohydrate intake is considered low and tennis players should increase their carbohydrate intake to 60 to 65%. Sufficient intake of carbohydrates and energy will provide fuel for the muscles and aid in the full restoration of muscle and liver glycogen stores. Players can consume complex carbohydrates in the forms of breads such as bagels, crackers, rice cakes, graham crackers and muffins, pasta, peas, beans such as kidney and navy, rice, and potatoes.

12.3.2 Fat

12.3.2.1 Description of Types

Fats are another major substrate used for energy during exercise. Fat is stored in the body as triglycerides within the fat cells, which are called adipocytes. A small percentage of triglycerides are stored in skeletal muscle and are also found circulating in the blood bound to albumin. Triglyceride is simply a glycerol molecule attached to three fatty acids. The major roles of fat in the body are: [24,30]

1. To provide and store energy
2. To protect and insulate the body's organs
3. To serve as a vitamin carrier and depress hunger
4. To provide essential fatty acids
5. To provide cellular structure.

12.3.2.2 Fat Measurement in Tennis

Few studies in tennis have researched fat metabolism.[27,31] Most studies investigating fat used as an energy substrate have focused on aerobic endurance and ultra-endurance activities. Free fatty acids are oxidized mainly during the rest and low-intensity phases of intermittent exercise. During match play of 2 hours, a slight increase in serum free fatty acids, pre- and post-match for young and old players (0.06 ± 0.02 to 0.85 ± 17 mmol·L^{-1} and 0.27 ± 0.09 to 1.50 ± 0.12 mmol·L^{-1}, respectively) was observed.[27] More research is needed on fat utilization during tennis play. Since tennis can be of moderate intensity if played recreationally and high intensity if played professionally and competitively, it appears that fat metabolism investigation may be of prime importance to the sport. This is especially true in the case of prolonged match play, which can last over 4 hours, and it would be necessary to determine the extent to which fatty acids contribute energy between points.

12.3.2.3 Recommendations

Since there is an almost endless supply of fat in body stores, players do not need to consume extra amounts in the diet. Less than 30% of total caloric intake of fat is recommended. Strength athletes should consume between 25 and 30%. Diets with a 25% fat intake will allow room for more carbohydrates to be consumed. In Grandjean's study, the 9 female Olympic athletes had an average fat intake of 68 g/d and 1.2 g/kg body weight, which accounted for 29% of total energy; this falls within the recommended range.[29] A diet high in fat can hinder carbohydrate intake, and fatigue can set in more quickly. Foods high in fat include fried foods, butter, creamy salad dressings, oils, mayonnaise, beef, pork, cheese, cheese sauces, whole milk, nuts, and potato chips. Complex carbohydrate foods are usually low in fat. Players should consume low-fat yogurt, skim milk, fruits, vegetables, bagels, and low-fat muffins.

12.3.3 Protein

12.3.3.1 Description of Types

Protein contributes very little energy during exercise. However, protein is utilized to a greater extent than initially thought and may be due to glycogen depletion rather than length of the exercise bout.[32] Amino acids are the form of protein that provides energy. Amino acids in excess of those needed to maintain normal daily physiological functions will be excreted. The primary amino acids involved in exercise are alanine, glutamine, and the branched-chain amino acids (BCAA) leucine, valine, and isoleucine. Protein has been shown to contribute energy during anaerobic conditions.[33] Protein utilization appears to increase during long-lasting interval exercise. When the body's carbohydrate reserves become low during exercise, protein breakdown will occur more frequently. As muscle glycogen is depleted during exercise, BCAAs enter the muscle and are oxidized. They may also function to donate an amino group for alanine synthesis from pyruvate. Protein utilization is not favored as the body must expend energy to pull off the nitrogen groups (an undesired waste of energy) and form ammonia, a metabolic by-product thought to be associated with fatigue.

12.3.3.2 Protein Measurement in Tennis

Protein utilization in tennis, like fat, has not been well researched. Nationally ranked tennis players subjected to 4 hours of continuous tournament tennis showed a 14% decrease in BCAAs.[18] Total time of play during the 4-hour match was 39.26 (± 2.27) minutes. The authors of this study concluded that most plasma amino acids will decrease during long-lasting interval exercise. A decrease in BCAAs indicates their involvement in muscle metabolism during interval activities.[18] More research is required to determine the amount of amino acid metabolism during highly intense interval activities. Most research involving amino acid utilization has focused on plasma BCAA changes during aerobic endurance activities and not during strength or power events.

12.3.3.3 Recommendations

Protein requirements for strength athletes are recommended at 1.4 to 1.8 g/kg/d.[34] The recommended dietary allowance (RDA) for the general population is 0.8 g/kg/d.[35] The 9 female Olympic tennis athletes in Grand-jean's study had an average protein intake of 80 grams per day (g/d) and 1.4 grams per kilogram of body weight (g/kg), providing 15% of total energy.[29] Strength athletes are most concerned with maximizing protein synthesis and minimizing protein catabolism. Ingesting adequate amounts of carbohydrate can have a protein-sparing effect. Table 12.1 lists gram weights of protein for some common foods. Players should consume protein in the forms of meat (beef, poultry, fish), soy analogues, egg whites, milk and cheeses, vegetables (green beans and peas, carrots and potatoes), fruits (bananas, oranges), and starches (macaroni, navy beans, and spaghetti). Players should specifically choose lean meat (broiled or grilled), cottage cheese, low-fat cheese, and low-fat milk, which can include frozen yogurt "smoothies").

TABLE 12.1

Protein Gram Weights of Common Foods

Common Food	Portion Size	Protein (g)
Beef, lean	3 ounces	24
Steak, lean	3 ounces	21
Chicken, breast	3 ounces	26
Egg/egg white	1	7
Milk, skim	1 cup	9
Beans, green	1 cup	2
Potato, baked	1	3
Banana	1	1
Orange	1	1
Bread, wheat	1 slice	3
Macaroni	1 cup	6
Navy beans, cooked	1 cup	14
Spaghetti with meat	1 cup	18

12.4 Training and Competition Nutrition

12.4.1 Pre-Match Nutrition

It is well established that consuming food immediately before exercise, conditioning, training, and competition will not benefit performance.[28] Depleted glycogen stores cannot be immediately replenished by a pre-exercise or pre-competition meal. However, pre-event meals, if timed appropriately, have the following benefits:[28]

1. To prevent hypoglycemia (low blood sugar), light-headedness, physical and mental fatigue

2. To help settle the stomach, absorb gastric juices, and diminish feelings of hunger

3. To stabilize glycogen stores (liver glycogen) and not adversely affect the energy supplies (especially with foods that can be stored as glycogen if they are consumed far enough in advance, usually 4 to 6 hours)

4. To help provide adequate amounts of water for the body.

Water should be consumed within 24 hours of training and competition. If weight is lost through sweat during an exercise bout, between 8 and 16 ounces of water should be ingested for each pound of body weight lost. Performance of high intensity and short duration can be diminished if individuals begin exercise with a fluid deficit.[36]

Complex carbohydrates should be consumed prior to training or competition but care should be taken that the consumption is not immediately prior to activity. The amount of time remaining before the event dictates the amount of food that should be ingested. If there are 4 or more hours between matches or training, players can consume large meals composed mainly of carbohydrates and small amounts of protein. If the time between is 2 to 4 hours, a smaller meal is needed comprised of breads (bagels and pita bread), vegetables, and fruit juices. A liquid meal or a sports drink can also be consumed during this time. Within 1 to a half hour of the event, players should ingest smaller snacks consisting of fruits (oranges, bananas), breads (crackers or slice of bread), and water. Carbohydrates should not be ingested within a half hour of the activity. Simple sugars, such as those found in non-diet soft drinks, candy, and large amounts of fruit juices should be avoided.

12.4.2   Nutrition and Hydration During Match Play

Tennis is played in a variety of climatic settings. Players often compete outdoors in sweltering conditions. Heat cramps, heat exhaustion, and heat stroke are major concerns for players who compete in high humidity and hot environments. During competition and training, fluid and carbohydrate intake will help to maintain hydration, prevent thermal injury, maintain oxidation of carbohydrates if glycogen depletion occurs, and delay fatigue. The American College of Sports Medicine has published guidelines for fluid replacement during exercise: [36]

1. Individuals should eat a balanced diet and consume adequate amounts of fluid within 24 hours of the event.
2. Individuals should drink about 500 ml of fluid about 2 hours prior to training/competition.
3. During the event, athletes need to drink early and at regular intervals in order to compensate for sweat loss.
4. Fluids should be cooler than ambient temperature (15 to 22°C or 59 to 72°F).
5. Carbohydrates and/or electrolytes should be added in appropriate amounts to a fluid replacement solution for events lasting longer than 1 hour.
6. For events lasting longer than 1 hour, carbohydrates should be consumed at a rate of 30 to 60 grams per hour; solutions should contain 4 to 8% carbohydrates.

7. Incorporating sodium in the rehydration solution is recommended for activities lasting longer than 1 hour.

Limited scientific information is available for guidelines for ingesting an appropriate fluid replacement beverage during intermittent exercise.[37] Water has been suggested as the best nutrient for exercise lasting less than 60 minutes, but sport nutritionists have increasingly recommended that benefits can occur with a diluted carbohydrate/electrolyte beverage. After 60 minutes, the purpose of consuming carbohydrates in a fluid replacement drink is to maintain blood glucose levels, enhance carbohydrate oxidation, increase the desire to drink, replace the amount of fluid lost through sweat, and replace electrolytes. Ingestion of carbohydrate becomes increasingly important as exercise is prolonged. Carbohydrate (CHO) feedings are beneficial during activities involving high-intensity intermittent exercise. In tennis there are conflicting reports as to whether carbohydrate fluid replacement drinks are beneficial. Two studies have reported that there may not be any benefit to performance through the consumption of commercially available fluid replacement drinks. In the first study, 12 competitive tennis players completed two 3-hour-long tennis matches during which they consumed 200 ml every 15 min^{-1} of either a 7.5% carbohydrate (7.5 g CHO·100 ml^{-1}) solution or a water placebo.[38] The ambient temperature was 27°C. Players completed a performance test: serve velocity, and a 183-meter shuttle run before and after each match. The study determined that there was no apparent benefit in including a CHO fluid replacement drink during 3 hours of tennis play for performance and fluid balance. In the second study, 16 tournament players participated in a 4-hour-long interrupted tennis match with 30 minutes of rest after 150 min.[39] The authors investigated the metabolic and ergogenic effects of carbohydrate and caffeine concentrations in commercially available beverages. A group of four male or female subjects played against each other in a round-robin format. The environmental conditions on the trial days were 28 ± 2°C and 42 ± 4% humidity. On three separate test dates, the players consumed either a placebo, a carbohydrate beverage, or a caffeine drink at court changeover and during the rest period, which was a 30-minute break after the second match. Players were tested on hitting accuracy, running speed, and perception. The authors concluded that CHO supplementation improved tennis-specific running speed but had no ergogenic effect on improving tennis performance. Caffeine improved glucose homeostasis, but did not have any effect on energy metabolism during continuous match play.

In contrast to the aforementioned research, two studies have reported that carbohydrate supplementation had performance-enhancing effects for tennis.[40,41] In the first study, on three separate occasions, 10 tennis players (5 males, aged 21 to 32 years and 5 females, aged 30 to 40 years) performed 2 hours of simulated tournament tennis.[40] The players had either no fluids (NF), a carbohydrate polymer drink (CHO), or water (W). Body weight, blood glucose levels, the Sargent jump test (power), and a tennis skills test were conducted before and after the 2 hours of tournament play. The tennis was played indoors at 23 to 25°C. Fluids were supplied prior to and throughout the tournament for the CHO and W trials at 15- to 20-minute intervals. Changes in body weight were more pronounced for the NF situation (–2.7%) compared to CHO (–0.4%) and W (–1.1%). Players who ingested CHO showed an 8.9% increase in plasma glucose, compared with a decrease of 11.6% and 7.3% in trials W and NF, respectively. The Sargent jump test showed relatively no change for the W trial, a 10.8% decrease for NF, and an 11.6% increase for CHO. After 2 hours of play, CHO displayed a slight decrease in skill performance compared with a 16.3% decrease with W and an 8.3% decrease with NF. The authors concluded that ingesting a CHO fluid can enhance athletic competition parameters, decrease errors in skill performance, and maintain fluid balance.

The second study[41] that showed CHO ingestion improved tennis performance involved 13 well-trained male tennis players (20 ± 1 years old). Twice at a 2-week interval, the players performed a 20-minute warm-up, followed by the Leuven Tennis Performance Test (LTPT, ± 50 minutes), a 70-meter shuttle run, 30 minutes of rest, and then a standardized 2-hour strenuous training session. After the training session, the LTPT and shuttle run were again administered to determine pre- and post-training changes. Performance was determined by evaluating the percentage of errors, ball velocity, distance to the sideline and baseline, first and second serve (followed by returning five balls programmed by a ball machine), and tactical strategies constituting match play: neutral, defensive, and offensive situations. During the entire protocol, the players ingested a solution containing 0.7 g CHO/kg/body wt/hr or an equal amount of a placebo drink (water) that was artificially sweetened and colored. A velocity-precision index was created to calculate the quality of a shot, which combines velocity and placement. Pretest scores were similar for both CHO and the placebo. During the testing protocol, the shuttle run and tennis performance for the first service and defensive rallies decreased in the placebo group. The first service, percentage of errors, and the quality of shots decreased more ($p<0.05$) in placebo than in the CHO group. There was no change for CHO or the placebo trails on stroke performance for the second serve, neutral rallies, and volleys. The researchers concluded that ingesting a CHO supplement during prolonged strenuous tennis play positively affects tennis performance for the first serve and in defensive situations.

Further research is needed for CHO replacement with either a lower CHO concentration and/or a high CHO concentration in more humid and hotter environments. Since maintaining blood glucose levels may not be needed via CHO replacement drinks, there are other benefits that tennis players may gain from consuming a carbohydrate fluid replacement drink during prolonged match play. These benefits might include inducing a player's desire to drink, preventing heat cramps,[42] and delaying fatigue.

Players can consume carbohydrates in the liquid and solid forms (fruits and energy bars) during match play, which are easily accessible due to the regular court changeovers. During changeovers, tennis players can also take advantage of ingesting fluids on a regular basis. Players should not wait until they are thirsty because the thirst mechanism is an unreliable indicator of fluid needs. Once thirst sets in, the athlete is already partially dehydrated.

12.4.3 Post-Match Nutrition

The post-match meal is important to replenish muscle and liver glycogen stores, rehydrate, and replace electrolytes lost during exercise. Athletes who participate in repeated and frequent exercise may require a fast carbohydrate recovery.[43] Within the first 2 hours after exercise, muscle glycogen resynthesis has been found to be enhanced the most.[44] Players should consume carbohydrates as quickly as possible after training or competition. Higher rates of synthesis have been shown to occur when smaller carbohydrate meals (0.4 g CHO/kg body weight) are consumed more frequently beginning immediately after exercise and every 15 minutes for 4 hours.[45] The recommended amount of carbohydrate replenishment is 1.5 g/kg body weight immediately and 2 hours after exercise. An athlete weighing 150 pounds could consume between 50 and 102 g/kg body weight. No additional benefits of glycogen restoration within the initial post-exercise hours occur when the consumption rate is doubled from 1.5 to 3.0 g/kg body weight.[46] A balanced diet stressing high carbohydrates, especially those with a high glycemic index (GI), seem to replenish glycogen stores the best and the quickest.[47,48] Table 12.2 displays common foods that have high and low mean glycemic values.[49] Glucose and sucrose are the forms of carbohydrate to choose for replenishment after exhaustive exercise. Fructose has a low glycemic response, and its consumption has been shown to result in lower rates of muscle glycogen resynthesis. After the first 24 hours of recovery, athletes should resume their normal high-carbohydrate diet. Nutritionally complete meals, which include complex CHO, fats, and protein, will also help to repair tissue damage and synthesize muscle protein.

12.5 Vitamins, Minerals, and Supplements

Research on the effects that vitamins, minerals, and supplements may have on tennis players is limited. Fifty-five percent of 9 Olympic-level athletes surveyed reported routine use of supplements.[29] There are 13 known vitamins that are classified as either fat-soluble or water-soluble. Vitamins A, D, E, and K are the fat-soluble vitamins. The water-soluble vitamins are: B_1 (thiamine), B_2 (riboflavin), B_6 (pyridoxine), B_{12} (cobalamin), biotin, folic acid, niacin, pantothenic acid, and vitamin C. Twenty-two elements have been identified as

TABLE 12.2

Common Foods With a Mean High Glycemic Index (GI)

Common Food	Mean GI	Glycemic Value
White bread*	100	High
Shredded wheat	97	High
Rice, white	83 ± 9	High
Potato, russett, baked	135 ± 2	High
Banana	79 ± 7	High
Raisins	93	High
Glucose	138 ± 3	High
Whole grain rye	58	Low
Buckwheat	74	Low
Potato, sweet	70	Low
Cherries	32	Low
Plum	34	Low
Milk, skim	46	Low
Yogurt	52	Low
Fructose	30	Low

* Foods are proportionally adjusted so that white bread has an equivalent of 100.
Source: Adapted from Jenkins, D. A., Wolever, T. M. S., Jenkins, A. L., Josse, R. G., and Wong, G. S., The glycaemic response to carbohydrate foods, *Lancet,* 2, 388, 1984.

minerals. Minerals are a part of vitamins, enzymes, and hormones and are located throughout the body in fluids, muscles, and connective tissues.

Excessive vitamin consumption will not enhance performance; however, vitamin deficiencies will decrease performance. Vitamin and mineral supplements will not cause increases in strength or aerobic endurance, prevent illness or injuries, build muscles, or provide energy.[22] Recently, however, vitamin E and creatine have been identified as nutrients that may enhance tennis performance.[50] Vitamin E serves as an antioxidant to prevent cell damage. Vitamin E is found in green leafy vegetables, whole wheat bread, nuts, peanut butter, margarines, and shortenings. The RDA is 7 to 13 mg. Creatine is purported to increase muscle size, muscle strength, improve athletic performance, and cause a quicker recovery time from intense muscle fatigue.[50] Creatine may be beneficial to activities of high intensity and short duration. Benefits of creatine use have been reported to:[51]

- Increase gains in strength performance (1 repetition maximum RM)
- Enhance peak power during isokinetic exercise
- Improve concentric and eccentric power, amplify vertical jump performance
- Increase maximal exercise capacity
- Improve single effort (6 second to 30 seconds) and/or repetitive sprint performance (recovery 30 sec to 5 min)

The sprint, power, vertical jump performance, and repetitive sprint performance enhancement would be of most interest to tennis players. However, side effects of creatine may be cramping, dehydration, water retention, and fatigue. Professional tennis players who used creatine have reported overheating and the inability to cool down during a tennis match.[52] Extreme care should be utilized when creatine is used because heat illnesses are a major concern for tennis players. Supplements are not necessary if the athlete consumes a well-balanced diet; however, many athletes do not know what a well-balanced diet is and may have poor eating habits. Athletes who know that nutrition is lacking and who decide to take vitamin or mineral supplements should consume a multivitamin with no more than 150% of the RDA for any particular nutrient.

12.6 Travel

Tennis players often travel to tournament sites regionally, nationally, and internationally. Eating nutritious meals while traveling can be difficult. It is very easy and inexpensive to eat at fast food or convenience stores if proper choices are made. Some guidelines for the traveling athlete are:

1. Prepare for the trip by determining nutritional goals in advance. Choose hotels with refrigerators and cooking facilities.
2. Select locations that are close to restaurants, supermarkets, and health food stores.
3. Take a food supply and, if possible, a cooler to store fruits and drinks.
4. High-fat foods found in restaurants include fried foods, regular salad dressings, oily dressings, high-fat desserts, creamed cottage cheese, high-fat cheeses, gravy, and cream sauces. Limit or avoid consumption of these high-fat foods.
5. Supermarkets, delicatessens, and health food stores can make healthy lunches or snacks to order and offer a variety of fruits, meats, and salad combinations.
6. Drink water, milk (skim or low-fat), and fruit juices.
7. Avoid alcohol and caffeine because they are diuretics and will lead to fluid loss.
8. Breakfast choices can include bagels and toast with low-fat or fat-free creams, jellies, oatmeal, cold cereal, pancakes, french toast or waffles with syrup, fresh fruit, and low-fat or nonfat yogurt.

9. Lunch can consist of roast beef, ham, chicken, or turkey sandwiches with low-fat mayonnaise and/or mustard, green leaf or fruit salads, non-cream or broth-based soups, baked potatoes, and fresh fruit.

10. For dinner, choices can be spaghetti or other pastas with tomato sauce, meat (roast beef, baked fish, or chicken and turkey), bread, crackers, rice, potatoes, vegetables, green leaf or fruit salad, fresh fruit, and low-calorie desserts.

11. Be clear and assertive about meeting nutritional needs. Do not abandon good eating habits because of boredom or be influenced by what others are eating.

12.7 Summary

Technological advances in tennis racquets and better physical conditioning of participants have increased the power and speed at which the sport of tennis is played. Strength, speed, and proper nutrition are essential components for the demands of tennis. Power and strength are important for most types of sports performance. Nutrient intake for sport activities depends upon which energy systems are primarily utilized during the activity. All substrates are used in producing ATP for energy. Time and intensity determine which systems are most activated. During tennis, energy is provided mainly by the ATP–CP or phosphagen system and the glycolytic/lactic acid system. Thus, the nutritional requirements for tennis are similar to those for athletes who strength train. A balanced diet emphasizing complex carbohydrates and low fat is the best choice for strength athletes. Adequate and appropriate intake of the macronutrients and fluids will enhance performance. Carbohydrate beverage supplementation may enhance tennis performance by sustaining blood glucose levels and encouraging players to drink, which helps to prevent dehydration. The requirements of travel need not include poor dietary choices which would diminish performance.

References

1. Gelberg, J. N., *The Big Technological Tennis Upset*, American Heritage of Invention and Technology, 12, 56, Spring 1997.
2. Navratilova, M. and Carillo, M., *Tennis My Way. A Complete Guide to Training and Playing*, Penguin Press, New York, 1984.
3. Lendl, I. and Mendoza, G., *Hitting Hot: Ivan Lendl's 14-Day Tennis Clinic*, Random House, New York, 1986.

4. Groppel, J. L., Loehr, J. E., Melville, D. S., and Quinn, A. M., Total fitness training for tennis, in *Science of Coaching Tennis*, Leisure Press, Champaign, IL, 1989, chap. 14.

5. Chu, D. A., *Power Tennis Training*, Human Kinetics Publishers, Champaign, IL, 1995.

6. Sale, D. G., Testing strength and power, in *Physiological Testing of the High-Performance Athlete*, 2nd ed., MacDougall, J. D., Wenger, H. A., and Green, H. J. (Eds.), Human Kinetics Publishers, Champaign, IL, 1991, chap. 3.

7. Behm, D., Strength and power conditioning for racquet sports, *Nat. Strength and Cond. J.*, 9, 37, 1987.

8. Kriese, C., Train physically for a purpose, in *Coaching Tennis*, Masters Press, Indianapolis, 1997, chap. 1.

9. Chu, D., Eccentric strength in tennis, in *USTA Sport Science for Tennis*, United States Tennis Association, Key Biscayne, FL, Fall 1995.

10. Roetert, P., Research grants reveal: athletes need quickness from head to toe, and strength training makes better tennis players, in *USTA Sport Science for Tennis*, United States Tennis Association, Key Biscayne, FL, Spring 1993.

11. Nishihara, M., Explosive speed for tennis, in *USTA Sport Science for Tennis*, United States Tennis Association, Key Biscayne, FL, Fall 1992.

12. Singer, R., Which comes first: speed or accuracy? in *USTA Sport Science for Tennis*, United States Tennis Association, Key Biscayne, FL., Winter 1993.

13. Jackson, C. G. R. and Simonson, S., The relationships between human energy transfer and nutrition, in *Nutrition for the Recreational Athlete*, Jackson, C. G. R. (Ed.), CRC Press, Boca Raton, FL, 1995, chap. 2.

14. Richers, T. A., Time-motion analysis of the energy systems in elite and competitive singles tennis, *J. Human Movement Studies*, 28, 73, 1995.

15. Fox, E. L., Bowers, R. W., and Foss, M. L., *The Physiological Basis of Physical Education and Athletics*, 4th ed., Wm. C. Brown Publishers, Dubuque, IA, 1989, chap 2.

16. Elliott, B., Dawson, B., and Pyke, F., The energetics of singles tennis, *J. Human Movement Studies*, 11, 11, 1985.

17. Chandler, T. J., Physiology of racquet sports, in *Exercise and Sports Science*, Garrett, Jr., W. E. and Kirkendall, D. T. (Eds.), Lippincott Williams and Wilkins, Philadelphia, 1999, chap. 58.

18. Strüder, H. K, Hollmann, W., Duperly, J., and Weber, K., Amino acid metabolism in tennis and its possible influence on the neuroendocrine system, *Br. J. Sp. Med.*, 29, 28, 1995.

19. Ainsworth, B. E., Haskell, W. L., Leon, A. S., Jacobs, Jr., D. R., Montoye, H. J., Sallis, J. F., and Paffenbarger, Jr., R. S., Compendium of physical activities: classification of energy costs of human physical activities, *Med. Sci. Sports Exerc.*, 25, 71, 1993.

20. American College of Sports Medicine, *Guidelines for Exercise Testing and Prescription*, 4th ed., Lea & Febiger, Philadelphia, 1991.

21. *Nutrition for Sport Success*, Swanson Center for Nutrition, Inc., Camden, NJ, 1984, 6.

22. Clark, N., *Nancy Clark's Sports Nutrition Guidebook*, Leisure Press, Champaign, IL, 1990.

23. Murray, R. and Horswill, C. A., Nutrient requirements for competitive sports, in *Nutrition in Exercise and Sport*, 3rd ed., Wolinsky, I. (Ed.), CRC Press, Boca Raton, 1998, chap. 22.

24. McArdle, W. D., Katch, F. I., and Katch, V. L., *Exercise Physiology: Energy, Nutrition, and Human Performance*, 3rd ed., Lea & Febiger, Philadelphia, 1991.

25. Hargreaves, M., Skeletal muscle carbohydrate metabolism during exercise, in *Exercise Metabolism*, Human Kinetics, Champaign, IL, 1995, chap 2.

26. Bergeron, M. F., Maresh, C. M., Kraemer, W. J., Abraham, A., Conroy, B., and Gabaree, C., Tennis: a physiological profile during match play, *Int. J. Sports Med.*, 12, 474, 1991.

27. Therminarias, A., Dansou, P., Chirpaz-Oddou, M.-F., Gharib, C., and Quirion, A., Hormonal and metabolic changes during a strenuous tennis match. Effect of ageing, *Int. J. Sports Med.*, 12, 10, 1991.

28. Williams, M. H., *Nutrition for Fitness and Sport*, 2nd ed., Wm. C. Brown Publishers, Dubuque, IA, 1988.

29. Grandjean, A. C. and Ruud, J. S., Olympic athletes, in *Nutrition in Exercise and Sport*, 2nd ed., Wolinsky, I. and Hickson, J. F. (Eds.), CRC Press, Boca Raton, 1994, chap. 18.

30. Murray, T. D., Squires, Jr., W. G., Hartung, G. H., and Bunger, J., Effects of diet and exercise on lipids and lipoproteins, in *Nutrition in Exercise and Sport*, 3rd ed., Wolinsky, I. (Ed.), CRC Press, Boca Raton, 1998, chap. 4.

31. Ferrauti, A., Weber, K., and Strüder, H. K., Effects of tennis training on lipid metabolism and lipoproteins in recreational players, *Br. J Sports Med.*, 31, 322, 1997.

32. Lemon, P. and Mullin, J., Effect of initial muscle glycogen levels on protein catabolism during exercise, *J. App. Physiol.: Resp., Env., Ex. Phys.*, 48, 624, 1980.

33. Hochachka, P. W. and Dressendorfer, R. H., Succinate accumulation in man during exercise, *Eur. J. Appl. Physiol.*, 35, 235, 1976.

34. Paul, G. L., Gautsch, T. A., and Layman, D. K., Amino acid and protein metabolism during exercise and recovery, in *Nutrition in Exercise and Sport*, 3rd ed., Wolinsky, I. (Ed.), CRC Press, Boca Raton, 1998, chap. 5.

35. Food and Nutrition Board, *Recommended Dietary Allowances*, 10th ed., National Academy of Sciences, Washington, D.C., 1989, 30.

36. American College of Sports Medicine, Position stand on exercise and fluid replacement, *Med. Sci. Sports Exerc.*, 28(1), i, 1996.

37. Shi, X. and Gisolfi, C. V., Fluid and carbohydrate replacement during intermittent exercise, *Sports Med.*, 25, 157, 1998.

38. Mitchell, J. B., Cole, K. J., Grandjean, P. W., and Sobczak, R. J., The effect of a carbohydrate beverage on tennis performance and fluid balance during prolonged tennis play, *J. Appl. Sport Sci. Research*, 6, 174, 1992.

39. Ferrauti, A., Weber, K., and Strüder, H.K., Metabolic and ergogenic effects of carbohydrate and caffeine beverages in tennis, *J. Sports Med. Phys. Fitness*, 37, 258, 1997.

40. Burke, E. R. and Ekblom, B., Influence of fluid ingestion and dehydration on precision and endurance performance in tennis, in *Current Topics in Sports Medicine. Proceedings of the World Congress of Sports Medicine*, Vienna 1982, Bachl, N., Prokop, L., and Suckert, R. (Eds.), Urban and Schwarzenberg, Wein, 1984.

41. Vergauwen, L., Brouns, F., and Hespel, P., Carbohydrate supplementation improves tennis performance, in *First Annual Congress of the European College of Sports Science: Frontiers in Sport Sciences*, Marconnet, P., Gaulard, J., Margaritis, I., and Tessier, F. (Eds.), May 28-31, Nice, 1996, pp. 700.

42. Bergeron, M. F., Heat cramps during tennis: a case report, *Int. J. Sport Nutr.*, 6, 62, 1996.
43. Doyle, J. A. and Papadopoulos, C., Simple and complex carbohydrates in exercise and sport, in *Energy-Yielding Macronutrients and Energy Metabolism in Sports Nutrition*, Driskell, J. A. and Wolinsky, I. (Eds.), CRC Press, Boca Raton, 2000, chap. 4.
44. Ivy, J. L., Katz, A. L., Cutler, C. L., Sherman, W. M., and Coyle, E. F., Muscle glycogen synthesis after exercise: effect of time of carbohydrate ingestion, *J. Appl. Physiol.*, 64, 1480, 1988.
45. Doyle, J. A., Sherman, W. M., and Strauss, R. L., Effects of eccentric and concentric exercise on muscle glycogen replenishment, *J. Appl. Physiol.*, 74, 1848, 1993.
46. Ivy, J. L., Lee, M. C., Brozinick, Jr., J. T., and Reed, M. J., Muscle glycogen storage after different amounts of carbohydrate ingestion, *J. Appl. Physiol.*, 65, 2018, 1988.
47. Wilkinson, J. G. and Liebman, M., Carbohydrate metabolism in sport and exercise, in *Nutrition in Exercise and Sport*, 3rd ed., Wolinsky, I. (Ed.), CRC Press, Boca Raton, 1998, chap. 3.
48. Burke, L. M., Collier, G. R., and Hargreaves, M., Muscle glycogen storage after prolonged exercise: effect of the glycemic index of carbohydrate feedings, *J. Appl. Physiol.*, 75, 1019, 1993.
49. Jenkins, D. A., Wolever, T. M. S., Jenkins, A. L., Josse, R. G., and Wong, G. S., The glycaemic response to carbohydrate foods, *Lancet*, 2, 388, 1984.
50. Johnson, P. L., Sports supplements: do they enhance tennis performance? in *USTA Sport Science for Tennis*, United States Tennis Association, Key Biscayne, FL, Winter, 1998.
51. Kreider, R. B., Creatine supplementation in exercise and sport, in *Energy-Yielding Macronutrients and Energy Metabolism in Sports Nutrition*, Driskell, J. A. and Wolinsky, I. (Eds.), CRC Press, Boca Raton, 2000, chap. 11.
52. Leand, A., Quick fix. Creatine use on the pro tour: wonder drug, or cramp waiting to happen?, in *Tennis*, Miller Publishing Group, New York, February 2000.

Appendix A

March 1998

Current Comment from the American College of Sports Medicine

Youth Strength Training

Fitness training has traditionally emphasized aerobic exercise such as running and cycling. More recently, the importance of strength training for both younger and older populations has received increased attention, and a growing number of children and adolescents are experiencing the benefits of strength training. Contrary to the traditional belief that strength training is dangerous for children or that it could lead to bone plate disturbances, the American College of Sports Medicine (ACSM) contends that strength training can be a safe and effective activity for this age group, provided that the program is properly designed and competently supervised. It must be emphasized, however, that strength training is a specialized form of physical conditioning distinct from the competitive sports of weightlifting and powerlifting in which individuals attempt to lift maximal amounts of weight in competition. Strength training refers to a systematic program of exercises designed to increase an individual's ability to exert or resist force.

Children and adolescents can participate in strength training programs provided that they have the emotional maturity to accept and follow directions. Many seven and eight-year-old boys and girls have benefitted from strength training, and there is no reason why younger children could not participate in strength-related activities, such as push-ups and sit-ups, if they can safely perform the exercises and follow instructions. Generally speaking, if children are ready for participation in organized sports or activities — such as Little League baseball, soccer, or gymnastics — then they are ready for some type of strength training.

The goal of youth strength training should be to improve the musculoskeletal strength of children and adolescents while exposing them to a variety of safe, effective, and fun training methods. Adult strength training guidelines and training philosophies should not be imposed on youngsters who are anatomically, physiologically, or psychologically less mature. Strength training should be one part of a well-rounded fitness program that also includes endurance, flexibility, and agility exercises.

Properly designed and competently supervised youth strength training programs may not only increase the muscular strength of children and adolescents, but may also enhance motor fitness skills (sprinting and jumping) and sports performance. Preliminary evidence suggests that youth strength training may also decrease the incidence of some sports injuries by increasing the strength of tendons, ligaments, and bone. During adolescence, training-induced strength gains may be associated with increases in muscle size, but this is unlikely to happen in prepubescent children who lack adequate levels of muscle-building hormones. Although the issue of childhood obesity is complex, youth strength training programs may also play an important role in effective weight loss strategies.

There is the potential for serious injury if safety standards for youth strength training such as competent supervision, qualified instruction, safe equipment, and age-specific training guidelines are not followed. All youth strength training programs must be closely supervised by knowledgeable instructors who understand the uniqueness of children and have a sound comprehension of strength training principles and safety guidelines (e.g., proper spotting procedures). The exercise environment should be safe and free of hazards, and all participants should receive instruction regarding proper exercise technique (e.g., controlled movements) and training procedures (e.g., warm-up and cool-down periods). A medical examination is desirable, though not mandatory, for apparently healthy children who want to participate in a strength training program. However, a medical examination is recommended for children with known or suspected health problems.

A variety of training programs and many types of equipment — from rubber tubing to weight machines designed for children — have proven to be safe and effective. Although there are no scientific reports that define the optimal combinations of sets and repetitions for children and adolescents, one to three sets of six to fifteen repetitions performed two to three times per week on nonconsecutive days have been found to be reasonable. Beginning with one set of several upper and lower body exercises that focus on the major muscle groups will allow room for progress to be made. The program can be made more challenging by gradually increasing the weight or the number of sets and repetitions. Strength training with maximal weights is not recommended because of the potential for possible injuries related to the long bones, growth plates, and back. It must be underscored that the overriding emphasis should be on proper technique and safety — not on how much weight can be lifted.

Proper training guidelines, program variation and competent supervision will make strength training programs safe, effective, and fun for children. Instructors should understand the physical and emotional uniqueness of children, and, in turn, children should appreciate the benefits and risks associated with strength training. If appropriate guidelines are followed, it is the opinion of ACSM that strength training can be an enjoyable, beneficial, and healthy experience for children and adolescents.

Written for the American College of Sports Medicine by Avery D. Faigenbaum, Ed.D. (Chair) and Lyle J. Micheli, M.D., FACSM. See also "Youth Resistance Training," *Sports Medicine Bulletin*, Vol. 32, Number 2, p. 28.

Current Comments are official statements by the American College of Sports Medicine concerning topics of interest to the public at-large.

Street Address: 401 W. Michigan St., Indianapolis, IN 46202-3233 USA
Mailing Address: P.O. Box 1440, Indianapolis, IN 46206-1440 USA
Telephone: (317) 637-9200; FAX: (317) 634-7817

[Used with permission.]

Appendix B

Note: The following has been excerpted from the full position stand so that only the section on strength training has been reproduced. The full position stand, including the references, can be found both in Medicine & Science in Sports & Exercise as noted in the summary and on the ACSM web site (http://www.acsm.org).

Medicine & Science in Sports & Exercise®

Volume 30, Number 6
June 1998

Position Stand

The Recommended Quantity and Quality of Exercise for Developing and Maintaining Cardiorespiratory and Muscular Fitness, and Flexibility in Healthy Adults

This pronouncement was written for the American College of Sports Medicine by: Michael L. Pollock, Ph.D., FACSM (Chairperson), Glenn A. Gaesser, Ph.D., FACSM (Co-chairperson), Janus D. Butcher, M.D., FACSM, Jean-Pierre Després, Ph.D., Rod K. Dishman, Ph.D., FACSM, Barry A. Franklin, Ph.D., FACSM, and Carol Ewing Garber, Ph.D., FACSM.

SUMMARY

ACSM Position Stand on The Recommended Quantity and Quality of Exercise for Developing and Maintaining Cardiorespiratory and Muscular

Fitness, and Flexibility in Adults. *Med Sci. Sports Exerc.*, Vol. 30, No. 6, pp. 975-991, 1998.

The combination of frequency, intensity, and duration of chronic exercise has been found to be effective for producing a training effect. The interaction of these factors provides the overload stimulus. In general, the lower the stimulus the lower the training effect, and the greater the stimulus the greater the effect. As a result of specificity of training and the need for maintaining muscular strength and endurance, and flexibility of the major muscle groups, a well-rounded training program including aerobic and resistance training, and flexibility exercises is recommended. Although age in itself is not a limiting factor to exercise training, a more gradual approach in applying the prescription at older ages seems prudent. It has also been shown that aerobic endurance training of fewer than 2 d·wk^{-1}, at less than 40-50% of V·O$_2$R, and for less than 10 min^{-1} is generally not a sufficient stimulus for developing and maintaining fitness in healthy adults. Even so, many health benefits from physical activity can be achieved at lower intensities of exercise if frequency and duration of training are increased appropriately. In this regard, physical activity can be accumulated through the day in shorter bouts of 10-min durations.

In the interpretation of this position stand, it must be recognized that the recommendations should be used in the context of participant's needs, goals, and initial abilities. In this regard, a sliding scale as to the amount of time allotted and intensity of effort should be carefully gauged for the cardiorespiratory, muscular strength and endurance, and flexibility components of the program. An appropriate warm-up and cool-down period, which would include flexibility exercises, are also recommended. The important factor is to design a program for the individual to provide the proper amount of physical activity to attain maximal benefit at the lowest risk. Emphasis should be placed on factors that result in permanent lifestyle change and encourage a lifetime of physical activity.

Introduction

Many people are currently involved in cardiorespiratory fitness and resistance training programs and efforts to promote participation in all forms of physical activity are being developed and implemented (242). Thus, the need for guidelines for exercise prescription is apparent. Based on the existing evidence concerning exercise prescription for healthy adults and the need for guidelines, the American College of Sports Medicine (ACSM) makes the following recommendations for the quantity and quality of training for developing and maintaining cardiorespiratory fitness, body composition, muscular strength and endurance, and flexibility in the healthy adult:

Muscular Strength and Endurance, Body Composition, and Flexibility

1. Resistance training: Resistance training should be an integral part of an adult fitness program and of a sufficient intensity to enhance strength, muscular endurance, and maintain fat-free mass (FFM). Resistance training should be progressive in nature, individualized, and provide a stimulus to all the major muscle groups. One set of 8-10 exercises that conditions the major muscle groups 2-3 d·wk^{-1} is recommended. Multiple-set regimens may provide greater benefits if time allows. Most persons should complete 8-12 repetitions of each exercise; however, for older and more frail persons (approximately 50-60 yr of age and above), 10-15 repetitions may be more appropriate.

2. Flexibility training: Flexibility exercises should be incorporated into the overall fitness program sufficient to develop and maintain range of motion (ROM). These exercises should stretch the major muscle groups and be performed a minimum of 2-3d·wk^{-1}. Stretching should include appropriate static and/or dynamic techniques.

Exercise Prescription for Muscular Strength and Muscular Endurance

The addition of resistance/strength training to the position statement results from the need for a well-rounded program that exercises all the major muscle groups of the body. Thus, the inclusion of resistance training in adult fitness programs should be effective in the development and maintenance of muscular strength and endurance, FFM, and BMD. The effect of exercise training is specific to the area of the body being trained (10,75,216). For example, training the legs will have little or no effect on the arms, shoulders, and trunk muscles, and *vice versa* (216). A 10-yr follow-up of master runners who continued their training regimen, but did no upper body exercise, showed maintenance of V·O$_2$max and a 2-kg reduction in FFM (197). Their leg circumference remained unchanged, but arm circumference was significantly lower. These data indicate a loss of muscle mass in the untrained areas. Three of the athletes who practiced weight training exercise for the upper body and trunk muscles maintained their FFM. A comprehensive review by Sale (216) documents available information on specificity of training.

Specificity of training was further addressed by Graves et al. (97). Using a bilateral knee extension exercise, these investigators trained four groups: group A, first half of the ROM; group B, second half of the ROM; group AB, full ROM; and a control group that did not train. The results clearly showed that the training result was specific to the ROM exercised, with group AB getting the best full range effect. Thus, resistance training should be performed through a full ROM for maximum benefit (97,142).

Muscular strength and endurance are developed by the progressive over-load principle, i.e., by increasing more than normal the resistance to move-ment or frequency and duration of activity (50,69,75,109,215). Muscular strength is best developed by using heavier weights (that require maximum or near maximum tension development) with few repetitions, and muscular endurance is best developed by using lighter weights with a greater number of repetitions (18,69,75,215). To some extent, both muscular strength and endurance are developed under each condition, but each loading scheme favors a more specific type of neuromuscular development (75,215). Thus, to elicit improvements in both muscular strength and endurance, most experts recommend 8-12 repetitions per set; however, a lower repetition range, with a heavier weight, e.g., 6-8, repetitions may better optimize strength and power (75). Because orthopaedic injury may occur in older and/or more frail participants (approximately 50-60 yr of age and above) when performing efforts to volitional fatigue using a high-intensity, low-to-moderate repetition maximum (RM), the completion of 10-15 repetitions or RM is recommended. The term RM refers to the maximal number of times a load can be lifted before fatigue using good form and technique.

Any magnitude of overload will result in strength development, but heavier resistance loads to maximal, or near maximal, effort will elicit a sig-nificantly greater training effect (75,109,156,158,215). The intensity and vol-ume of exercise of the resistance training program can be manipulated by varying the weight load, repetitions, rest interval between exercises and sets, and number of sets completed (75). Caution is advised for training that emphasizes lengthening (eccentric) contractions, compared with shortening (concentric) or isometric contractions, as the potential for skeletal muscle soreness and injury is increased particularly in untrained individuals (8,125).

Muscular strength and endurance can be developed by means of static (iso-metric) or dynamic (isotonic or isokinetic) exercises. Although each type of training has its advantages and limitations, for healthy adults, dynamic resis-tance exercises are recommended as they best mimic everyday activities. Resistance training for the average participant should be rhythmical, per-formed at a moderate-to-slow controlled speed, through a full ROM, and with a normal breathing pattern during the lifting movements. Heavy resistance exercise can cause a dramatic acute increase in both systolic and diastolic blood pressure (150,157), especially when a Valsalva maneuver is evoked.

The expected improvement in strength from resistance training is difficult to assess because increases in strength are affected by the participant's initial level of strength and their potential for improvement (75,102,109,171). For example, Mueller and Rohmert (171) found increases in strength ranging from 2% to 9% per week depending on initial strength levels. Also, studies involving elderly participants (73,74) and young to middle-aged persons using lumbar extension exercise (198) have shown greater than 100% improvement in strength after 8-12 wk of training. Although the literature reflects a wide range of improvement in strength with resistance training pro-grams, the average improvement for sedentary young and middle-aged men and women for up to 6 months of training is 25-30%. Fleck and Kraemer (75), in a review of 13 studies representing various forms of isotonic training, reported an average improvement in bench press strength of 23.3% when subjects were tested on the equipment with which they were trained and 16.5% when tested on special isotonic or isokinetic ergometers (six studies). These investigators (75) also reported an average increase in leg strength of 26.6% when subjects were tested with the equipment that they trained on (six studies) and 21.2% when tested with special isotonic or isokinetic ergometers (five studies). Improvements in strength resulting from isometric training have been of the same magnitude as found with isotonic training (29,75,96,97).

In light of the information reported above, the following guidelines for resistance training are recommended for the average healthy adult. A minimum of 8-10 exercises involving the major muscle groups (arms, shoulders, chest, abdomen, back, hips, and legs) should be performed 2-3 d·wk^{-1}. A minimum of 1 set of 8-12 RM or to near fatigue should be completed by most participants; however, for older and more frail persons (approximately 50-60 yr of age and above), 10-15 repetitions may be more appropriate. These recommendations for resistance training are based on three factors. First, the time it takes to complete a comprehensive, well-rounded exercise program is important. Programs lasting more than 60 min per session appear to be associated with higher dropout rates (186). Also, Messier and Dill (165) reported that the average time required to complete 3 sets of a weight-training program was 50 min compared with only 20 min for 1 set. Second, although greater frequencies of training (29,75,91) and additional sets or combinations of sets and repetitions may elicit larger strength gains (18,50,75,109), the difference in improvement is usually small in the adult fitness setting. For the more serious weight lifter (athlete), a regimen of heavier weights (6-12 RM) of 1-3 sets using periodization techniques usually provides greater benefits (75). Third, although greater gains in strength and FFM can be attained when using heavy weights, few repetitions (e.g., 1-6 RM), and multiple set regimens, this approach may not be suitable for adults who have different goals than the athlete. Finally, from a safety standpoint, these types of programs may increase the risk of orthopaedic injury and precipitation of a cardiac event in middle-aged and older participants (43,199)

Research appears to support the minimal standard that is recommended for the adult fitness/health model for resistance training. A recent review by Feigenbaum and Pollock (72) clearly illustrated that the optimal frequency of training may vary depending on the muscle group. For example, Graves et al. (98) found that 1 d·wk^{-1} was equally as effective in improving isolated lumbar extension strength as training 2 or 3 d·wk^{-1}. DeMichele et al. (51) found 2 d·wk^{-1} of torso rotation strength training to be equal to 3 d·wk^{-1} and superior to 1 d·wk^{-1}. Braith et al. (29) found that leg extension training 3 d·wk^{-1} elicited a greater effect than exercising 2 d·wk^{-1}. Others have found that chest press exercise 3 d·wk^{-1} showed a greater improvement in strength than 1 or 2 d·wk^{-1} (72). In summary, it appears that 1-2 d·wk^{-1} elicits optimal gains in strength for the spine and 3 d·wk⁻¹ for the appendicular skeletal regions of the body. Also, the 2 d·wk⁻¹ programs using the arms and legs showed 70-80% of the gain elicited by the regimens using a greater frequency.

In the same review mentioned above, Feigenbaum and Pollock (72) compared eight well-controlled studies and found that no study showed that 2 sets of resistance training elicited significantly greater improvements in strength than 1 set and only one study showed that a 3-set regimen was better than 1 or 2 sets. Berger (18) using the bench press exercise found 3 sets to elicit a 3-4% greater increase in strength ($P < 0.05$) than the 1- or 2-set groups. None of the studies reported was conducted for more than 14 wk; thus, it is possible that various multiple set programs may show greater strength gains when conducted over a longer time span. Program variation may also be an important factor in improving resistance training outcomes but must be verified by additional research (75). Considering the small differences found in the various programs relating to frequency of training and multiple versus single-set programs, the minimal standard recommended for resistance training in the adult fitness setting seems appropriate for attaining most of the fitness and health benefits desired in fitness and health maintenance programs.

Although resistance training equipment may provide better feedback as to the loads used along with a graduated and quantitative stimulus for determining an overload than traditional calisthenic exercises, calisthenics and other resistive types of activities can still be effective in improving and maintaining muscular strength and endurance (86,109,195).

Appendix C

Note: The following has been excerpted from the full position stand so that only the section on strength training has been reproduced. The full position stand, including the references, can be found both in *Medicine & Science in Sports & Exercise* as noted in the summary and on the ACSM web site (http://www.acsm.org).

Medicine & Science in Sports & Exercise®

Volume 30, Number 6
June 1998

Position Stand

Exercise and Physical Activity for Older Adults

This pronouncement was written for the American College of Sports Medicine by: Robert S. Mazzeo, Ph.D., FACSM (Chair), Peter Cavanagh, Ph.D., FACSM, William J. Evans, Ph.D., FACSM, Maria Fiatarone, Ph.D., James Hagberg, Ph.D., FACSM, Edward McAuley, Ph.D., and Jill Startzell, Ph.D.

Summary

ACSM Position Stand on Exercise and Physical Activity for Older Adults. *Med. Sci. Sports. Exerc.*, **Vol. 30, No. 6, pp. 992-1008, 1998.**

By the year 2030, the number of individuals 65 yr and over will reach 70 million in the United States alone; persons 85 yr and older will be the fastest growing segment of the population. As more individuals live longer, it is imperative to determine the extent and mechanisms by which exercise and physical activity can improve health, functional capacity, quality of life, and independence in this population. Aging is a complex process involving many variables (e.g., genetics, lifestyle factors, chronic diseases) that interact with one another, greatly influencing the manner in which we age. Participation in regular physical activity (both aerobic and strength exercises) elicits a number of favorable responses that contribute to healthy aging. Much has been learned recently regarding the adaptability of various biological systems, as well as the ways that regular exercise can influence them.

Participation in a regular exercise program is an effective intervention/modality to reduce/prevent a number of functional declines associated with aging. Further, the trainability of older individuals (including octo- and nonagenarians) is evidenced by their ability to adapt and respond to both endurance and strength training. Endurance training can help maintain and improve various aspects of cardiovascular function (as measured by maximal $V \cdot O_2$, cardiac output, and arteriovenous O_2 difference), as well as enhance submaximal performance. Importantly, reductions in risk factors associated with disease states (heart disease, diabetes, etc.) improve health status and contribute to an increase in life expectancy. Strength training helps offset the loss in muscle mass and strength typically associated with normal aging. Additional benefits from regular exercise include improved bone health and, thus, reduction in risk for osteoporosis; improved postural stability, thereby reducing the risk of falling and associated injuries and fractures; and increased flexibility and range of motion. While not as abundant, the evidence also suggests that involvement in regular exercise can also provide a number of psychological benefits related to preserved cognitive function, alleviation of depression symptoms and behavior, and an improved concept of personal control and self-efficacy.

It is important to note that while participation in physical activity may not always elicit increases in the traditional markers of physiological performance and fitness (e.g., $V \cdot O_2 max$, mitochondrial oxidative capacity, body composition) in older adults, it does improve health (reduction in disease risk factors) and functional capacity. Thus, the benefits associated with regular exercise and physical activity contribute to a more healthy, independent lifestyle, greatly improving the functional capacity and quality of life in this population.

Introduction

Aging is a complex process involving many variables (e.g., genetics, lifestyle factors, chronic diseases) that interact with one another, greatly influencing the manner in which we age. Participation in regular physical activity (both aerobic and strength exercises) elicits a number of favorable responses that contribute to healthy aging. Much has been learned recently regarding the adaptability of various biological systems, as well as the ways that regular exercise can influence them.

Although it is not possible to be all-inclusive regarding the influence of exercise and physical activity on aging, this position stand will focus on five major areas of importance. These topics include: (i) cardiovascular responses to both acute and chronic exercise; (ii) strength training, muscle mass, and bone density implications; (iii) postural stability, flexibility, and prevention of falls; (iv) the role of exercise on psychological function; and (v) exercise for the very old and frail.

It is estimated that by the year 2030 the number of individuals 65 yr and over will reach 70 million in the U.S. alone; persons 85 yr and older will be the fastest growing segment of the population. Thus, as more individuals live longer, it is imperative to determine the extent and mechanisms by which exercise and physical activity can improve health, functional capacity, quality of life, and independence in this population.

Strength Training

Loss of muscle mass (sarcopenia) with age in humans is well documented. The excretion of urinary creatinine, reflecting muscle creatine content and total muscle mass, decreases by nearly 50% between the ages of 20 and 90 yr (238). Computed tomography of individual muscles shows that after age 30, there is a decrease in cross-sectional areas of the thigh, decreased muscle density, and increased intramuscular fat. These changes are most pronounced in women (96). Muscle atrophy may result from a gradual and selective loss of muscle fibers. The number of muscle fibers in the midsection of the vastus lateralis of autopsy specimens is significantly lower in older men (age 70-73 yr) compared with younger men (age 19-37 yr) (121). The decline is more marked in Type II muscle fibers, which decrease from an average of 60% in sedentary young men to below 30% after the age of 80 yr (113), and is directly related to age-related decreases in strength.

A reduction in muscle strength is a major component of normal aging. Data from the Framingham (100) study indicate that 40% of the female population aged 55-64 yr, 45% of women aged 65-74 yr, and 65% of women aged 75-84 yr were unable to lift 4.5 kg. In addition, similarly high percentages of women in this population reported that they were unable to perform some aspects of normal household work. It has been reported that isometric and dynamic strength of the quadriceps increases up to the age of 30 yr and decreases after the age of 50 yr (116). An approximate 30% reduction in strength between 50 and 70 yr of age is generally found. Much of the reduction in strength is due to a selective atrophy of Type II muscle fibers. It appears that muscle strength losses are most dramatic after the age of 70 yr. Knee extensor strength in a group of healthy 80 yr old men and women studied in the Copenhagen City Heart Study (40) was found to be 30% lower than a previous population study (7) of 70 yr old men and women. Thus, cross-sectional as well as longitudinal data indicate that muscle strength declines by approximately 15% per decade in the 6th and 7th decade and about 30% thereafter (40,84,114,161). While there is some indication that muscle function is reduced with advancing age, the overwhelming majority of the loss in strength results from an age-related decrease in muscle mass.

Strength and functional capacity. The decline in muscle strength associated with aging carries with it significant consequences related to functional capacity. A significant correlation between muscle strength and preferred walking speed has been reported for both sexes (12). A strong relationship between quadriceps strength and habitual gait speed in frail institutionalized men and women above the age of 86 yr supports this concept (63). In older, frail women, leg power was highly correlated with walking speed, accounting for up to 86% of the variance in walking speed (13). Leg power, which represents a more dynamic measurement of muscle function, may be a useful predictor of functional capacity in the very old. This suggests that with the advancing age and very low activity levels seen in institutionalized patients, muscle strength is a critical component of walking ability.

Protein needs and aging. Inadequate dietary protein intake may be an important cause of sarcopenia. The compensatory response to a long-term decrease in dietary protein intake is a loss in lean body mass. Using the currently accepted 1985 WHO (242) nitrogen-balance formula on data from four previous studies, the combined weighted averages yielded an overall protein requirement estimate of 0.91 ± 0.043 g-kg^{-1}-d^{-1}. The current Recommended Dietary Allowance (RDA) in the United States of 0.8 g-kg^{-1}-d^{-1} is based on data collected, for the most part, on young subjects. Recent data (29) suggest that the safe protein intake for elderly adults is 1.25 g-kg-1-d-1. On the basis of the current and recalculated short-term nitrogen-balance results, a safe recommended protein intake for older men and women should be set at 1.0-1.25 g of high quality protein-kg^{-1}-d^{-1}. As discovered in one study, approximately 50% of 946 healthy free-living men and women above the age of 60 yr living in the Boston, Massachusetts area consumed less than this amount of protein, and 25% of the elderly men and women in this same survey consumed less than 0.86 g and less than 0.81 g protein-kg^{-1}-d^{-1}, respectively (85). A large percentage of homebound older adults consuming their habitual dietary protein intake (0.67 g mixed protein-kg^{-1}-d^{-1} have been shown (26) to be in negative nitrogen-balance.

Energy metabolism. Daily energy expenditure declines progressively throughout adult life (146). In sedentary individuals, the main determinant of energy expenditure is fat-free mass (185), which declines by about 15% between the third and eighth decade of life, contributing to a lower basal metabolic rate in older adults (37). Twenty-four hour creatinine excretion (an index of muscle mass) is closely related to basal metabolic rate at all ages (238). Nutrition surveys of those over the age of 65 yr show a very low energy intake for men (1400 kcal/d; 23 kcal/kg/d). These data indicate that the preservation of muscle mass and the prevention of sarcopenia can help prevent the decrease in metabolic rate. Body weight increases with advancing age up to 60 yr, and an age-associated increase in relative body fat content has been demonstrated by a number of investigators. The increased body fatness results from a number of factors, but chief among them are a declining metabolic rate and activity level coupled with an energy intake that does not match this declining need for calories (190).

In addition to its role in energy metabolism, age-related skeletal muscle alterations may contribute to such age-associated changes as reduction in bone density (17,209,214), insulin sensitivity (110), and aerobic capacity (67). For these reasons, strategies for preserving muscle mass with advancing age, as well as for increasing muscle mass and strength in the previously sedentary elderly, may be an important way to increase functional independence and decrease the prevalence of many age-associated chronic diseases.

Strength training. Strength conditioning is generally defined as training in which the resistance against which a muscle generates force is progressively increased over time. Muscle strength has been shown to increase in response to training between 60 and 100% of the 1 RM (129). Strength conditioning results in an increase in muscle size, and this increase in size is largely the result of an increase in contractile protein content.

It is clear that when the intensity of the exercise is low, only modest increases in strength are achieved by older subjects (8,115). A number of studies have demonstrated that, given an adequate training stimulus, older men and women show similar or greater strength gains compared with young individuals as a result of resistance training. Two to threefold increases in muscle strength can be accomplished in a relatively short period of time (3-4 mo) in fibers recruited during training in this age population (71,72).

Heavy resistance strength training seems to have profound anabolic effects in older adults. Progressive strength training improves nitrogen-balance, which greatly improves nitrogen retention at all intakes of protein, and for those on marginal protein intakes, this may mean the difference between continued loss or retention of body protein stores (primarily muscle). A change in total food intake or, perhaps, selected nutrients, in subjects beginning a strength-training program can affect muscle hypertrophy (150).

Strength training may be an important adjunct to weight loss interventions in the elderly. Significant increases in resting metabolic rate with strength training have been associated with a significant increase in energy intake required to maintain body weight in older adults (29). The increased energy expenditure included increased resting metabolic rate and the energy cost of resistance exercise. Strength training is, therefore, an effective way to increase energy requirements, decrease body fat mass, and maintain metabolically active tissue mass in healthy older people. In addition to its effect on energy metabolism, resistance training also improves insulin action in older subjects (152).

Regularly performed aerobic exercise has positive effects on bone health in healthy, postmenopausal women (77,163). The effects of a heavy resistance strength training program on bone density in older adults can offset the typical age-associated declines in bone health by maintaining or increasing bone mineral density and total body mineral content (164). However, in addition to its effect on bone, strength training also increases muscle mass and strength, dynamic balance, and overall levels of physical activity. All of these outcomes may result in a reduction in the risk of osteoporotic fractures. In contrast, traditional pharmacological and nutritional approaches to the treatment or prevention of osteoporosis have the capacity to maintain or slow the loss of bone but not the ability to improve balance, strength, muscle mass, or physical activity.

Recommendations. In summary, it is clear that the capacity to adapt to increased levels of physical activity is preserved in older populations. Regularly performed exercise results in a remarkable number of positive changes in older men and women. Because sarcopenia and muscle weakness may be an almost universal characteristic of advancing age, strategies for preserving or increasing muscle mass in the older adult should be implemented. With increasing muscle strength, increased levels of spontaneous activity have been seen in both healthy, free-living older subjects and very old and frail men and women. Strength training, in addition to its positive effects on insulin action, bone density, energy metabolism, and functional status, is also an important way to increase levels of physical activity in the elderly.

Appendix D

Note: The following is the summary from the full position stand. The full position stand, including the references, can be found both in *Medicine & Science in Sports & Exercise* as noted in the summary and on the ACSM web site (http://www.acsm.org).

American College of Sports Medicine Position Stand

Osteoporosis and Exercise

Summary

American College of Sports Medicine Position Stand on Osteoporosis and Exercise. *Med. Sci. Sports Exerc.,* **Vol. 27, No. 4, pp. i-vii, 1995.**

Osteoporosis is a disease characterized by low bone mass and microarchitectural deterioration of bone tissue leading to enhanced bone fragility and a consequent increase in fracture risk. Both men and women are at risk for osteoporotic fractures. However, as osteoporosis is more common in females and more exercise-related research has been directed at reducing the risk of osteoporotic fractures in women, this Position Stand applies specifically to women. Factors that influence fracture risk include skeletal fragility, frequency and severity of falls, and tissue mass surrounding the skeleton. Prevention of osteoporotic fractures, therefore, is focused on the preservation or enhancement of the material and structural properties of bone, the prevention of falls, and the overall improvement of lean tissue mass. The load-bearing capacity of bone reflects both its material properties, such as density and modulus, and the spatial distribution of bone tissue. These features of bone strength are all developed and maintained in part by forces applied to bone during daily activities and exercise. Functional loading through physical activity exerts a positive influence on bone mass in humans. The extent of this

influence and the types of programs that induce the most effective osteogenic stimulus are still uncertain. While it is well-established that a marked
decrease in physical activity, as in bedrest for example, results in a profound
decline in bone mass, improvements in bone mass resulting from increased
physical activity are less conclusive. Results vary according to age, hormonal
status, nutrition, and exercise prescription. An apparent positive effect of
activity on bone is more marked in cross-sectional studies than in prospective studies. Whether this is an example of selection bias or differences in the
intensity and duration of the training programs is uncertain at this time. It
has long been recognized that changes in bone mass occur more rapidly with
unloading than with increased loading. Habitual inactivity results in a
downward spiral in all physiologic functions. As women age, the loss of
strength, flexibility, and cardiovascular fitness leads to a further decrease in
activity. Eventually older individuals may find it impossible to continue the
types of activities that provide an adequate load-bearing stimulus to maintain bone mass.

Fortunately, it appears that strength and overall fitness can be improved at
any age through a carefully planned exercise program. Unless the ability of
the underlying physiologic systems essential for load-bearing activity are
restored, it may be difficult for many older women to maintain a level of
activity essential for protecting the skeleton from further bone loss. For the
very elderly or those experiencing problems with balance and gait, activities
that might increase the risk of falling should be avoided. There is no evidence
at the present time that exercise alone or exercise plus added calcium intake
can prevent the rapid decrease in bone mass in the immediate postmenopausal years. Nevertheless, all healthy women should be encouraged to exercise regardless of whether the activity has a marked osteogenic component in
order to gain the other health benefits that accrue from regular exercise.
Based on current research, it is the position of the American College of Sports
Medicine that: 1. Weight-bearing physical activity is essential for the normal
development and maintenance of a healthy skeleton. Activities that focus on
increasing muscle strength may also be beneficial, particularly for non-
weight-bearing bones. 2. Sedentary women may increase bone mass slightly
by becoming more active but the primary benefit of the increased activity
may be in avoiding the further loss of bone that occurs with inactivity. 3.
Exercise cannot be recommended as a substitute for hormone replacement
therapy at the time of menopause. 4. The optimal program for older women
would include activities that improve strength, flexibility, and coordination
that may indirectly, but effectively, decrease the incidence of osteoporotic
fractures by lessening the likelihood of falling.

Appendix E

Note: The following has been excerpted from the full position stand so that only the two summary sections have been reproduced. The full position stand, including the references, can be found both in *Medicine & Science in Sports & Exercise* as noted and on the ACSM web site (http://www.acsm.org).

American College of Sports Medicine Position Stand

Reference: *Medicine and Science in Sports and Exercise,* **Volume 15, Number 1, 1983, pp. ix-xiii.**

Proper and Improper Weight Loss Programs

Millions of individuals are involved in weight reduction programs. With the number of undesirable weight loss programs available and a general misconception by many about weight loss, the need for guidelines for proper weight loss programs is apparent.

Based on the existing evidence concerning the effects of weight loss on health status, physiologic processes and body composition parameters, the American College of Sports Medicine makes the following statements and recommendations for weight loss programs.

For the purposes of this position stand, body weight will be represented by two components, fat and fat-free (water, electrolytes, minerals, glycogen stores, muscular tissue, bone, etc.):

1. Prolonged fasting and diet programs that severely restrict caloric intake are scientifically undesirable and can be medically dangerous.

2. Fasting and diet programs that severely restrict caloric intake result in the loss of large amounts of water, electrolytes, minerals, glycogen stores, and other fat-free tissue (including proteins within fat-free tissues), with minimal amounts of fat loss.

3. Mild calorie restriction (500-1000 kcal less than the usual daily intake) results in a smaller loss of water, electrolytes, minerals, and other fat-free tissue, and is less likely to cause malnutrition.

4. Dynamic exercise of large muscles helps to maintain fat-free tissue, including muscle mass and bone density, and results in losses of body weight. Weight loss resulting from an increase in energy expenditure is primarily in the form of fat weight.

5. A nutritionally sound diet resulting in mild calorie restriction coupled with an endurance exercise program along with behavioral modification of existing eating habits is recommended for weight reduction. The rate of sustained weight loss should not exceed 1 kg (2 lb) per week.

6. To maintain proper weight control and optimal body fat levels, a lifetime commitment to proper eating habits and regular physical activity is required.

Therefore, a desirable weight loss program is one that:

1. Provides a caloric intake not lower than 1200 kcal·d^{-1} for normal adults in order to get a proper blend of foods to meet nutritional requirements. (**Note:** this requirement may change for children, older individuals, athletes, etc.).

2. Includes foods acceptable to the dieter from the viewpoints of sociocultural background, usual habits, taste, cost, and ease in acquisition and preparation.

3. Provides a negative caloric balance (not to exceed 500-1000 kcal·d^{-1} lower than recommended), resulting in gradual weight loss without metabolic derangements. Maximal weight loss should be 1 kg·wk^{-1}.

4. Includes the use of behavior modification techniques to identify and eliminate dieting habits that contribute to improper nutrition.

5. Includes an endurance exercise program of at least 3 d/wk, 20-30 min in duration, at a minimum intensity of 60% of maximum heart rate (refer to ACSM Position Statement on the Recommended Quantity and Quality of Exercise for Developing and Maintaining Fitness in Healthy Adults, *Med. Sci. Sports* 10:vii, 1978).

6. Provides that the new eating and physical activity habits can be continued for life in order to maintain the achieved lower body weight.

Appendix F

Selected Web Sites

American College of Sports Medicine
  http://www.acsm.org

American Journal of Clinical Nutrition
  www.faseb.org/ajcn

Center for Nutrition in Sport and Human Performance at the University of
Massachusetts
  http://www.umass.edu/cnshp/index.html

Gatorade Sports Science Institute
  http://www.gssiweb.com

National Library of Medicine: MEDLINE
  www.nlm.nih.gov

Appendix G

List of Nutrients

Arsenic
Biotin
Boron
Calcium
Carbohydrates
Carnitine
Carotenoids
Chloride
Choline
Chromium
Copper
Energy
Fiber
Fluoride
Folate
Iodine
Iron
Lipids
Magnesium
Manganese
Molybdenum
Niacin

Nickel
Other trace elements
Pantothenic Acid
Phosphorus
Phytochemicals
Potassium
Protein
Riboflavin
Selenium
Silicon
Sodium
Thiamin
Vanadium
Vitamin A
Vitamin B_{12}
Vitamin B_6
Vitamin C
Vitamin D
Vitamin E
Vitamin K
Zinc

Appendix H

May 1998

Current Comment from the American College of Sports Medicine

Vitamin and Mineral Supplements and Exercise

People who engage in physically active lifestyles are frequently targets of advertisements proclaiming the need for vitamin and mineral supplements. These advertisements presume that athletes, ranging from international competitors to week end participants in recreational activities, are at risk of developing nutritional deficiencies and subsequent impairments in performance and health.

Surveys of athletes indicate the success of these advertisements; the prevalence of use of vitamin and mineral supplements is widespread. Estimates indicate that more than 50% of elite, female endurance athletes and about 40% of non-elite male athletes regularly consume vitamin and mineral supplements. Use of daily supplements is also prevalent among other groups of athletes as 56% of male and 33% of female high school and collegiate athletes report using vitamin and mineral supplements. Consumption of these supplements, however, is not limited to athletes; results of the National Health and Nutrition Examination Survey (1976-1980) indicate that a considerable fraction of women (25%) and men (16%) ingest vitamin and mineral supplements daily. Proponents of vitamin and mineral supplementation argue that daily consumption of these supplements enhances performance, provides a source of energy and prevents illness and injury. Scientific evidence to support these claims is lacking.

Physical activity may increase the need for some vitamins and minerals. However, the increased requirement generally can be attained by consuming a balanced diet based on a variety of foods. Individuals at risk for low vitamin and/or mineral intake are those who consume a low energy diet for extended periods of time. These individuals are at risk of developing a marginal, subclinical nutrient deficiency. Although vitamin and mineral supplementation may improve the nutritional status of an individual who consumes marginal amounts of nutrients and may enhance the physical performance of those athletes with overt nutrient deficiencies, there is no scientific evidence to support the general use of vitamin and mineral supplements to improve athletic performance. The increased energy intake of physically active individuals should provide the additional vitamins and minerals needed if a wide variety of foods is included in the diet.

Estimates of nutrient requirements for physically active people are based on population standards. Commonly used estimates are the recommended daily allowance (RDA) and the estimated safe and adequate daily dietary intake (ESADDI). These estimates are calculated to meet the needs of nearly all members of the U.S. population, with the exception of pregnant women and people with medical problems. Although population standards, such as RDA and ESADDI, were not derived for individuals participating in strenuous physical activity, they provide a reasonable approximation of the vitamin and mineral needs of physically active people.

Vitamins

Vitamins are essential organic compounds that function as regulators of protein, carbohydrate and fat metabolism. Although vitamins are necessary to transform the potential energy in food to chemical energy for work, they are not direct sources of energy.

Scientific evidence for an ergogenic benefit of vitamin supplements in individuals who consume a well-balanced diet is lacking. Furthermore, any improvement in physical performance attributed to vitamin supplement use in an adequately nourished individual is likely the result of a placebo effect.

A recent issue is the use of antioxidant vitamins to enhance performance and promote health. These vitamins include vitamins C and E, along with beta carotene (a precursor of vitamin A). Preliminary evidence suggests a potential, indirect, beneficial effect of supplementation with these vitamins on performance by reducing skeletal muscle damage and enhancing some aspects of immune function. These provocative findings await confirmation in well-designed clinical trials.

Minerals

Minerals are inorganic elements and act as cofactors for enzymes that influence all aspects of energy metabolism. Minerals are not sources of energy. Mineral nutritional status may be impaired among individuals who restrict their energy intake for performance or aesthetic reasons. In particular, girls and women participating in ballet, gymnastics and endurance running may be prone to inadequate intakes of calcium and iron. Low dietary calcium may increase the risk of stress fractures in athletes. Although it is not known if supplemental calcium will enhance performance, additional calcium, preferably from food, may be beneficial in achieving optimal peak bone mass in girls and young women and reducing bone loss in the elderly.

Reduced body iron status may alter physical performance. Among female athletes, decreased serum ferritin, an index of body iron stores, is common, but anemia is infrequent (5%). Decreased body iron stores may be attributed to low iron intake or increased iron loss due to menstruation, gastrointestinal bleeding, and sweating. Supplemental iron is beneficial in improving iron status of athletes with reduced body iron stores and improving endurance performance of anemic athletes. The effects of iron supplementation on performance of non-anemic athletes is equivocal.

Foods With High Vitamin and Mineral Content

As physically active individuals seek to maximize essential nutrient intakes, proper food selection is necessary. In some cases, foods that have a high content of minerals are also significant sources of B vitamins. Some examples of readily available foods that contribute significantly to the individual's vitamin and mineral requirements are summarized below:

Minerals	B Vitamins	Vitamins A, C & E
Beef, lean	Beef, lean	Carrots
Pork, lean	Pork, lean	Milk, skim
Chicken, skinless	Chicken	Peanuts
Tuna, water-packed	Tuna	Orange juice
Kidney beans	Refried beans	Broccoli
Milk, skim	Milk, skim	Spinach
Yogurt	Yogurt	Strawberries

Effects of Vitamin and Mineral Supplementation

Indiscriminate use of vitamin and mineral supplements in individuals without nutrient deficiency can result in detrimental effects. Chronic ingestion of large doses of ascorbic acid can produce physiologic disturbances. Some examples include renal stone formation, decreased coagulation time, erythrocyte hemolysis, and gastrointestinal disturbances. It was recently suggested that the iron-overload induced cardiac deaths of three athletes may have been precipitated by megadose supplements of vitamin C. Thus, a genetic predisposition among some individuals to develop iron overload should limit daily vitamin C ingestion to 500 milligrams. Similarly, luxuriant intakes of supplemental zinc will induce a secondary copper deficiency and decrease high density lipoprotein cholesterol concentrations.

Among otherwise well-nourished individuals, long-term consumption of vitamin and mineral supplements in amounts exceeding RDA or ESADDI can result in adverse effects on other nutrients. Thus, vitamin and mineral supplement usage should be viewed judiciously, if at all, in healthy individuals.

Conclusion

Because of their interest in maximizing performance, athletes may seek to use dietary supplements to gain competitive advantages. However, the athletes should be aware of the following critical points:

- Performance will not be improved if individuals consuming nutritionally adequate diets use nutritional supplements.
- Only athletes with a defined nutrient deficiency or deficiencies will benefit from supplementation of the limiting nutrient(s).
- Concerns about the nutritional adequacy of an individual's diet should be evaluated by a registered dietitian experienced in counseling athletes.
- Athletes should consume a diet that includes a variety of foods to optimize vitamin and mineral intakes rather than use nutritional supplements.
- Use of megadoses of vitamins and minerals is not recommended because of potential adverse interactions among nutrients and toxicity.
- Physically active people who intermittently use vitamin and mineral supplements as a prophylaxis should use a product that does not exceed the RDA or ESADDI for essential nutrients.

Written for the American College of Sports Medicine by Henry C. Lukaski, Pli.D., FACSM (Chair); Emily Haymes, Ph.D., FACSM; and Mitch Kanter, Ph.D., FACSM. The contribution of Kristin Ewing, LRD, is gratefully acknowledged.

Current Comments are official statements by the American College of Sports Medicine concerning topics of interest to the public at-large.

Street Address: 401 W. Michigan St., Indianapolis, IN 46202-3233 USA
Mailing Address: P.O. Box 1440, Indianapolis, IN 46206-1440 USA
Telephone: (317) 637-9200; FAX: (317) 634-7817

Appendix I

Note: The following is the introductory summary from the full position stand. The full position stand, including the references can be found both in *Medicine & Science in Sports & Exercise* as noted and on the ACSM web site (http://www.acsm.org).

American College of Sports Medicine Position Stand

Reference: *Medicine and Science in Sports and Exercise,* **Volume 19, Number 5, 1987, pp. 534-539.**

The Use of Anabolic/Androgenic Steroids in Sports

Based on a comprehensive literature survey and a careful analysis of the claims concerning the ergogenic effects and the adverse effects of anabolic-androgenic steroids, it is the position of the American College of Sports Medicine that:

1. Anabolic-androgenic steroids in the presence of an adequate diet can contribute to increases in body weight, often in the lean mass compartment.

2. The gains in muscular strength achieved through high-intensity exercise and proper diet can be increased by the use of anabolic-androgenic steroids in some individuals.

3. Anabolic-androgenic steroids do not increase aerobic power or capacity for muscular exercise.

4. Anabolic-androgenic steroids have been associated with adverse effects on the liver, cardiovascular system, reproductive system, and psychological status in therapeutic trials and in limited research on athletes. Until further research is completed, the poten-

tial hazards of the use of the anabolic-androgenic steroids in athletes must include those found in therapeutic trials.

5. The use of anabolic-androgenic steroids by athletes is contrary to
   the rules and ethical principles of athletic competition as set forth
   by many of the sports governing bodies. The American College of
   Sports Medicine supports these ethical principles and deplores the
   use of anabolic-androgenic steroids by athletes.

This document is a revision of the 1977 position stand of the American College of Sports Medicine concerning anabolic-androgenic steroids (4).

Appendix J

April 1999

Current Comment from the American College of Sports Medicine

Anabolic Steroids

The use of drugs to enhance strength and endurance has been observed for thousands of years. Today, individuals, including adolescents, continue to employ a variety of drugs, such as anabolic steroids, in hope of improving their athletic performance and appearance. Anabolic steroids are not mood altering immediately following administration. Instead, the appetite for these drugs has been created predominantly by our societal fixations on winning and physical appearance.

Anabolic steroids are synthetic versions of the primary male sex hormone, testosterone. Testosterone, produced primarily by the testes, is responsible for the masculinization and muscle growth during male adolescence. Anabolic steroids are administered primarily in the oral and injectable forms, and needle sharing has been reported, especially among adolescents. These drugs are usually obtained from black market sources, which often include distributors of other illegal drugs.

Individuals who use anabolic steroids, particularly those experienced in weight training, will experience increases in strength and muscle significantly beyond those observed from training alone. Regardless, the use of anabolic steroids is not without negative consequences. First, steroid use is illegal and in violation of state and federal laws. Second, it's considered cheating! To protect the health of the athletes and to maintain the spirit of fair competition, virtually all organizations overseeing athletic competitions, including the National Federation of State High School Associations, oppose the use of anabolic steroids. However, many adolescents who use anabolic steroids do not participate in school-sponsored sports. Third, adolescent steroid users are exposing themselves to potentially serious health problems during the physically and emotionally vulnerable period when their own hormonal cycles are changing. Physical health concerns associated with steroid use include liver and heart disease, and stroke, while physiological effects consist of drug dependence and increased aggression.

In females, anabolic steroids have been associated with a number of adverse effects, some of which appear to be permanent even when drug use is stopped. These include menstrual abnormalities, deepening of voice, shrinkage of breasts, male-pattern baldness, and an increase in sex drive, acne, body hair, and clitoris size. Younger steroid users, both male and female, are at risk of permanently halting their linear growth, which could result in shorter stature than nature had intended.

It is becoming increasingly obvious that anabolic steroid use is not just confined to collegiate, professional, and Olympic athletes. There is a growing body of evidence that high school and even junior high school students are using steroids.

Lifetime prevalence rates for steroid use among male adolescents generally range between 4 and 12 percent, and between .5 and 2 percent for female adolescents. A review of national-level studies of adolescent steroid use shows a mixed trend between 1989 and 1996. In one national study using 1989 steroid usage rates for males and females as a benchmark, a significant decline in use occurred between 1989-1996. However, since 1991, steroid use by males, as measured by 2 of 3 national surveys, has been generally stable. Furthermore, since 1991, data from these same three national surveys point to a significant increase in anabolic steroid use among adolescent females. The 1995 Youth Risk and Behavior Surveillance System showed that of 9th to 12th graders in public and private high schools in the U.S., 4.9% of males and 2.4% of females have used anabolic steroids at least once in their lives. Based on 1995 estimates of high school students, these prevalence rates translate to approximately 375,000 adolescent males and 175,000 female steroid users. It should also be noted that the use of anabolic steroids by adolescents is not limited to the United States. Studies in Canada, South Africa, England, and Sweden have reported overall levels of steroid use for high school-age students similar to those in the United States.

Only a partial profile can be created to characterize the adolescent steroid user. Steroid users are more likely to be males and to use other illicit drugs, alcohol, and tobacco. Student athletes are also more likely than non-athletes to use steroids; football players, wrestlers, weightlifters, and bodybuilders have significantly higher prevalence rates than students in other activities. However, the effects of age, race, gender, and grade level on steroid use are not fully understood. In addition, several other areas, such as academic performance and socioeconomic status, require further investigation before associations can be made with a reasonable degree of confidence.

During the past decade, several strategies have been employed to fight anabolic steroid use among adolescents. These activities have focused primarily on the passage of federal and state laws prohibiting the use of anabolic steroids, as well as the implementation of numerous prevention, education, and intervention programs. Only a handful of high schools have elected to employ drug tests as a deterrent to steroid use, most likely because of the prohibitive costs of such tests (~$120/test). While law enforcement has had some impact, it is not the complete answer, especially given the rise in steroid use among adolescent females. Prevention programs need to be multifaceted. A consistent message against steroid use needs to come from parents, teachers, and coaches on a continual basis. Adolescents need to learn refusal skills as well as to be provided with the latest and most accurate information on sports nutrition, strength training, conditioning, and the use of supplements. Most importantly, young people need a strong moral and ethical compass that establishes clear boundaries that will not be crossed in pursuit of victory.

Written for the American College of Sports Medicine by Charles E. Yesalis, Sc.D., FACSM (Chair) and Michael S. Bahrke, Ph.D., FACSM.

Current Comments are official statements by the American College of Sports Medicine concerning topics of interest to the public at-large.

Street Address: 401 W. Michigan St., Indianapolis, IN 46202-3233 USA
Mailing Address: P.O. Box 1440, Indianapolis, IN 46206-1440 USA
Telephone: (317) 637-9200; FAX: (317) 634-7817

[Used with permission.]

Appendix K

Note: The following is the summary from the full position stand. The full position stand, including the references, can be found both in *Medicine & Science in Sports & Exercise* as noted in the summary and on the ACSM web site (http://www.acsm.org).

Medicine & Science in Sports & Exercise®

Volume 28, Number 1
January 1996

Position Stand

Exercise and Fluid Replacement

This pronouncement was written for the American College of Sports Medicine by Victor A. Convertino, Ph.D., FACSM (Chair); Lawrence E. Armstrong, Ph.D., FACSM; Edward F. Coyle, Ph.D., FACSM; Gary W. Mack, Ph.D.; Michael N. Sawka, Ph.D., FACSM; Leo C. Senay, Jr., Ph.D., FACSM; and W. Michael Sherman, Ph.D., FACSM.

Summary

American College of Sports Medicine. Position Stand on Exercise and Fluid Replacement. *Med Sci. Sports Exerc.,* **Vol. 28, No. 1, pp. i-vii, 1996.**

It is the position of the American College of Sports Medicine that adequate fluid replacement helps maintain hydration and, therefore, promotes the health, safety, and optimal physical performance of individuals participating in regular physical activity. This position statement is based on a comprehensive review and interpretation of scientific literature concerning the influence of fluid replacement on exercise performance and the risk of thermal injury associated with dehydration and hyperthermia. Based on available evidence, the American College of Sports Medicine makes the following general recommendations on the amount and composition of fluid that should be ingested in preparation for, during, and after exercise or athletic competition:

1. It is recommended that individuals consume a nutritionally balanced diet and drink adequate fluids during the 24-h period before an event, especially during the period that includes the meal prior to exercise, to promote proper hydration before exercise or competition.

2. It is recommended that individuals drink about 500 ml (about 17 ounces) of fluid about 2 h before exercise to promote adequate hydration and allow time for excretion of excess ingested water.

3. *During* exercise, athletes should start drinking early and at regular intervals in an attempt to consume fluids at a rate sufficient to replace all the water lost through sweating (i.e., body weight loss), or consume the maximal amount that can be tolerated.

4. It is recommended that ingested fluids be cooler than ambient temperature [between 15° and 22°C (59° and 72°F)] and flavored to enhance palatability and promote fluid replacement. Fluids should be readily available and served in containers that allow adequate volumes to be ingested with ease and with minimal interruption of exercise.

5. Addition of proper amounts of carbohydrates and/or electrolytes to a fluid replacement solution is recommended for exercise events of duration greater than 1 h since it does not significantly impair water delivery to the body and may enhance performance. During exercise lasting less than 1 h, there is little evidence of physiological or physical performance differences between consuming a carbohydrate–electrolyte drink and plain water.

6. During intense exercise lasting longer than 1 h, it is recommended that carbohydrates be ingested at a rate of 30-60 $g \cdot h^{-1}$ to maintain oxidation of carbohydrates and delay fatigue. This rate of carbohydrate intake can be achieved without compromising fluid delivery by drinking 600-1200 $ml \cdot h^{-1}$ of solutions containing 4-8% carbohydrates ($g \cdot 100\ ml^{-1}$). The carbohydrates can be sugars (glucose or sucrose) or starch (e.g., maltodextrin).

7. Inclusion of sodium (0.5-0.7 $g \cdot l^{-1}$ of water) in the rehydration solution ingested during exercise lasting longer than 1 h is recommended since it may be advantageous in enhancing palatability,

promoting fluid retention, and possibly preventing hyponatremia in certain individuals who drink excessive quantities of fluid. There is little physiological basis for the presence of sodium in an oral rehydration solution for enhancing intestinal water absorption as long as sodium is sufficiently available.

Index